Essential Postgraduate Surgery

Edited by

Louis Fligelstone MB BCh FRCS(Eng) FRCS(Gen)
Consultant General and Vascular Surgeon,
Morriston Hospital, Swansea NHS Trust, Swansea

Alun Huw Davies MA DM FRCS(Eng)
Reader and Honorary Consultant in Surgery,
Deputy Head of Division (Teaching),
Division of Surgery, Anaesthetics and Intensive Care,
Imperial College School of Medicine,
Charing Cross Hospital, London

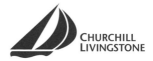

CHURCHILL
LIVINGSTONE

EDINBURGH LONDON NEW YORK PHILADELPHIA ST LOUIS SYDNEY TORONTO 2001

CHURCHILL LIVINGSTONE
An imprint of Harcourt Publishers Limited

First published 2001

ISBN 0 443 060258

British Library Cataloguing in Publication Data
A catalogue record for this book is available from the British
Library

Library of Congress Cataloging in Publication Data
A catalog record for this book is available from the Library of
Congress

Note
Medical knowledge is constantly changing. As new information
becomes available, changes in treatment, procedures,
equipment and the use of drugs become necessary. The editors,
contributors and the publishers have, as far as it is possible,
taken care to ensure that the information given in this text is
accurate and up to date. However, readers are strongly advised
to confirm that the information, especially with regard to drug
usage, complies with the latest legislation and standards of
practice.

The
publisher's
policy is to use
paper manufactured
from sustainable forests

Printed in China
NPCC/01

Preface

We have produced this book with the aim of providing a distillation of essential, current knowledge required for success in the postgraduate examinations for the MRCS. These exams are the required entry to the Specialist Registrar grade. It should also be of benefit to the more able medical students approaching their Final MB examinations. It may also be of use for the Intercollegiate Fellowship FRCS as a quick review text.

This is *not* a complete surgical text, but a concise review of the main components of general surgery and orthopaedics. The information is up to date, concise and presented in a format to encourage systematic review of subjects both for revision and to provide a working knowledge that is useful in the day to day management of patients. This has been helped, where appropriate, by clear algorithms.

In most chapters short recommended reading lists are provided to guide the interested reader.

We believe that the information and systems for presenting knowledge, and advice regarding viva techniques in Chapter 1 will be reassuring and improve the chances of success in any examination.

Louis Fligelstone
Alun H. Davies   2000

Contents

Contributors

Neil Bugg MB BS BSc FRCA
Specialist Registrar in Anaesthetics, Chelsea and Westminster Hospital, London, UK

Christopher R. Darby MB BS MD FRCS
Consultant Transplant Surgeon, Churchill Hospital, Oxford, UK

Alun Huw Davies MA DM FRCS(Eng)
Reader and Honorary Consultant in Surgery, Deputy Head of Division (Teaching), Division of Surgery, Anaesthetics and Intensive Care, Imperial College School of Medicine, Charing Cross Hospital, London

Julie Dunn MD FRCS
Consultant General Surgeon, Royal Devon and Exeter Hospital, UK

Stephen Eckersall MB BS FRCA
Consultant Anaesthetist, Lister Hospital, Stevenage, UK

Sean Elliott MB ChB FRCA
Consultant Anaesthetist, Queen Alexandra Hospital, Portsmouth, UK

Louis Fligelstone MB BCh FRCS(Eng) FRCS(Gen)
Consultant General and Vascular Surgeon, Morriston Hospital, Swansea NHS Trust, Swansea, Wales, UK

John Hines FRCS(Urol)
Consultant in Urology, Whipps Cross Hospital, London, UK

Eleanor A. Ivory MA MRCGP FRCSEd
Specialist Registrar in Accident and Emergency Medicine, John Radcliffe Hospital, Oxford, UK

Michelle E. Lucarotti MD FRCS
Consultant General Surgeon, Gloucester Royal Hospital, Gloucester, UK

Contributors

Neil Moat MB BS MS FRCS
Consultant Cardiac Surgeon, Royal Brompton and Harefield
Hospital; Honorary Senior Lecturer, The Imperial College School of
Medicine, London, UK

Terry O'Kelly MD FRCS
Consultant Colorectal Surgeon, Aberdeen Royal Infirmary,
Aberdeen, Scotland, UK

Tim Owen FRCS
Consultant Surgeon, Orthopaedic Department, Royal Glamorgan
Hospital, Ynysmaerdy, Wales, UK

Paul Peters MS FRCS(CTH)
Senior Registrar in Cardiothoracic Surgery, Royal Brompton and
Harefield Trust, London, UK

Gillian L. Smith MA FRCS
Specialist Registrar in Urology, Lister Hospital, Stevenage, UK

Mark Vipond MS FRCS
Consultant General Surgeon, Gloucester Royal Hospital,
Gloucester, UK

Adam L. Widdison BA BM BCh MA DM FRCS
Consultant in Surgical Gastroenterology, Royal Cornwall Hospitals
Trust, Treliske Hospital, Truro, UK

1. General introduction

Louis Fligelstone

The practice of surgery demands a logical, methodical approach that requires a sound knowledge of anatomy and applies the basic principles of physiology and pathology for the management of any condition encountered. These principles applied to differing clinical presentations leads to a clear management plan and successful outcome. Presentation of information in a format that shows understanding of the condition and its management will produce success in the examination setting and, more importantly, when dealing with patients.

Application of proven systems are useful for the acquisition of knowledge and provides a systematic approach for the description of conditions and their management. Outlined below are several tried and tested systems that are of use for describing a pathological condition, treatment options, complications of a condition or procedure, obtaining a full history of pain, causes of obstruction to a viscus and how to describe an operation.

PATHOLOGY

The basis of all pathological processes requires a clear definition of the condition. A good example is that of a tumour which has been described as 'an abnormal growth of tissue, that continues long after the stimulus that initially caused the growth has ceased to be present'. This definition can cover all tumours, both benign and malignant.

Following the definition, features of the condition need to be described. The mnemonic '**I**n a **S**urgeon's **G**own, a **P**hysician **M**ight **M**ake **S**ome **P**rogress' is useful:

Incidence
Age
Sex
Geography
Aetiology
Pathology
Macroscopic/Microscopic appearance
Management
Staging/Spread
Prognosis

Using this mnemonic, any pathological condition can be described in a very clear manner.

The term **management** describes the process of diagnosis (history/examination), confirmation (specific tests) and subsequent treatment. Whenever asked about a condition, it is important to stress that 'a full history and examination' forms the basis of the initial assessment followed by general tests, e.g. full blood count, urea and electrolytes and urine dip testing, and then more specific tests, e.g. liver function tests in a patient with a history of gallstone disease. Investigations should be scaled from cheap and non-invasive to more expensive and more invasive, e.g. the assessment of a patient with a history of cholecystitis would include full blood count to assess the white cell count for ongoing inflammation or infection, urea and electrolytes, as patients may vomit with gallbladder pathology, may become dehydrated or, if the patient is jaundiced, they may suffer the hepato-renal syndrome with incipient renal failure. Urine dip testing for urobilinogen and bilirubin to assess the difference between acholuric jaundice and obstructive jaundice. Specific tests would include liver function tests which look for the level of bilirubin and abnormalities of the enzyme systems pointing towards bile duct obstruction or hepatocellular jaundice. The next specific investigation would be an ultrasound scan of the upper abdomen to assess the gallbladder and biliary tree for the presence of mural gallbladder inflammation and presence of calculi casting echogenic shadows, and the presence or otherwise of calculi within the biliary tree or dilatation of the biliary tree secondary to a stone obstructing the common bile duct. Furthermore, invasive investigation may include an endoscopic retrograde cholangio pancreaticogram (ERCP) and occasionally percutaneous transhepatic cholangiogram (PTC) or in patients where there are health reasons or the above have failed, a magnetic resonance cholangio pancreaticogram (MRCP). ERCP and PTC may be therapeutic as well as diagnostic.

When discussing the **therapy** for any condition, one should consider prevention and education. They are not mutually exclusive. Good examples are self breast examination in the early detection of breast lumps, and avoidance of smoking for coronary and peripheral vascular disease. When discussing the treatment of a condition, one can sometimes discuss this under the following headings:

GENERAL MEASURES

Rest
Resting may be mental or physical. Examples would include rest following a sprain or resting the gut after a resection to allow healing of the anastomosis.

Hygiene
General hygiene, e.g. handwashing, has proven very important in the prevention of transmission of infection or, e.g. in those that are kept nil by mouth, oral toilet can prevent overgrowth with candida or other oral bacteria.

Diet
Provision of adequate nutrition is essential and alternative routes of administration may be required, e.g. total parenteral nutrition in inflammatory bowel disease. Avoidance of harmful substances such as alcohol, opiates and smoking are also of benefit.

Pharmacological agents
These may be in the form of anti-inflammatory, antibacterial, antiviral, antimitotics. Antibiotics are a special case as they may be used as prophylaxis, i.e. to prevent infection or therapeutic to treat an established infection.

Other therapeutic modalities
These include radiotherapy, high frequency ultrasound, extracorporeal shock waves for lithotripsy and, in the future, genetic manipulation.

ESSENTIAL SUPPORT SERVICES

Nursing
Specific nursing instructions and agreed management plans are essential for the rapid recovery of the patient.

Physiotherapy, speech therapy, occupational therapy
These are all essential and should not be forgotten when considering the management of a patient. Without these facilities, patients may not make a full recovery.

Surgical
Procedures in surgery may be curative, palliative, preventative.

Follow-up
A structured follow-up plan is useful, as it shows an understanding of the pathological process. Routine follow-up of patients, however, is frowned upon, especially with the limited resources within the National Health Service. The value of long-term follow-up is currently under question, even for conditions such as colorectal cancer.

SURGICAL SIEVE

When considering any condition or physical sign, one can use the surgical sieve when looking for a differential diagnosis or cause.

Classically the surgical sieve is divided into congenital causes and acquired causes. Acquired causes can be remembered using the order

INDICATIVE PM

- Infective
- Neoplastic
- Drugs
- Iatrogenic
- Collagenosis
- Autoimmune
- Traumatic
- Idiopathic
- Vascular
- Endocrine or Environmental
- Psychological
- Metabolic.

Infective processes can be further sub-divided into bacterial, viral, fungal, parasitic, spirochaetal, ricketsial, retroviral or prion-induced.

When considering **complications** of a condition or process, one should discuss them in terms of general and specific. The general complications that should always be mentioned are those of bleeding, infection and failure to heal. Specific complications are those restricted to the procedure carried out or the condition. A good example of specific complications are those of peptic ulceration:

1. **Bleeding** – Presenting as haematemesis or malaena.
2. **Perforation**
   a. Perforation into the general peritoneal cavity causing peritonitis
   b. Perforation into the latter sac causing back pain and limited peritonism.
3. **Penetration** – Posteriorly into the pancreas.
4. **Stricture** – Gastric outlet obstruction due to pyloric scarring or dysphagia due to oesophageal stricture formation.
5. **Malignant change**.

CONSENT

Consent is currently very topical. It is an opportunity for the surgeon and patient to discuss the condition in order that the patient understands the procedure that is to be carried out and the risks associated with it. It is currently accepted that the complications that have an incidence of 1% or greater should be clearly described to the patient and recorded on the consent form. Failure to obtain informed consent can lead to general complaints or even charges of battery. Care with consent can save considerable waste of resources by not having to deal with complaints. Attention to general and specific complications is considered essential.

THE HISTORY OF PAIN

Using the mnemonic, SOCRATES, when taking the history of pain, one should clearly define:

Site
Onset/offset – time/dates
Character
Radiation
Associations
Timing (duration, frequency, change, progression, etc.)
Exacerbating/relieving factors
Severity

One should always ask the patient what they believe the pain is due to, as this can often unmask unrealistic anxieties or even lead to the diagnosis.

CAUSES OF OBSTRUCTION TO A VISCUS

Obstruction may be due to mechanical factors:

a. These may be due to a lesion within the lumen, e.g. a foreign body
b. In the wall, e.g. a tumour, or polyp causing intussusception
c. Extrinsic compression
e. Functional obstruction may be neurogenic, e.g. paralytic ileus or pharmacological, e.g. anticholinergic agents.

DESCRIPTION OF AN OPERATIVE PROCEDURE

When describing an operation, one may be asked to describe the procedure alone, or more commonly, when asked to describe an operation, one should mention preoperative preparation, those manoeuvres prior to incision, then the procedure and subsequent postoperative management.

PREOPERATIVE PREPARATION

Full history and examination, tests to confirm the diagnosis, informed consent, marking the **site**, marking the **side** and special preparation. Special preparation would include bowel preparation for colonic surgery, betablockade for patients with thyrotoxicosis and the cross-matching of blood products. It is important not to forget prophylaxis; this includes antibiotics for prophylaxis of wound infection and thromboembolic prophylaxis (Mini-Hep, TED stockings, mechanical compression devices perioperatively). The placement of tubes preoperatively, e.g. an intravenous cannula for resuscitation, rehydration; a nasogastric tube to decompress the stomach; a urinary catheter to decompress the bladder and monitor urine output. The perioperative medical management of conditions such as diabetes, hypertension, ischaemic heart disease and chronic obstructive pulmonary disease should also be addressed.

Pre-incision
Description of the anaesthetic technique to be used, either local, regional or general anaesthesia. The position of the patient, e.g. supine, prone, Lloyd Davies or jack-knife positions.

Skin preparation
Anti-sepsis, depilation and towelling. The position of the surgeon and the assistants. This can be described pre-incision and adjustments made during the procedure. The choice of incision, e.g. midline, paramedian, Kochers, etc.

The procedure
One should mention the approach remembering important surgical and anatomical landmarks. Entering appropriate tissue planes should be stressed. It is always important to assess and confirm the pathology and to assess for any coexisting pathologies. The general principles of confirming the diagnosis, mobilising the part to be operated on and, in bowel surgery, the resection to include comments on vascular supply, adequate en block resection and basic principles of anastomosis. When describing the operation, using phrases such as 'I would incise the peritoneum, I would use 3/0 vicryl ligatures; whilst mobilising the structure, I would be careful to avoid injuring adjacent structures', shows recognition of potential pitfalls and how to prevent them rather than waiting on the examiner presenting you with an injury and asking you how to deal with it! One should then describe closure with details of haemostasis, drainage and suture material. It is important that the surgeon and scrub nurse have a dialogue to confirm that the swab and instrument check is correct.

Postoperative management
A postoperative management plan needs to be written at the time of the operation and also communicated to the nurses who will care for the patient. This includes:

- Timing for the removal of drains, sutures and changing of dressings
- Specific instructions regarding certain types of nursing care, e.g. the frequency and nature of observations such as pulse, blood pressure, temperature, urine output

- Administration of antibiotics or other drugs
- Timing of postoperative checks for haemoglobin and appropriate levels for transfusion
- Records of specimens for histology and microbiology are essential. Postoperative blood tests and their timing are important
- Any further radiology, e.g. to check the position of a central line that was placed during the procedure.

Finally, comments on recognised complications specific to the procedure, broken down into those that may occur early and late, should be included.

APPROACH TO THE EXAM

Currently all examinations in surgery are entrance examinations; the MRCS is an entry qualification required to obtain a Specialist Registrar post, and the Intercollegiate FRCS is required prior to gaining the Certificate of Completion of Specialist Training (CCST), which is required prior to being appointed to a Consultant post. These examinations are not to be feared as they assess you on work and conditions that are common place. The exam should be approached calmly and with a positive, mature attitude. Nearly all candidates will pass, especially with the advent of special courses, e.g. the STEP distance learning course. The examinations are more standardised than previously, and information is more widely available. The attitude of examiners for the MRCS is that they are looking for candidates who would be suitable for entry to the Specialist Registrar programme and who they would feel happy to have as their Registrar. Certain courses are required prior to appointment to a Specialist Registrar post, such as the Basic Surgical Skills Course and the Advanced Trauma Life Support Course. Details of the examinations for the surgical colleges can be obtained easily. One should contact the college early and discuss career aspirations with your local college tutor, and access to basic surgical training courses should be sought at the earliest possible opportunity. Motivated candidates who practise cases in the out-patient setting and on the wards develop a practised confident air. The use of higher surgical trainees for mock vivas and for practising examination skills is to be commended. Luck may occasionally play a part but is no substitute for hard work.

VIVA TECHNIQUES

The viva situation can be a terrifying ordeal. However, with appropriate practice and a positive mental attitude, they can be an enjoyable challenge rather than an ordeal. The viva starts with an initial impression which can be improved by wearing a sober suit, smart shirt, tie and clean shoes. A haircut should be conventional and carried out 2 weeks before the viva to allow things to settle. One should sit up, lean slightly forward, do not slouch or lounge in the chair. If one is nervous and tempted to fiddle with your hands or wave them in the air whilst talking, it is a good idea to clasp them together. Do not cross your arms or legs as this displays a negative attitude *or* shows that one feels threatened. Good quality eye contact is neither too short as this appears to be shifty and shows that confidence is lacking, nor too long, which would be intimidating or suggest poor social skills. Talk and look at the examiner who has asked the question. Modulate your voice to stress important points. Speak clearly and slowly. When one is anxious, there is a temptation to speak too quickly and the examiner may not be able to understand the points one is making.

It is important that one should not speak without engaging the brain first. The pressure to answer a question is great, but it is important not to fill a silence with nonsense. Filling a silence can lead to a situation from which it is difficult to recover. Remember the adage that if one digs a hole, the best thing to do is to stop digging if one wishes to get out.

The acronym PLANT can be used to help with answering any question:

Pause after the question to give yourself time to think.
Listen. Ensure that you have listened to the question. If you have not heard it clearly, ask for the question to be repeated.
Analyse the question that has been asked.
Note the points that you wish to include in your answer and then order them appropriately.
Talk.

You should speak clearly, addressing the points in the order that you wish to, e.g. if asked the causes of an abnormality, list them starting with the commonest, ending with the least frequent. Do not automatically repeat the question, as the examiner will have asked the question several times before and this becomes tiresome and is known to be a delaying tactic. Remember that you will be examined by two examiners; address the examiner that asks the question, as the second examiner scores the answer. You will have your chance to speak to the other examiner in due course. Do not ramble. Explain clearly and feel comfortable to stop at the end of the answer and await a further question. You may find that you are able to guide the direction of the viva, but beware that you do not lead into an area with which you are unfamiliar. In exceptional circumstances, you may realise that you have said something foolish, that is clearly incorrect. In this situation, using a phrase such as 'I would like to correct what I have just said as I realise it is incorrect', can show the examiner that you have seen the error of your ways and allow you to recoup the situation. If you are asked a question that you have absolutely no idea about, then admit it. However, doing this frequently will show that you have obviously not prepared. Do not be put off by the examiner that has a gruff appearance or abrupt manner, as people have many different characteristics and it may not be anything to do with your particular viva performance. It is important to be open and present a professional appearance.

2. Orthopaedic surgery

Tim Owen

OSTEOARTHRITIS

Any synovial joint may be affected by 'wear and tear' degenerative arthritis, but it is more common in the load-bearing joints such as the hip and the knee. Osteoarthritis (OA) is more common in the Western world than in developing countries.

Aetiology

- Primary osteoarthritis has no known cause
- Secondary osteoarthritis
  1. Congenital abnormalities, e.g. congenital dislocation of the hip joint
  2. Trauma, e.g. fractures involving a joint surface
  3. Infection, e.g. pyogenic or tuberculous arthritis
  4. Connective tissue disorders, e.g. rheumatoid arthritis.

Radiological features

- Loss of joint space
- Sclerosis of joint margins
- Bone cyst formation
- Osteophytes.

Principles of management

Conservative management

- Weight reduction
- Walking aids, e.g. walking stick or frame
- Analgesics
- Non-steroidal anti-inflammatory drugs
- Physiotherapy including hydrotherapy
- Aids in the house supplied by the occupational therapist.

Surgical treatment

- Total replacement arthroplasty, e.g. total hip replacement, total knee replacement
- Osteotomy, e.g. upper femoral, upper tibial osteotomy

- Arthrodesis, e.g. ankle, subtalar and mid-tarsal joints
- Excision arthroplasty, e.g. Keller's arthroplasty for hallux rigidus.

SURGICAL TREATMENT OF OSTEOARTHRITIS OF HIP JOINT

Total replacement arthroplasty

Total replacement arthroplasty is now the most common surgical procedure for osteoarthritis of the hip. Approximately 40 000 total hip arthroplasties are performed per year in the UK. This is one of the most successful surgical operations performed which improves quality of life.

The high density polyethylene acetabular component and the titanium or cobalt chrome femoral component are fixed in situ with methylacrylic cement.

Complications include infection, loosening and recurrent dislocation. Infection rates should be less than 1%. The hip replacements with the longest 'track records' are the Charnley, Stanmore and Exeter total hip replacement, which have survival rates of approximately 90% at 20 years following implantation.

Upper femoral osteotomy

Suitable for younger patients without femoral head collapse and with a reasonable range of movements of the hip joint. Either a varus or valgus osteotomy may be performed. The principle is to realign the weight-bearing area of the hip joint.

Arthrodesis

Now rarely accepted by patients. Occasionally appropriate for severe osteoarthritis secondary to trauma in young male patients.

SURGICAL TREATMENT OF OSTEOARTHRITIS OF THE KNEE JOINT

Upper tibial osteotomy

Valgus osteotomy of the upper tibia is performed for medial compartmental disease. The principle is to realign the load-bearing surface of the knee joint. For best results, the degenerative changes should be confined to the medial compartment, the knee joint should flex to at least 90°, and the patient should be under 65 years of age.

Arthrodesis of the knee joint

The principle is to convert a stiff, painful joint into a totally stiff, painless joint. The ipsilateral hip joint should show no signs of degenerative disease.

Total knee replacement

It has been considerably more difficult to design prostheses for knee replacement than for hip replacement because of the inherent instability of the knee joint and the design of replacements for the cruciate ligaments. Modern knee replacements are very much improved on the earlier models. Emphasis is now on resurfacing prostheses which allow normal movements at the knee joint and maintain stability.

ARTHROPLASTY

Arthroplasty is the surgical refashioning of a joint designed to relieve pain and/or improve joint mobility.

Types of arthroplasty

* Excision arthroplasty – both joint surfaces are excised and not replaced, e.g. Girdlestone's operation, Keller's operation
* Interposition arthroplasty – insertion of a liner or spacer into the joint, e.g. Silastic spacer
* Hemiarthroplasty – excision and replacement of one joint surface, e.g. Austin Moore hemiarthroplasty
* Total replacement arthroplasty – excision and replacement of bone joint surfaces, e.g. total hip replacement.

Features of an *ideal* replacement arthroplasty

* Provides complete pain relief
* Produces an adequate range of movement without compromising joint stability
* Is capable of bearing the loads required
* Has a low coefficient of friction
* Has a low rate of wear
* Made from materials which are tissue compatible in the formed or wear product state
* In the event of component failure or complications, the design of the prosthesis should allow for revision surgery.

Materials used for joint replacement

Ultra-high molecular weight polyethylene (UHMWPE)
Used as a weight-bearing surface against metal with the following characteristics:

* Decreased friction
* Decreased metal wear products
* Decreased wear resistance as compared to metal on metal
* Most common material for the acetabular component of most hip replacements.

Titanium

* A very strong alloy containing aluminium and vanadium
* Low incidence of allergic reaction and is therefore used in patients with a history of metal allergy

- Good bio-compatibility
- Requires anodising to prevent excessive wear
- It is expensive
- Titanium is used in a number of the tibial components of total knee joint replacements
- Poor wear qualities
- In combination with a polyethylene acetabular component causes excessive wear and is not now commonly used for the head of the prosthesis.

Cobalt-chrome alloys

- Several types are available containing differing amounts of nickel, molybdenum and titanium
- Very corrosion resistant
- Manufactured by casting
- High tensile strength but quite expensive.

Silicone elastomers

- A very flexible material which is quite inert
- Poor load-bearing characteristics
- Ideal for use as a spacer in the finger joints and for replacing the first metatarso-phalangeal joint.

Polymethylmethacrylate

- Cold-polymerising plastic compound used as a cement to secure prosthetic components of a conventional joint replacement
- Antibiotics may be added to the cement to reduce the incidence of infection, especially in revision surgery.

Complications of replacement arthroplasties

Infection
Infection of a prosthesis is a disaster that requires removal of the foreign material, combined with a salvage procedure to preserve function. The infection rate should be less than 1%. Incidence of infection can be reduced by:

- Prophylactic antibiotics
- Antibiotic-loaded cement
- Laminar air flow ventilation in operating theatres and the use of space suits
- Stringent aseptic technique.

Mechanical loosening
Breakdown of the bond between the bone and the cement results in loosening of the components and eventually loss of bone. Incidence of loosening of the components is decreased by improved cementation techniques:

- Dry operative field
- Lavage systems
- Cement guns to introduce cement under pressure
- Cement restrictors.

When loosening occurs, early revision is now advocated, the revision being performed before loss of the bone occurs. Morbidity and mortality of revision surgery are significantly higher and the long-term results poorer than those of primary hip replacement.

Component failure
With some early designs and materials, femoral stem fractures were seen. With the introduction of better designs and improved materials, these problems are now extremely rare.

Metal sensitivity
This is thought to be the occasional cause of loosening in implants that contain nickel.

Dislocation
Most commonly occurs with total hip replacements. Recurrent dislocation is nearly always due to surgical error in implantation and orientation of the prosthesis

Individual joints

Hip joint

1. Most commonly performed joint replacement
2. Hemi-replacement arthroplasty (Thompson's hemiarthroplasty) in which only the femoral head is replaced is most frequently performed for subcapital femoral neck fractures
3. With conventional cemented total hip replacement arthroplasty, the emphasis is now on a cemented cobalt chrome alloy stem and a cemented high-density polyethylene acetabular component
4. Metal-backed polyethylene-cemented acetabular components are no longer used because of the high rates of loosening of these components
5. Improved cementation techniques have decreased the incidence of mechanical loosening, but this still remains a significant problem in the younger patient
6. Uncemented implants were developed in the hope of eliminating the problems of mechanical loosening, especially in the younger patient, e.g. porous-coated components which are press fit components initially and then rely on bone ingrowth between the pores for stability. The bone ingrowth has been improved by the application of hydroxyapatite to the pores to obtain increased strength of fixation. Results for these uncemented components have now exceeded 10 years of

clinical follow-up, and there are excellent results with a number of types of component (e.g. AML, Furlong).

The principle of resurfacing replacement is to resurface the femoral head with minimal resection of bone. The results of resurfacing replacements have so far been poor and the technique is not widely performed.

Excision arthroplasty is most commonly performed as a salvage procedure for failed total hip replacement arthroplasty, especially if a component has become infected.

Knee joint

1. Unconstrained resurfacing total knee replacement
   a. Allow for minimal bone resection; in the event of failure, may be converted to a revision semi-constrained prosthesis or rarely an arthrodesis
   b. Stability is dependent on the collateral ligaments
   c. All normal movements can occur at the joint, thus reducing the incidence of mechanical loosening
   d. Precise surgical technique is required for the implantation of the prosthesis
   e. Long-term results greater than 10 years are excellent
2. Semi-constrained knee replacement
   a. Loose link between the femoral and the tibial components allow for inherent stability
   b. Once popular but now rarely used
3. Hinged knee replacement
   a. Ease of insertion and rapid postoperative rehabilitation are achieved, but the rate of mechanical loosening is extremely high, and their use is confined for difficult revision cases in the elderly, low demand patient
   b. Allows for flexion and extension only, due to torsional stresses, this type of replacement has a high rate of mechanical loosening
   c. Used in the treatment of severely incapacitated rheumatoid arthritic patients with multiple joint involvement and who are low demand
   d. Also used in revision joint replacement surgery
4. Unicompartmental knee replacement surgery
   a. Introduced as an alternative to osteotomy when disease is confined to either the medial or the lateral compartment of the knee joint
   b. Results in selected cases are extremely good, e.g. the Oxford Knee.

Shoulder joint

1. Replacement arthroplasty is now widely used
2. The main indication is pain relief

3. Total replacement arthroplasty may be indicated in patients with severe rheumatoid arthritis or avascular necrosis of the humeral head
4. Problems have been encountered with the fixation of the glenoid component but new prostheses are much improved
5. Design of the humeral component should ideally prevent proximal migration of the humeral component
6. The most important factor governing the end result is good postoperative rehabilitation. Scrupulous attention should be paid to repairing the rotator cuff
7. Hemi-replacement'arthroplasty in which only the humeral head is replaced may be indicated in patients with severe humeral neck fractures, such as four-part fractures, and patients with avascular necrosis of the humeral head.

Elbow joint

1. Excision arthroplasty may produce useful function and pain relief in a severely diseased joint
2. Hinged prosthetic total elbow replacement arthroplasty does not have a particularly good long-term result due to mechanical loosening
3. Resurfacing of the humerus and olecranon is no more encouraging.

Finger joints

1. Metacarpophalangeal joints may need to be replaced in cases of severe rheumatoid arthritis. A hinged or elastomer spacer is used
2. Correction of deformity, by tendon balancing or soft tissue release, prior to insertion of the implants is essential
3. Preoperative hand function must be carefully assessed
4. Cosmetic appearance is not an indication for arthroplasty
5. Arthroplasty of the proximal and distal interphalangeal joints is rarely indicated.

Wrist joint

1. Excision arthroplasty of individual carpal bones, e.g. trapezium for osteoarthritis of the first carpometacarpal joint
2. Excision of individual bones and replacement of silastic spacer, e.g. scaphoid or lunate for a vascular necrosis
3. Excision of distal ulnar styloid for mal-united Colles' fracture or in combination with synovectomy for rheumatoid arthritis.

RHEUMATOID ARTHRITIS

This is the commonest form of inflammatory joint disease, having an incidence of 1% of the population, being more common in females (3:1), typically occurring in the third to fifth decades. This condition is characterised by an asymmetrical, erosive, deforming polyarthritis affecting both the small and large peripheral joints. The cause of rheumatoid arthritis (RA) remains obscure.

Diagnosis

The diagnosis is made in patients with clinical features of inflammatory arthritis for at least 6 weeks, with four or more of the following criteria:

1. Morning stiffness greater than 1 hour
2. Arthritis of three or more joints
3. Arthritis of hand joints
4. Symmetrical arthritis
5. Rheumatoid nodules
6. Rheumatoid factor
7. Radiological changes.

Serological tests

Rheumatoid factor may be detected using the latex or the Rose–Waaler tests. Antinuclear factor is positive in 30%. Other markers of the disease that can be used are anaemia, thrombocytosis, raised C-reactive protein, increased plasma viscosity or increased erythrocyte sedimentation rate. They can be used to follow disease activity.

1. Synovial fluid analysis – this excludes joint infection or crystal arthropathy
2. Synovial biopsy is non-specific
3. Plain radiography is used to follow progression of erosive joint disease.

Pathology

- Rheumatoid arthritis is characterised by both extravascular immune complex disease and disordered cell-mediated immunity producing chronic inflammation, granuloma formation and joint destruction
- There is an initial synovitis, with infiltration by T-lymphocytes, plasma cells and macrophages followed by hypertrophy of the synovium and pannus formation. The pannus spreads across the joint surface, destroying the underlying cartilage and subchondral bone
- Bone erosions occur earliest at the sites of synovial reflection. The joint capsule and its associated ligaments are progressively weakened by the inflammatory process
- Muscle adjacent to the affected joints atrophy. The result is progressive destruction of the joint with instability and subluxation

- Subcutaneous 'rheumatoid nodules', with characteristic central fibrinoid necrosis and granulomata, occur over bony prominences in 20% of cases.

Clinical symptoms and problems

- Onset of the disease is usually insidious with joint pain, stiffness and symmetrical swelling of the peripheral joints. Typically, the small joints of the hands and the feet are the first to be affected
- In 20% of cases, the onset of the disease is that of an acute polyarthritis with severe systemic symptoms
- In 10%, often middle-aged men, the disease may be more insidious with fatigue, malaise and weight loss without joint symptoms
- Distinguishing it from chronic infection or from malignant disease may be difficult
- The extra-articular manifestations of rheumatoid disease may be haematological, lymphatic, ocular, cardiac, pulmonary and neurological.

Management
Because the aetiology of RA is unknown, its treatment is empirical and consists of symptom relief, suppression of active disease and maintenance of function to allow integration in society.

Splintage
In acute exacerbations, particularly at the wrist, elbow and knee, splintage may help to prevent or correct deformity. Immobilisation in a cast is helpful for acute painful synovitis.

Physiotherapy
Exercise and correction of early fixed flexion can prevent permanent deformity (e.g. quadriceps exercises can prevent posterior subluxation of the knee).

First-line medication
NSAIDs and simple analgesics are used to relieve pain and stiffness but do not alter the course of the disease process.

Second-line medication
These are disease-modifying drugs and used for more aggressive disease, e.g. antimalarial, sulphasalazine, penicillamine and parenteral gold.
Steroids are used systemically in severe exacerbations which fail to respond to first-line therapy or in life- or sight-threatening visceral disease, e.g. pericarditis, polyarteritis or scleritis. Prednisolone is the corticosteroid of choice.

Steroid injection
Intra-articular injections are effective in the control of acute synovitis in large joints.

Immunosuppressive therapy
These drugs may have dangerous side-effects and their indications are limited, including life-threatening extra-articular rheumatoid manifestations with active joint disease which has failed to respond to high-dose steroids. Such drugs include azathioprine, cyclophosphamide and methotrexate.

INFECTION IN RHEUMATOID ARTHRITIS

Septic arthritis can complicate rheumatoid arthritis. In debilitated or immunosuppressed individuals, the normal signs and indices of infection may be absent. *Staphylococcus aureus* is the usual organism. Rheumatoid disease is the commonest cause of secondary amyloidosis.

SURGICAL TREATMENT

Hip joint

- The hip joints are involved in 50% of patients at 10 years following onset of the disease. It is a late manifestation of the disease and a small group of patients may deteriorate rapidly
- When patients develop symptoms, consideration should be made for early surgery to maintain mobility and prevent problems with other joints such as flexion contractures
- Hip replacement relieves pain in over 90% of patients with RA at 10 years. It should be anticipated that the functional requirements are less than patients with OA. Mechanical loosening of the acetabular component is higher than that in patients with OA, and the infection risk is nearly twice that of OA because of immunosuppression and poor wound healing.

Knee joint

- The knee is affected in 90% of patients with longstanding RA. Often there are fixed flexion deformities, and instability because of damage to the ligaments or bone or both
- Synovectomy early in the disease process in young patients with RA has good results, with over 70% of patients sustaining good results at 2 years following chemical synovectomy with Yttrium
- Arthroscopic surgical synovectomy or open synovectomy produces a similar improvement of the patient's symptoms, but is more invasive than chemical synovectomy
- Total knee replacement surgery has a success rate at over 10 years follow-up. Consideration should be made to perform

this early when patients have appreciable symptoms and non-operative treatment is not controlling pain relief and function. Semi-constrained knee replacements are needed when there are severe deformities, e.g. valgus deformity and subluxation

THE RHEUMATOID FOOT

The foot is involved in over 75% of patients with RA. Surgery of the severely affected foot can be very beneficial. The patient's functional needs and expectations should be assessed. Clinical problems in the rheumatoid foot include pain and valgus deformity in the ankle, hindfoot valgus and subtalar arthritis, collapse of the medial longitudinal arch, pronation of the forefoot, and dorsal subluxation of the lesser toes and metatarsalgia.

Management

- Modification of footwear involves providing surgical shoes with medial arch supports, calipers with an inside T-strap if the ankle is involved, the provision of a high toe box to avoid pressure over the PIP joints of the toes and a metatarsal dome may help relieve motatarsalgia. Initially non-operative treatment should be performed in the majority of all patients with RA because surgical treatments have a high rate of complications in the foot because of poor wound healing and often an associated vasculitis in the foot
- Non-steroidal anti-inflammatory drugs (NSAIDs) and local injections of steroid and brief spells of immobilisation may relieve acute synovitis
- Surgical treatment involves either ankle fusion or ankle replacement. Ankle fusion has a high rate of non-union and ankle replacement has a high rate of mechanical loosening, despite good pain relief from both procedures
- Surgical procedures for the hindfoot are triple arthrodesis, surgical procedures for the forefoot can be treated by a variety of operations, the majority of which carry out excision arthroplasty of the subluxed and dislocated metatarsophalangeal joints.

RHEUMATOID SHOULDER

Assessment of the whole of the upper limb is important when planning treatment. Non-operative treatment involves the use of physiotherapy and the use of NSAIDs. Surgical treatment involves joint replacement surgery. This can be either total joint replacement if there is enough glenoid remaining to insert a glenoid component, or a hemiarthroplasty (only replacement of the humeral head with a stemmed surface replacement).

RHEUMATOID WRIST

Involvement of the wrist occurs in greater than 90% of patients with longstanding disease. A pain-free, stable wrist is essential for optimal hand function. Rheumatoid disease of the wrist presents with pain, swelling and deformity. Secondary effects on the median nerve, extensor or flexor tendons may necessitate surgical intervention.

Clinical problems

- Disease affecting the whole of the wrist joint causing pain and volar subluxation. The head of the ulna becomes prominent, producing the piano key sign, the ligaments of the wrist capsule become stretched and weakened. The wrist becomes unstable
- Synovitis may produce rupture of the flexor or extensor tendons, or entrapment of the median nerve.

Assessment

- Assessment of the whole of the upper limb is important when planning treatment
- Non-operative treatment involves referral to a rheumatologist regarding the provision of drug treatment, the use of steroid injections and use of splints to rest the joints in positions of function
- Surgical treatment involves the use of synovectomy when there is proliferative synovial disease which has resulted in, or might predispose to, tendon rupture and when it is causing carpal tunnel syndrome by compression of the median nerve
- For end-stage disease of the wrist, the gold standard treatment is to perform an arthrodesis of the wrist joint to provide a painless, stable wrist. Wrist joint replacement is used, but long-term results reveal a high rate of mechanical loosening.

THE RHEUMATOID HAND

Involvement of the hand in the patient with RA causes functional problems and is frequently mutilating. The combination of joint, muscle and tendon involvement gives rise to zig zag deformities.

- The clinical problems with hand involvement of RA include subluxation and dislocation of the metacarpophalangeal joints, associated with intrinsic muscle tightness of the small muscles of the hand with resultant ulnar deviation of the fingers
- Swan neck deformities (hyperextension of the PIPJ and flexion of the DIPJ) and boutonnière deformities (hyperextension of the DIPJS and flexion of the PIPJS) occur in the thumb and fingers. The thumb can also develop Z deformity
- The main clinical problem with the thumb is that it becomes frail

- Other clinical problems of the hand include flexor synovitis which, because of swelling, restricts motion
- Other problems include flexor and extensor tendon rupture and carpal tunnel syndrome.

THE RHEUMATOID NECK

Up to 90% of patients with RA have radiological signs of involvement of the cervical spine. Deformity and instability occur as a result of rheumatoid involvement of the joints and the ligaments. They are most often seen in patients who have severe nodular disease, a high rheumatoid factor, corticosteroid and longstanding disease. This can lead to various forms of instability of the atlanto-occipital, atlanto-axial and subaxial joints. In the severest form, this can lead to a rapid onset of cervical myelopathy with progressive neurological involvement, paralysis and death. Treatment can be by the provision of cervical collars or for the more severe forms of instability including myelopathy for decompression of the spinal cord and fusion of the involved vertebra.

CHILDHOOD HIP CONDITIONS

SLIPPED UPPER FEMORAL EPIPHYSIS (SUFE)

The incidence of this condition is 2 per 100 000 and is more common in boys than girls (3:2). Individuals often have delayed bone age. The reported incidence of bilateral disease in symptomatic cases is 10%, and up to 40% when a second asymptomatic hip is identified.

Experimental evidence shows that oestrogen can increase the strength of the growth plate and that growth hormone can decrease it. In both sexes, the strength of the growth plate is at its lowest at puberty. The slip occurs through the hypertrophic layer of cells. There is a clinical association between SUFE and some endocrine conditions such as hypothyroidism, pituitary dysfunction and hypogonadism.

- The presenting clinical symptoms are usually of pain in the groin, thigh or knee, and a limp
- X-rays should include an AP X-ray and a frog lateral X-ray, otherwise the SUFE may be missed
- There is no place for non-operative treatment
- Operative treatment involves fixation of the SUFE in situ with cannulated screws as soon as it is diagnosed, to prevent progression
- Salvage surgical procedures may be required in severe instances of avascular necrosis of the bone or chondrolysis not controlled by conservative means. This includes osteotomy, total joint replacement or arthrodesis.

PERTHES' DISEASE

This is an osteochondritis of the hip which occurs as a result of ischaemic necrosis of the upper femoral epiphysis. It occurs most commonly between 4 and 8 years of age (2–16 years). It is commoner in boys than girls (4:1), and is bilateral in 10% of cases. Occasionally there is a family history, but there is no evidence that this is an inherited disorder. There is slightly increased risk with breech delivery and in lower socio-economic groups: it is more common in urban populations. Children with Perthes' disease have a lower mean birth weight and a delayed bone age. The aetiology is unknown. Up to 3% of children with irritable hips have Perthes' disease, but there is no evidence that 'benign transient synovitis' is a causative factor.

The onset of the condition is usually insidious with a limp with pain on activity. Pain is in the groin, thigh or the knee. Examination reveals a restricted range of movements of the hip. There may be a true leg length discrepancy.

The diagnosis and the disease are monitored on plain X-rays of the hips. These reveal the extent of the epiphyseal involvement and the radiological stage of the disease. Certain clinical and radiological factors determine the prognosis of the hip. These include deformity of the femoral head, joint incongruity, age of onset of the disease, protracted course of the disease, type and timing of treatment. Partial involvement or anterior femoral head involvement favours a good prognosis.

Treatment

Since the primary cause of Perthes' disease is not known, treatment is aimed at minimising the secondary changes. Initially, the child with acute pain is treated on bed rest with traction until symptoms subside.

Non-operative treatment

- Patients with early disease and children under 4 years of age need no treatment, but are reviewed clinically and radiologically every 3 months
- Treatment of patients in other groups depends on the presence of 'at risk' signs
- Treatment aims to contain the femoral head in the acetabulum to minimise deformity while spontaneous healing occurs. In the majority, this means splintage in abduction/internal rotation braces.

Surgery

- Reserved for those over 6 years of age and with severe disease or in failure of conservative treatment
- Involves the use of an osteotomy to enable the femoral head to be contained within the acetabulum.

IRRITABLE HIP

This is a common condition of childhood, characterised by an acutely painful hip. The aetiology is unknown. There are no specific diagnostic tests. The diagnosis is therefore one of exclusion and made in retrospect on the clinical course of the condition. The diagnosis is made once other conditions have been excluded by routine tests and clinical observation.

Differential diagnosis

1. Perthes' disease
2. Septic arthritis
3. Osteomyelitis
4. Slipped upper femoral epiphysis
5. Trauma
6. Rheumatoid arthritis
7. Rheumatic fever.

Diagnosis

- There is no predilection for side; however, bilateral disease is rare (approximately 1%).
- Age range is between 2 and 12 years (mean 6 years)
- Male to female ratio is 2:1
- The child presents with pain and a limp, and is often unable to weight bear
- In the majority, the history is short (less than 48 hours). There may be a history of similar episodes of pain
- A history of recent infection, often of the respiratory tract, can be elicited in 30%
- On examination, the hip movements are restricted and the hip is tender to palpation in the groin
- Blood tests and plain X-rays are normal, and exclude other conditions
- Ultrasound scan of the hip is useful. This will determine if an effusion of the hip joint is present and has the advantage of being non-invasive
- If severe symptoms are present, then aspiration of the effusion can be performed and sent for microbiology and culture and sensitivity to exclude septic arthritis of the hip
- If septic arthritis has been excluded, the treatment is bed rest
- A proportion may require bed rest or if the diagnosis is in doubt. Then when the symptoms improve, the patient is allowed to weight bear
- There is no evidence that an irritable hip which has been correctly diagnosed gives rise to complications
- It is widespread practice to re-X-ray the hip 6 weeks later to exclude any other pathology, such as Perthes' disease.

DEVELOPMENT DYSPLASIA OF THE HIP (DDH)

- The incidence of this condition is 1 per 1000 live births, and is four times more common in females
- The left hip is more frequently involved than the right (0:1)
- Bilateral DDH is more common than that of the right side alone
- Risk factors include a breech delivery, being first born, a positive family history and Caesarean section
- There *is* an association with other musculoskeletal abnormalities (e.g. congenital torticollis and congenital foot deformities)
- Possible aetiological factors include mechanical influences, hormone-induced joint laxity, primary acetabular dysplasia and polygenetic inheritance.

Neonatal screening

All babies are examined for hip instability in the first week of life. The range of hip movements, particularly reduction of abduction in flexion, abnormal skin contours, leg length inequality, and the results of the Ortolani (to detect a dislocated but reducible hip) and Barlow tests (to detect a dislocatable hip) should be recorded. Most dysplastic hips are diagnosed at this stage. Correct diagnosis and treatment will result in a 95% cure rate.

The **unstable dislocatable hip** at this stage needs no immediate treatment, and may be reviewed at 3 weeks of age. If it has stabilised, no further action is taken until 3–4 months when radiographs are taken to confirm a satisfactory position.

The **dislocated hip** is reduced and held in a Pavlik harness or Van Osen splint. Ultrasound scan confirms reduction. Splintage should be for a period of 3 months. The child is reviewed regularly, clinically and by X-ray, until the patient is skeletally mature.

If the **dysplastic hip** is diagnosed between the ages of 6 and 18 months, the dislocated hip is no longer reducible by simple abduction of the hip. Bilateral hip dislocation may be difficult to detect. Surgery is usually necessary because of established secondary changes. Preoperative skin traction is necessary to get the femoral head at the level of the acetabulum. Then either closed reduction or open reduction is performed to relocate the femoral head in the acetabulum. Surgery is followed by the application of a hip spica for a period of 3–6 months.

Patients with a DDH that is diagnosed between 18 months and 3 years are established walkers with a waddling (Trendelenburg) gait and hyperlordosis of the lumbar spine. These children require open reduction. A period of preoperative traction is required. The types of operation are: femoral osteotomy, pelvic osteotomy, a combination of femoral and acetabular osteotomy. The principle of the operations is to place the femoral head in the developing acetabulum so that the acetabulum will develop normally.

If DDH is diagnosed between the ages of 3 and 8 years, treatment is difficult. Often secondary changes in the soft tissues and in both the femoral head and in the pelvis have occurred. Surgery involves various types of pelvic osteotomies, femoral shortening procedures and soft tissue reconstructions. Bilateral disease up to the age of 5 years is treated in the same way. Surgery is not recommended over the age of 5 years. Individuals are normally mobile without pain, but may require reconstructive arthroplasty in adulthood.

LOW BACK PAIN

This is the commonest complaint affecting the back. There are many aetiologies for this condition:

1. Spinal causes
2. Mechanical causes
   a. Degeneration and displacement (prolapse) of intervertebral disc
   b. Spondylosis
   c. Spondylolisthesis
   d. Scoliosis
   e. Instability syndromes
3. Tumours
   a. Secondary bone tumours, especially from primary tumours of the breast, lung, prostate, thyroid, kidney and the gastrointestinal tract
   b. Multiple myeloma
   c. Primary bone tumours
   d. Neural tumours
4. Infection
5. Discitis
6. Osteomyelitis, pyogenic or tuberculous
7. Ankylosing spondylitis
8. Central spinal stenosis
9. Soft tissue ligamentous injuries
10. Referred back pain
    a. Pain experienced in the back but due to a pathology other than the spinal column
    b. Infection of the urinary, biliary or female genital tracts
    c. Neoplasms of the abdomen or the pelvis
    d. Abdominal aortic aneurysm.

TREATMENT OF PROLAPSED INTERVERTEBRAL DISC

A tear in the annulus fibrosis allows herniation of the nucleus pulposus and is usually secondary to a flexion-rotational injury. The L4/L5 and the L5/S1 disc levels are the most commonly affected.

Signs of L5 nerve root compression

- Decreased sensation in the L5 dermatome
- Weakness of extensor hallucis longus
- Weakness of dorsiflexion of the ankle
- Wasting of extensor digitorum brevis.

Signs of S1 nerve root compression

- Decreased sensation in the S1 dermatome
- Weakness of plantarflexion of the ankle
- Weakness of eversion of the subtalar joint
- Absent or diminished ankle jerk.

Patients usually present with low back pain, pain in the leg in the L5 or S1 nerve root distribution, and tension signs in the leg with limitation of straight leg raising and a positive sciatic stretch test.

Treatment

Conservative or non-operative
Successful in the majority of cases. Most patients settle with conservative treatment, currently it is recommended that the patient should remain mobile. Bed rest is now thought to increase morbidity and prolong symptoms. This is complemented with NSAIDs, analgesics, muscle relaxants, physiotherapy and epidural analgesia.

Surgical
Indications for surgery are:

- Failure to respond to non-operative treatment
- Recurrent acute episodes with loss of work
- Large central disc prolapse causing sphincter disturbance
- Prior to surgery, MRI or CT scanning are required to confirm the site of the disc protrusion
- Operative treatment involves either fenestration, discectomy or microdiscectomy.

Chemonucleolysis
Certain centres use an extract of papain called chymopapain in the treatment of early disc prolapse. This proteolytic enzyme is injected directly into the disc. Anaphylactic reactions have been reported following its use.

Treatment of nerve root entrapment syndrome

Entrapment of the nerve roots in the lateral gutter may be due to osteophytic lipping from the posterior facet joints. The presenting features are of sciatic pain in an L5 or S1 nerve root distribution. Straight leg raising is normal with absent tension signs. There is often evidence of chronic nerve root denervation.

Conservative treatment

- Weight loss
- NSAIDs
- Physiotherapy
- Lumbar support corset.

Surgical treatment

- Surgery aims to relieve leg pain in emotionally stable patients who fail to respond to conservative measures
- Patients should be investigated by preoperative nerve conduction studies, MRI or CT scans if necessary
- Nerve root decompression is performed with undercutting facetectomies.

Treatment of central spinal canal stenosis

Central compression of the cauda equina may be due to hypertrophy of the ligamentum flavum, shingling of the lamina or osteophytic lipping. Patients present with pain in the legs which is enhanced by walking and associated with muscle weakness. Symptoms tend to abate after resting for 10–15 *minutes* and especially by *sitting*. Intermittent claudication due to peripheral vascular disease (PVD) is an important differential diagnosis, especially as this condition often affects middle-aged to elderly patients. A normal ankle brachial pressure index (ABPI) in the absence of diabetes mellitus excludes PVD as a cause. In central spinal stenosis, the proximal muscle groups tend to be wasted.

1. Conservative treatment consists primarily of wearing a lumbar support corset
2. Surgery usually involves decompressive laminectomy.

SYMPTOMS VIRTUALLY PATHOGNOMONIC OF A PROLAPSED DISC

Compression of the L5 nerve root causes pain in the buttock, lateral thigh and anterolateral calf, radiating across the dorsum of the foot to the hallux and second toe, with numbness and tingling in the same distribution. There may be weakness of the extensor hallucis longus and sometimes the tibialis anterior.

Compression of the S1 nerve root causes pain in the lateral aspect of the thigh and calf, which radiates to the lateral aspect of the foot and the lateral three toes. Plantar flexion may be weak, and the ankle jerk is diminished or absent.

Compression of the L4 nerve root causes pain in the posterolateral aspect of the thigh and the anteromedial part of the leg. The quadriceps femoris may be weak and the leg feel unstable, the knee jerk may be diminished or absent. **Acute massive 'central disc' prolapse is rare, but is a surgical emergency.**

The onset is sudden following herniation of a massive amount of disc material into the spinal canal. Pain is felt in the back and radiates down the back of both thighs and legs, with numbness in the same distribution, often extending into the soles of the feet and perineum (saddle anaesthesia). The ankles are weak or paralysed, as are the sphincters of the bladder and the bowel. The ankle jerks are absent.

Management

- The majority of patients can be managed without surgery
- In 90% of patients, symptoms resolve within 3–6 months
- There is a trend for maintaining mobility and avoiding bed rest as this may lead to a shorter period of disability
- Investigations aim to confirm the clinical diagnosis
- Only if all the clinical signs, symptoms and investigations localise a disc protrusion to a specific site and level is the disc protrusion likely to be the cause of the patient's pain. Failure to appreciate this fact is responsible for much unnecessary and inappropriate surgery
- If patients have failed conservative treatment and require surgery, investigation should include a plain X-ray, scan or magnetic resonance imaging (MRI) scan or computed tomography (CT) scan to confirm the level of the lesion and to exclude congenital abnormalities of the spine and other pathology
- Myelography is very rarely used today.

Surgical treatment

- Chemonucleolysis involves the percutaneous injection of chymopapain into the nucleus pulposus. Moderate improvement may be seen in up to 75% of patients. There is a 0.04% risk of death due to anaphylaxis. There is concern over the number of patients who have residual low back pain
- Microdiscectomy yields excellent results in 90–95% of patients.

ACUTE CERVICAL DISC DISEASE

Cervical disc protrusions can be described as both 'soft' and 'hard'.

1. A soft disc protrusion is the result of a prolapse of nuclear material through a tear in the annulus fibrosis. It is comparable to acute lumbar disc protrusion and its aetiology is thought to be the same. Soft discs occur at a single level of the cervical spine

2. A hard disc is an osteophyte or osteophytic bar and may be part of a generalised degenerative disc disease of the cervical spine. These may present at several levels. Acute prolapse of a cervical disc occurs most commonly in the fourth decade of life and affects men more than women (2:1). It is associated with heavy lifting, cigarette smoking. The levels most commonly affected are C6/C7 (70%) and C5/C6 (24%), where the bending movements and weight carried are maximal.

Presentation

- Neck and shoulder pain may be the only presenting feature
- Nerve root compression when it occurs is usually unilateral, and causes pain accompanied by numbness, tingling and weakness in the distribution of the affected nerve root
- Myelopathy may be of sudden onset
- The corticospinal tracts are commonly affected, causing increased tone, hyperreflexia, clonus and upgoing plantar (Babinski) responses
- There may be weakness and loss of proprioception in the lower limbs
- **The acute onset of cervical myelopathy is a surgical emergency**.

Management

1. An accurate history and examination is followed by plain radiographs and MRI scan (the investigation of choice) to confirm the clinical diagnosis before surgery or if the clinical diagnosis is in doubt
2. Non-operative treatment includes analgesics, NSAIDs and gentle physiotherapy which are helpful in the acute phase. Cervical spine traction may be of benefit to relieve pain and spasm when the acute pain is severe
3. Operative treatment is indicated in the acute situation or when conservative treatment has failed to control severe pain or there is increasing neurological deficit or myelopathy:
   a. The disc compressing the nerve root is resected, either by an anterior or posterior approach
   b. Cervical spine fusion at the same time as decompression of the nerve root is controversial
   c. Anterior fusion with grafting allows the disc height to be restored
4. Operations of the wrong level, which is a frequent reason surgery is unsuccessful, can be avoided by meticulous identification of the level by pre- and intra-operative imaging, either by fluoroscopy or most accurately with plain X-rays in the operating theatre.

OSTEOMYELITIS

Acute osteomyelitis is most often due to haematogenous infection from a primary source elsewhere in the body in neonates and in children. Haematogenous osteomyelitis is caused by a single infection. In neonates and children, *Staphylococcus aureus* is the commonest organism; streptococci and Gram-negative organisms are seen less commonly. In children under 2 years of age, streptococci and *Haemophilis influenzae* are commonly seen.

1. Bacterial osteomyelitis is commonest in children. The infection localises in the metaphysis as it has a rich blood supply. The combination of medullary spread and periosteal stripping leads to necrosis of the infected cortical bone
2. In adults, the commonest cause is secondary to a compound fracture, but infection may also be blood-borne. Exogenous infection may be mixed and not confined to a single organism
3. Sickle cell disease is a special case where infection with salmonella is often the case; however, in adults, staphylococci predominate
4. Childhood osteomyelitis occurs most commonly in young boys aged 6–9 years of age. The overall incidence appears to be declining. Often there is a history of injury, a febrile illness, or an infective focus
   a. The child presents with pain in the limb and a reluctance to use it
      - He may be toxic
      - The earliest physical sign is metaphyseal tenderness
      - Erythema occurs much later
      - Local swelling indicates subperiosteal pus, and fluctuance an abscess
   b. In neonates, the diagnosis is difficult: 75% of neonates with osteomyelitis are not acutely unwell at presentation
   c. Disseminated staphylococcal infection is of rapid onset, with multisystem involvement
   d. Most patients become rapidly toxic and shocked
   e. The mortality is over 10% and over a third have long-term complications
   f. Subacute osteomyelitis has an insidious onset with short history of pain, but minimal loss of function
   g. Clinically, patients have pain but no signs of toxicity.

Investigation

1. Blood tests
   a. Full blood count – white cell count *usually* elevated (neonates may have normal counts)
   b. ESR – usually elevated

   c. Blood cultures (multiple times and sites) identifies organism in 50% of cases

   d. Anti-staphylococcal and anti-streptococcal titres

2. Swabs
   a. Throat swab
   b. Three early morning MSU and sputum cultures (requesting assessment for acid fast bacilli)

3. Radiology
   a. Plain X-rays of the affected bone, note this may be normal for up to 2 weeks after the onset of the symptoms therefore:
     • Isotope bone scan especially useful in pelvis and spine, positive in up to 80% of cases
     • Chest X-ray excludes TB.

The differential diagnosis includes trauma, tumour, cellulitis and erysipelas.

Treatment
This varies according to the age and presentation of the condition.

Neonatal osteomyelitis

• The patient is often septicaemic and requires doses of parenteral antibiotics such as erythromycin and fusidic acid
• If there is no marked improvement within 24 hours, surgical exploration and drainage is required to prevent diaphyseal ischaemia.

Older children and adults
There are proponents for and against early surgery. Advantages of early surgery include:

1. Early confirmation of the clinical diagnosis
2. Pus is obtained for culture and determination of antibiotic sensitivities
3. Early surgical decompression reduces the risk of subsequent ischaemic bone damage
4. Disadvantages of early surgery are as follows:
   a. Operation is frequently unnecessary for simple subperiosteal infections
   b. Exploration of the medullary cavity may potentially spread a localised infection
   c. The patient's general condition may be poor, surgery may be best postponed until the patient's general condition improves.

Suggested management
Once the diagnosis is suspected, and the appropriate investigations done, high-dose parenteral antibiotics are commenced. First-line antibiotic therapy is with a combination of

erythromycin and fusidic acid. If after 48 hours there are no signs of improvement on clinical assessment (pulse, temperature and ESR) surgical exploration and decompression are performed. Antibiotics altered to suit the sensitivities of the organism isolated. Antibiotics should be continued for 3 months.

Complications of osteomyelitis

1. Septicaemia, which may prove fatal if untreated
2. Acute suppurative arthritis
3. Chronic osteomyelitis, which itself has several serious complications including
   a. chronic discharging sinuses
   b. sequestrum formation
   c. bone deformity
   d. pathological fractures
   e. amyloidosis.

Treatment of chronic osteomyelitis

Osteomyelitis may become chronic as a result of inadequate treatment, a highly virulent organism, or impaired host resistance. A chronic Brodie's abscess containing thick pus and fragments of necrotic bone (sequestrum) develops in a cavity surrounded by sclerosed bone. Separating the diseased bone from normal tissues is new bone (involucrum) laid down by the periosteum. Defects in the involucrum (cloacae) allow the continued leakage of pus, which may result in sinus formation.

- Treatment is mainly conservative with antibiotic therapy for acute symptoms
- Sequestrectomy may be indicated for a persistent discharging sinus
- Brodie's abscess is seen on X-ray as a cavity with sclerotic margins; treatment is by surgical excision and curettage of the cavity, leaving sloping margins in an attempt to prevent further collections of pus
- Gentamicin beads or gentamicin-impregnated collagen (e.g. Collatemp) are now used in chronic bone infection. Slow release of gentamicin produces high concentrations of antibiotic at the site of the infection. A chain of beads is usually removed after 2 weeks, but may be left longer in a cavity. The advantage of impregnated collagen is that it provides a higher local dose of gentamicin and biodegrades, therefore avoiding the necessity of removal, which can be painful in the case of gentamicin beads.

Treatment of osteomyelitis in the vertebral column
This is a special case.

- Infection may be pyogenic, caused by *Staph. aureus, Escherichia coli, Klebsiella, Proteus* or *Pseudomonas* sp. Brucella infection should also be excluded in high-risk groups such as farm workers and vets

- The vertebral column is also a common site for tuberculous infection
- Treatment initially is conservative with bed rest and large doses of parenteral antibiotics, even in the presence of neurological impairment
- A needle biopsy is useful to identify the causative organism and determine its sensitivities
- Patients should remain on bed rest for 6 weeks followed by mobilisation wearing a plaster jacket
- Surgical exploration and decompression is only indicated if conservative measures fail
- Antibiotics should be continued for 3 months.

SEPTIC ARTHRITIS

Usually this is due to blood-borne infection from a primary focus elsewhere, but may be due to a penetrating injury of the joint cavity, or secondary to adjacent intraosseous infection. *Staph. aureus* is the most frequent infective agent. The investigation is as for osteomyelitis but should also include aspiration of the affected joint with fluid sent for microscopy for crystals, organisms, culture and sensitivity. Aspiration of deeper joints is often carried out under ultrasound guidance.

If pus is present on aspiration or organisms seen in the aspirate, surgical drainage and irrigation of the joint must be performed immediately. There is no place for conservative treatment alone, once a diagnosis of septic arthritis has been made.

Rest the affected joint in a position of function. High doses of parenteral antibiotics are given. Erythromycin and fusidic acid are given until the organism and its sensitivities have been identified. Antibiotic therapy should be continued for up to 3 months.

BONE TUMOURS

All primary bone tumours are rare. The commonest bone tumour is metastatic spread from a primary malignant tumour at another site. The common sites of tumours with secondary spread to bone are:

- Lung
- Breast
- Adrenal
- Kidney
- Prostate
- Thyroid
- Gastrointestinal.

Classification of primary bone tumours

- Tumour-like lesions, e.g. aneurysmal bone cyst, fibrous dysplasia, eosinophilic granuloma
- Bone-forming tumours, e.g. osteoma, osteoblastoma, osteosarcoma
- Cartilage-forming tumours, e.g. enchondroma, echondroma, chondroblastoma, chondrosarcoma
- Giant cell tumours
- Bone marrow tumours, e.g. myeloma, Ewing's tumour
- Vascular tumours, e.g. haemangioma, angiosarcoma
- Nervous tissue tumours, e.g. neurofibroma, neurilemmoma
- Other connective tissue tumours, e.g. lipoma, liposarcoma, fibroma, fibrosarcoma.

Investigation of patients with bone tumours should include the following:

1. Plain X-rays of the affected bone, chest X-ray, CT scan of the chest where appropriate. Full blood count, ESR, liver function tests
2. Serum electrophoresis if myeloma is suspected. Serum acid phosphatase
3. Bone biopsy
   a. If the diagnosis is in doubt, a biopsy is indicated
   b. Incision site of the biopsy must be carefully planned with consideration to any further surgery which may be undertaken once the diagnosis is confirmed. Biopsy now should only be taken in specialist centres by the surgeon who is going to perform the definitive surgical procedure after confirmation of the diagnosis. The exact diagnosis of a tumour may be difficult and it is essential that an experienced pathologist looking at bone tumours in a specialised centre is used, and it is still common that samples are sent to a panel of pathologists for a consensus opinion
4. Isotope bone scan
5. MRI of the affected bone which provides a very accurate assessment of the extent of the tumour and will detect skip lesions.

BENIGN BONE TUMOURS

Tend to occur in adolescents and young adults. Radiologically the lesions demonstrate clearly defined margins. Benign tumours are usually pain-free unless complicated by a pathological fracture. Curettage and bone grafting procedures may be required to prevent pathological fracture.

MALIGNANT BONE TUMOURS

Primary malignant bone tumours are rare and account for less than 1% of all deaths from malignant disease. In the UK there are fewer than 350 new cases per year. They are listed below in the order of most to least frequent:

- Osteosarcoma
- Chondrosarcoma
- Ewing's sarcoma
- Malignant fibrous histiocytoma.

Primary malignant bone tumours are often very aggressive. The most common presenting features are pain and swelling. The pain is non-mechanical and worsens with time. Commonly the tumour arises adjacent to a joint and may restrict its movement. Pathological fracture is unusual. They tend to occur in adolescents and young adults.

Exceptions include osteogenic sarcoma complicating Paget's disease, chondrosarcoma and malignant giant cell tumours. Characteristically, the patient complains of pain; in patients with vertebral motastases, pain at night is typical. Radiologically the lesions appear aggressive with ill-defined margins In most cases, radiographs will confirm the diagnosis.

Differential diagnosis
Principally from:

- Metastatic disease
- A benign tumour of bone
- Osteomyelitis
- Lymphomas or multiple myeloma
- A simple cyst
- Fibrous dysplasia
- Paget's disease
- Eosinophilic granuloma.

Treatment
Multimodality treatment is now favoured.

1. Chemotherapy is often given both before and after surgery
2. In those cases where there is little invasion of adjacent soft tissues, amputation is often not required. Limb preservation involves resection of that part of the bone which contains tumour followed by reconstruction using an individually tailored and often extensive prosthesis
3. Adjuvant radiotherapy is important in those patients in which tumour clearance is minimal.

Treatment of osteogenic sarcoma

Osteosarcoma is the commonest of all primary malignant bone tumours, accounting for about 20% of all bone sarcomas. It occurs at all ages, but is commonest in the second decade of life. The commonest sites are in the distal femur and proximal tibia, followed by the proximal humerus and the proximal femur. Three-quarters arise in the long bones usually of the lower limb, and at the site of a metaphysis. The radiographic features are those of a sclerotic intramedullary lesion of the metaphysis, which expands and destroys bone. More than 90% of the tumours have penetrated the cortex at the time of penetration. Periosteal bone at the edge of the tumour provokes reactive bone formation (Codman's triangle).

The disease-free survival rate for all osteosarcomas improved rapidly in the 1980s from 25% at 5 years to just over 70%. This was directly related to the introduction of effective adjuvant chemotherapy and, to a lesser extent, resection of lung metastases.

Before the advent of cytotoxic chemotherapy, the natural history of osteogenic sarcoma was that 80% of the patients would develop pulmonary metastases within a few months of the diagnosis. Cade proposed that the primary tumour be treated by radiotherapy and amputation delayed for 6 months and only be performed if no pulmonary metastases appeared. The discovery that osteogenic sarcoma is sensitive to high-dose methotrexate (HDMTX) with folinic acid has changed the treatment fundamentally.

Staging of the tumour should be carried out prior to bone biopsy. The aim is to determine the local extent and distant spread of the tumour. Local extent is best demonstrated by MRI scans. These should image the whole of the bone to exclude 'skip' lesions and the adjacent soft tissues. Distant spread is assessed using bone scans, plain X-rays of the chest and CT scan of the lungs.

After incision biopsy to confirm the clinical diagnosis, the patient is treated with three courses of chemotherapy, which varies in different centres but always includes HDMTX. Neoadjuvant chemotherapy is an essential part of the modern management of osteosarcoma. Most regimens are based on HDMTX. After these investigations, it is possible to stage the tumour using the system devised by Enneking. This combines tumour *grade* (I = low grade: II = high grade: III = low or high grade with distant spread) and *site* (A = intercompartmental: B = extracompartmental) to give a descriptor which has been shown to correlate well with the prognosis for the commonest types of bone tumour.

After confirming the absence of secondary deposits, surgery is then performed. Various possibilities exist:

1. For tumours in the long bones, en bloc wide excision and endoprosthetic replacement is often feasible, provided extensive marrow or adjacent soft tissue involvement are

not present. A local excision leaves a large defect in the skeleton. There are a variety of ways in which these can be reconstructed. Bone grafts can be used, or alternatively, a modular or custom-made endoprosthetic replacement may be used. The choice of method depends on the age, activity and life expectancy of the patient, the type of tumour, the need for adjunctive therapy, the availability of prostheses and allografts, and the individual experience of the operating surgeon

2. If prosthetic replacement is contraindicated, limb amputation is required. Amputation must not be performed through the involved bone

3. Various dispensable bones such as the scapula and the ribs can usually be resected without too much functional impairment.

The tumour specimen is carefully examined to determine the percentage of viable tumour cells. If the tumour is largely or totally destroyed by the preoperative chemotherapy, the same regimen is continued postoperatively for a further three courses and the patient falls into a favourable prognostic group. If the majority of the tumour cells appear viable, the chemotherapy is changed to a second-line regimen and the patient falls into a poor prognostic group. The patients with primary bone tumours should be managed in specialist centres. The complications of allograft and endoprosthetic replacement of large bone defects carry with them all the problems of joint replacement, but on a larger scale and with greater significance to life and limb. In specialist centres, the infection rate is in the region of 7%. There is no place for the general orthopaedic surgeon in treating primary bone tumours.

MISCELLANEOUS CONDITIONS

CARPAL TUNNEL SYNDROME

This is caused by compression of the median nerve at the wrist as it passes through the fibro-osseous tunnel in the wrist. Symptoms classically cause tingling, numbness and pain and discomfort in the radial three and a half digits. Symptoms are characteristically worse at night, often waking the patient from sleep. The patient often shakes or elevates the hand to try and ease the symptoms. The symptoms may cause a decrease in the patient's ability to perform fine manipulative tasks such as writing and sewing.

The condition is most common in middle-aged women and is idiopathic. Other causes include pregnancy, rheumatoid arthritis, acromegaly, diabetes, post-Colles fracture and following peri-lunate fracture dislocation of the wrist. Local causes include lipomas and ganglions in the carpal tunnel.

Clinical signs include wasting of the thenar muscles, a positive Tinel's sign and a positive Phalen's test (wrist flexion).

Pitfalls in the diagnosis are that the clinical symptoms of carpal tunnel syndrome vary widely in practice in both its distribution and in its severity.

Treatment
Treatment is both non-operative and operative.

Non-operative
Non-operative treatment includes splintage of the wrist at night to avoid flexion of the wrist and causation of symptoms, avoiding activities which exacerbate the symptoms. Injection of steroid should be avoided because of the risk of infection, intra-neural neuromas of the median nerve and damage to the median nerve.

Operative
Operative treatment involves decompression of the carpal tunnel by dividing the superficial transverse carpal ligament. This can be performed as a day case and can be performed under local anaesthesia. It is also now being performed endoscopically in some centres. The idea of this method of treatment is to try and avoid the symptoms of thenar pain and scar discomfort that can occur after standard carpal tunnel decompression. This technique is not widely performed in the UK at present.

ENTRAPMENT OF THE ULNAR NERVE

This is the second most common site of peripheral nerve entrapment after carpal tunnel syndrome.

Entrapment may occur by compression beneath the aponeurotic arch of flexor carpi ulnaris (cubital tunnel syndrome) or result from an isolated injury to the nerve, compression by bony deformity or scarring or recurrent subluxation of the nerve around the medial epicondyle. Patient symptoms include numbness and tingling in the ulnar nerve distribution, followed by pain in the elbow and forearm and may disturb sleep. Motor signs include weakness of pinch grip, a positive Froment's sign and weakness of adductor pollicis, weakness of grip due to paresis of flexor digitorum profundus to the ring and little fingers, weakness of the interossei/lumbrical muscles, small muscle wasting of the hand and varying degrees of ulnar claw hand.

Treatment
Treatment may be non-operative or operative.

Non-operative
Non-operative treatment involves splintage of the elbow at rest and at night, and the use of NSAIDs.

Operative
Operative treatment involves surgical release:

- A simple (Osborne) release
- A release and medial epicondylectomy
- An anterior transposition of the ulnar nerve.

The ulnar nerve can also be trapped more distally in the arm and can become trapped at the level of the wrist in Guyon's canal. (Guyon's canal is the canal bounded by the transverse carpal ligament, the volar carpal ligament, the hook of hamate and the pisiform. It also contains the ulnar artery and the vein.) The commonest cause of entrapment of Guyon's canal is a ganglion arising from one of the radiocarpal joints or occurring as a result of an occupational injury. Either the motor or the sensory branches may be affected as they both pass through the canal and division of the nerve into these two branches occurs in this canal. (The dorsal sensory branch is spared as it arises more proximally.)

TENOSYNOVITIS

This condition follows rapid repetitive movements which are either unaccustomed or resumed after a break from work or a holiday. Pain and swelling are located to the tendon sheath (usually the 2nd and 3rd dorsal compartments). Clinically there is swelling and tenderness over the area of the tendon sheath. Stretching of the affected tendons and contraction of the tendon against resistance reproduce the pain. Crepitus is occasionally felt or heard. The symptoms settle rapidly after a few days' rest or a change in the work routine.

DE QUERVAIN'S TENOSYNOVITIS

Fibrosis and stenosis may occur after inflammation of a tendon sheath. De Quervain's stenosing tenovaginitis affects the long abductor and the short extensor of the thumb. Pain and tenderness is located to the first dorsal compartment, and Finkelstein's test confirms the diagnosis in the absence of osteoarthritis of the first metacarpal. This condition has also been described with the extensor pollicis longus tendon and that of the extensor digiti minimi.

TENDINITIS

This is similar to tenosynovitis except that the condition affects the tissues around the tendon proximal to the tendon sheaths. Pain, swelling and tenderness are found at that point, where the long abductor and the short extensor of the thumb cross over the radial extensors of the wrist. There is frequently crepitus and therefore the condition is referred to as peritendinitis crepitans. The clinical course is the same as for tenosynovitis.

DUPUYTREN'S DISEASE

This is a common condition characterised by contractures of the palmar and digital fascia. It is twice as common in men and the incidence rises with age. It is thought to affect in the region of 25% of the male population over the age of 70 years in the UK. The incidence is subject to considerable geographical variation, and is greater in Westernised societies.

Dupuytren's disease is associated with knuckle (Garrod's) pads, plantar fibromatosis in the feet, Peyronie's disease, alcoholism and epilepsy-treatment with phenytoin, Epanutin or phenobarbitone. A history of trauma is frequently elicited, but it is debatable whether blunt trauma and manual work are causative. It is likely that genetic predisposition is the most important factor and that the other factors determine the age of onset of the disease.

The disease affects the palmar fascia and its associated ligamentous structure producing firm bands. Contractures then occur and are thought to occur either by contraction of the myofibroblast or by progressive loss of extension as more collagen is laid down. The digits most commonly affected are the ring and little fingers, followed by the middle finger and the thumb. The earliest sign of palmar disease is nodule formation. Pit formation is caused by contracture of the vertical fibres of the affected fascia.

Management

Splintage
Splintage may delay progression of the disease, but will not reverse it. The simplest way to decide if surgery is indicated is to ask the patient to place the hand flat on a table. If the patient is unable to do so, then surgery is indicated. Surgery involves fasciectomy of the involved fascia. The wounds are closed with the introduction of Z plasties of the skin to prevent contraction of the scar. If correcting severe deformities, skin grafts may be required during wound closure.

Fasciotomy
Fasciotomy (simple division of a fibrous band without fasciectomy) may be indicated in very elderly patients with severe contractures who have developed skin maceration as a prelude to further fasciectomy. Amputation may be indicated in the elderly or infirm. It may also be required in the treatment of patients with severe fixed flexion of the proximal interphalangeal joint of the little finger.

Postoperative
Immediate postoperative care involves physiotherapy to maintain joint movement and prevent contractures. Postoperative splints may be worn between periods of exercise to prevent recurrence of

contractures. If skin grafts have been used, prolonged splintage may be necessary. Disease may recur locally or new disease may occur at a neighbouring site. Careful surgical technique should minimise digital nerve injury and skin necrosis.

HALLUX VALGUS

This deformity consists of lateral deviation of the big toe at the first metatarsophalangeal joint with medial deviation of the first metatarsal. The first metatarsolphalangeal joint may be subluxed or dislocated. A hallux valgus angle greater than 15° and an intermetatarsal angle greater than 9° are abnormal.

Pronation of the great toe may occur when the hallux valgus angle exceeds 30°. The aetiology of this condition is uncertain but there appears to be a familial tendency, and race and the wearing of Western footwear are strongly implicated.

Treatment

Treatment may be non-operative or operative.

- Non-operative treatment includes the modification of footwear. A young patient with a prominent medial eminence with a relatively normal hallux valgus angle and intermetatarsal angle, should have their existing footwear modified. If their symptoms persist despite this, then often a surgical simple exostectomy and soft tissue procedure will help
- In mild to moderate hallux valgus in young people (less than 55 years of age) with a hallux valgus angle of 20–35° and with an intermetatarsal angle less than 15°, if conservative treatment has failed, then the surgical options are bunionectomy and a soft tissue correction (McBride's procedure) or a distal metatarsal osteotomy (Mitchell's osteotomy, Wilson's, Chevron) are indicated
- In severe hallux valgus deformity in young patients (less than 55 years of age with a hallux valgus angle greater than 35° and with an intermetatarsal angle greater than 10°, it is often necessary to perform a proximal basal metatarsal osteotomy. In patients with very high functional demands and with osteoarthritis at the metatarsophalangeal joint, the surgeon should consider performing an arthrodesis of the joint which is likely to serve the patient better
- In older patients with hallux valgus (greater than 65 years of age), the operation of choice is a Keller's procedure (excision arthroplasty of the metatarsophalangeal joint). This is a good operation in the low demand patient as the speed of recovery from the procedure is rapid. In the older patient with high functional demands, or if the patient has preoperative forefoot metatarsalgia, then the surgeon should consider performing an arthrodesis of the joint

- The most difficult age group of patient to treat hallux valgus is between 55 years and 65 years of age
- The management and assessment of hallux valgus should take account of the pain, footwear problems, functional limitation and cosmetic factors. Conservative treatment involves wearing capacious footwear
- Bunionectomy is successful when symptoms are totally related to the bony eminence, but minimal deformity and when combined with a soft tissue procedure.

HALLUX RIGIDUS

This is a condition characterised by painful limitation of movement of the metatarsophalangeal joint of the great toe and with osteoarthritis of the joint.

- The main problems for the patient with this condition are pain and stiffness of the joint. Women complain because of the lack of movement of the joint that they are unable to wear high-heeled shoes. Young patients complain that they get pain at the push-off phase of running. This condition tends to present in early to middle adult life when patients are physically active. High heels and flexible shoes cause pain.
- Non-operative management involves modification of footwear with wearing of a flat shoe, avoiding high heels. The application of a stiff sole avoids movement of the joint and eases symptoms
- Injection of the joint with corticosteroid and manipulation of the joint under anaesthetic often helps in selected cases
- Surgical options include cheilectomy in young patients (involves excision of the dorsal osteophytes to achieve an approximate range of 70° of passive dorsiflexion), and osteotomy of the proximal phalanx of the great toe to increase the range of dorsiflexion in young patients
- Operations in the older patient are Keller's procedure, or arthrodesis of the metatarsophalangeal joint in the patient with high functional demands or with preoperative forefoot metatarsalgia.

SOFT TISSUE DISORDERS OF THE ELBOW AND FOREARM

Elbow pain arising in the soft tissues occurs in 1–3% of the general population and is very common in sportsmen, manual workers and in industrial workers who perform repetitive tasks.

TENNIS ELBOW (LATERAL EPICONDYLITIS)

This is commonest in the 4th and 5th decades and may be related to degenerative change in the soft tissues. It is also seen in amateur tennis players, where it is related to their backhand stroke, and in professionals in relation to their serve. The pain is of gradual origin and is usually well localised, but it may radiate to the extensor aspect of the forearm. Patients often complain of a weak grip and of dropping objects. Tenderness is usually localised to the lateral epicondyle and supracondylar ridge. The pathology is uncertain, but is probably that of a degenerative or traumatic tear of the tendo-periosteal attachment of extensor carpi radialis brevis and the common extensor origin.

Treatment

- Non-operative treatment, including rest, steroid injections, epicondylar clamps and physiotherapy will settle over 90% of cases of tennis elbow
- Surgical treatment involves release of the common extensor origin. Results are best in those patients with a short history. Surgery is successful in approximately 70%.

OLECRANON BURSITIS

Inflammation of the bursa between the insertion of the triceps and the subcutaneous tissue is supposedly common in students as a result of resting on the elbow. Treatment of acute bursitis involves the use of NSAIDs, rest and occasionally aspiration. It may become infected. In chronic olecranon bursitis, if the remaining bursa which becomes hard due to fibrosis causes problems with resting on the elbow, surgical removal is indicated.

FRACTURES

It is essential to understand the principles of management. The principles have been supported by the development of new techniques to achieve more effective application of these basic principles:

1. Reduction of fracture
2. Maintenance of fracture reduction
   a. Skeletal or skin traction
   b. External splintage (plaster of Paris, external fixation)
   c. Rigid internal fixation
3. Rehabilitation, physiotherapy and mobilisation.

INTERNAL FIXATION

Indications

- Failure to achieve or maintain adequate reduction by external means, e.g. unable to control the position of the fracture in plaster

- Fracture involving a joint surface which requires very accurate anatomical reduction (elbow fractures and ankle fractures). This allows immediate movement of the joint thereby preventing joint stiffness and loss of function, e.g. supracondylar fracture of the elbow joint
- Multiple long bone fractures or ipsilateral fractures in one limb, e.g. the 'floating knee' syndrome with ipsilateral fractures of the femoral and tibial shafts. The patient's survival is significantly increased if after initial resuscitation based on ATLS principles, the patient is taken to theatre and the long bone fractures internally fixed. If they are not fixed, the patients have a much higher risk of developing fat emboli and multiple system organ failure including shock lung and disseminated intravascular coagulation (DIC)
- Pathological fractures. These fractures of long bones should be fixed with intramedullary nails which are 'locked' by both screws proximally and distally which pass through the nail to provide the most stable fixation. This allows immediate weight bearing, mobilisation of the patient and pain relief. The patient can then have radiotherapy when the wound has healed from surgery, with minimum delay if this is thought necessary by the treating physician
- Hip fractures for early mobilisation in elderly patients in the 1970s were treated with traction and bed rest. Because of the increasing numbers of the elderly population and the increasing number of hip fractures, internal fixation has revolutionised the treatment of these fractures, so that patients can be mobilised immediately full weight bearing after surgery and can either be discharged home, to rehabilitation, or to nursing homes. If fractures are rigidly fixed, pain from the fracture site is abolished and eases nursing for the patient with no pain on lifting or turning
- Fractures with neurovascular complications, e.g. a femoral shaft fracture associated with a rupture of the femoral artery. This requires stabilisation of the fracture by internal fixation and then vascular repair of the damaged artery.

Complications of internal fixation

- Infection. This should be less than 1%. Perioperative antibiotics, usually a cephalosporin, should be used
- Delayed union
- Non-union (hypertrophic and atrophic non-union)
- Fracture of implant due to metal fatigue. When fractures heal, essentially the fixation device (be it an intramedullary nail or plate) 'holds' the fracture in place until the fracture has healed. If the patients place excessive loads across the fracture site before the fracture unites, the metalwork will fatigue and then break. The same applies if, for instance, the fracture is delayed healing

or has not united, placing increased length of reliance and stress on the metalwork which eventually results in fatigue of the metalwork and failure of the metalwork
- Failure of the fixation due to poor surgical technique or osteoporotic bone

Complications of fracture healing
Definition of these complications is important as it determines subsequent approaches to management.

- Mal-union is union of a fracture with an angular or rotational deformity or unacceptable shortening, i.e. not an anatomical fixation
- Delayed union represents a delay in the normal time for fracture healing to have occurred; there is no radiological evidence of non-union
- Atrophic non-union is characterised radiologically by sclerosis at the bone ends; bony union will not occur without further surgery or bone grafting or both procedures
  1. Hypertrophic non-union is characterised by proliferative new bone around the fracture ends to give the typical 'elephant boot' appearance radiologically
  2. Atrophic non-union is characterised by atrophied bone ends which have a spiked appearance.

Causes of mal-union, delayed union and non-union

- Poor blood supply to the bone fragments, e.g. fractures of the distal third of the tibia, and waist of the scaphoid. This can be caused as a result of the initial fracture with stripping of the soft tissues and periosteum from the bone at the time of the injury or by poor surgical technique with unnecessary stripping of the soft tissue from the bone devascularising the fracture site
- Segmental fracture of a long bone. This implies a more severe energy injury to the bone with increased soft tissue damage
- Wide separation of the fracture surfaces, e.g. loss of bone substance in gunshot wounds, excessive muscle retraction of bone fragments, excessive traction leading to over distraction
- Severe compound fracture with major soft tissue damage
- Infection. If a deep infection occurs following internal fixation, this can result in an infected atrophic non-union. This results in a very difficult situation to deal with and often requires very complicated surgery in specialised centres. (This can involve excision of the bone with chronic infection in it and the bone transport and bone grafting procedures using circular external fixators.) There is still a high risk of amputation with an infected non-union
- Interposition of soft tissue such as muscle and periosteum between the fracture surfaces.

Treatment of non-union

- Hypertrophic non-unions respond well to bone grafting procedures with or without external fixation. Hypertrophic non-unions must be stabilised for the fracture to unite. In theory, they do not need to be bone grafted for the bone to unite. The hypertrophied bone is trying to heal but needs to be stabilised by internal or external fixation
- Atrophic non-unions are more difficult to treat than hypertrophic non-unions as bone grafting is frequently unsuccessful. (It is always necessary to bone graft atrophic non-unions in an attempt to get these to unite.)
  1. Vascularised bone grafts may be indicated in some difficult cases, e.g. vascularised fibula grafts can be used and this type of surgery needs to be performed in specialised centres with orthopaedic and plastic surgeons with an interest in the subject
  2. Bone transport can be used by the application of external fixators which move segments of bone into the bone defect at the site of the non-union, particularly if there is a large bone loss from the fracture site. This type of surgery is complicated, takes several months to perform, requires an understanding patient to comply with the treatment and has a high incidence of complications
  3. In some cases, despite all attempts to enable the fracture to unite, there is no alternative to amputation.

COMPOUND FRACTURES

All compound fractures of bones should be treated as surgical emergencies. The patients should be taken to the operating theatre within 6 hours of the accident (not 6 hours from the arrival to hospital), as this has been shown to decrease the rate of colonisation of the wound by bacteria and decrease the infection rate of the fracture, which is vital. Compound fractures are graded by the Gustilo and Anderson classification which grades the severity of the fracture, the severity of the skin and soft tissue damage, and whether there is any neurovascular deficit. This is important regarding the final prognosis for the patient.

1. Immediate treatment
   a. Resuscitation with intravenous fluids and blood transfusion. Advanced Trauma Life Support (ATLS) principles should be used by all medical personnel in the treatment of these injuries
   b. Analgesics
   c. Systemic antibiotics should include broad-spectrum agents with specific sensitivity against *Staph. aureus*. In highly contaminated injuries or agricultural farmyard injuries, an aminoglycoside and metronidazole should be added. At this point it is extremely useful to photograph the wounds before

covering them with saline-soaked swabs before the patient is taken to the operating theatre. This prevents personnel constantly removing the dressings, thereby increasing the risk of contamination of the wounds and is a permanent record
   d. Anti-tetanus prophylaxis is needed
   e. External splintage at the scene with inflatable or plastic splints.
2. Surgical treatment
   a. Surgical debridement must be performed within 6 hours of the injury
   b. Thorough wound toilet is followed by excision of all dead tissue. Large amounts of normal saline (9 litres) are used to mechanically flush out the debris and bacteria in the contaminated wound
   c. Adjacent tissues are examined to ensure that structures such as tendons and nerves are intact
   d. Fasciotomy may be required to prevent impairment of the distal circulation. If the limb is swollen or there is any doubt about compartment syndrome, a fasciotomy should be performed
   e. Primary wound closure should never be performed. In such cases, the wound is always left open. The wound is then inspected at 48 hours and this debrided again if there is any necrotic tissue remaining. When the wound is clean and granulating, the wound can either be closed secondarily at 3–5 days, or if there is enough local skin and soft tissue. If there is not enough skin, a split skin graft applied or the wound closed with a local flap, or when there is a large defect including fascia, muscle and with bone exposed, a free flap applied by the plastic surgeons
   f. Internal fixation is contraindicated
   g. The fracture is often best controlled by the use of an external fixator so that the soft tissue can be treated appropriately. Often the treatment of the soft tissues is just as important as the bone injuries.

KNEE JOINT INJURIES

Collateral ligament injuries
These occur as a direct result of a valgus or varus injury to the knee joint. They may occur in isolation or in conjunction with a cruciate ligament or meniscal injury. The treatment is dependent on the severity of the injury.

Simple sprain

- All of the ligament fibres remain in continuity
- Treatment includes analgesics and NSAIDs
- Physiotherapy and hydrotherapy are also very useful.

Partial tear

- Only a portion of the ligament fibres remain in continuity
- More pain and bruising are present than after a simple sprain, but there is no clinical or radiological evidence of joint instability
- Physiotherapy is performed as soon as the acute swelling has subsided.

Complete tear

- Complete disruption of the ligament fibres occurs, often with an associated capsular tear
- The knee joint is clinically unstable
- Diagnosis is confirmed by examination under anaesthetic and stress radiographs
- The injury may be associated with an internal derangement of the knee joint
- Following a complete tear, the ligament fibres retract and the defect is filled by scar tissue if repair is not undertaken
- Conservative treatment often causes the ligament to heal with some laxity, resulting in an unstable joint: such treatment which involves immobilisation in a plaster cylinder for 6 weeks may be appropriate in some elderly patients
- Immediate surgical repair is normally indicated in younger patients.

Anterior cruciate ligament injuries
Anterior cruciate ligament injury is the commonest cause of a haemarthrosis in an adult. Fifty percent of knees with an acute haemarthrosis have a tear of the anterior cruciate ligament. Anterior cruciate ligament is taut in full flexion and internal rotation of the tibia. It may be ruptured in isolation by forced flexion and internal rotation of the tibia or in combination with collateral ligament injury. The injury is suggested by the presence of a haemarthrosis with a positive anterior drawer sign, a positive Lachman sign and a positive pivot shift test.

A radiograph of the injured knee occasionally shows an avulsed fragment of bone detached from the site of insertion of the avulsed ligament.

Arthroscopy identifies the degree of injury and the site of the rupture; it also allows lavage of the haemarthrosis. In an ideal world, all patients with an acute haemarthrosis of the knee following trauma should have an examination under anaesthetic of the knee to test stability of the knee and arthroscopy of the knee to make an accurate initial diagnosis and to plan the appropriate initial treatment of the knee. This provides a rapid system of dealing with these patients. If the ligament has been avulsed from bone at either end, surgical repair is indicated, especially in young patients. Repair of the anterior cruciate ruptured at its mid part cannot adequately be performed and should not be performed. If surgery is thought to be indicated, then an anterior cruciate ligament reconstruction should be performed.

Long-term complication of anterior cruciate rupture is anterolateral knee joint instability, resulting in a positive jerk or pivot shift test.

Reconstruction of the anterior cruciate ligament is most commonly performed using the central third of the patella tendon. Other methods involve the use of the gracilis and semitendinosus tendons for construction of the graft, and by synthetic grafts or a combination of tendon and synthetic grafts. The procedure is now regularly performed arthroscopically in several centres. This provides less morbidity from the procedure and quicker recovery from the operation. Rehabilitation is long and requires intensive physiotherapy, and a return to sport after the procedure is in the order of 6 months to 1 year following surgery.

Posterior cruciate ligament injury

Posterior cruciate ligament may be damaged by a blow on the anterior aspect of the flexed knee or in combination with collateral ligament injuries. Positive posterior drawer sign confirms the diagnosis. Treatment is conservative unless a bone fragment at the site of insertion into the tibia has been avulsed.

Meniscal injuries

Meniscal injury is caused by rotatory force on the weight-bearing flexed knee. Various types of tear are recognised:

- Bucket handle tear
- Anterior horn tag tear
- Posterior horn tag tear
- Peripheral detachment
- Horizontal cleavage tear.

Symptoms

- Local pain, swelling
- Feeling of joint instability, i.e. the knee gives way, mechanical locking of the knee joint.

Physical signs

- Joint effusion
- Quadriceps wasting
- Joint line tenderness
- Extension block (locked knee)
- Positive McMurray test.

Investigations

- Plain radiographs of the knee joint excludes other pathology, followed by MRI scan, the test of choice, due to its very high

accuracy and non-invasive nature with absence of harmful X-irradiation
• Arthrography may yield a positive diagnosis, but this is now virtually obsolete.

Surgical management
Complete removal of the torn meniscus is usually avoided if at all possible. Arthroscopic menisectomy has the great advantage over open operation of rapid rehabilitation and return to work. The torn part of the meniscus is excised and the major portion of the cartilage remains in situ to minimise the development of degenerative changes in the knee joint.

In the Accident and Emergency Departments, owing to the frequency of this condition, it is important to remember a working differential diagnosis of a locked knee:

1. Loose intra-articular body
2. Osteophyte formation secondary to osteoarthritis
3. Osteochondral fracture
4. Osteochondritis dissecans
5. Synovial osteochondromatosis
6. Meniscal tear.

3. Trauma

Eleanor A. Ivory

The Royal College of Surgeons report on the management of patients with major injury (1988) found that up to 33% of deaths due to major trauma in their study were potentially preventable. The main causes of these deaths were:

- Haemorrhage – spleen, lung, liver
- Hypoxia
- Subdural haemorrhage
- Pulmonary embolism
- Misdiagnosis and inappropriate treatment.

The current Major Trauma Outcome Study (MTOS) continues to audit and monitor trauma care.

Mortality and morbidity of trauma victims are significantly reduced if management is logical and well planned in the initial phase. This so called 'golden hour' is a critical time during which the application of a didactic system that is universally understood and practised provides for an optimum outcome. Trauma care aims 'to provide oxygenated blood to the tissues, and to do no further harm'.

INITIAL MANAGEMENT OF THE MULTIPLY INJURED PATIENT

Takes place in three stages:

1. Preparation and triage
2. Primary survey
3. Secondary survey.

PREPARATION AND TRIAGE

Preparation is essential. A team leader is agreed, and available staff assigned specific roles. Based on the patient's pre-hospital history, essential equipment is prepared and final checks made. Resuscitation staff wear protective clothing, gloves and eye protection – universal precautions.

Triage means sorting of patients. In major trauma it may take two forms:

- Number of expected casualties does not exceed the facilities – all critically injured are treated
- Number of casualties exceeds facilities – critically injured most likely to survive are treated first.

PRIMARY SURVEY

Rapid and repeated assessment to diagnose and simultaneously treat existing or potentially life-threatening conditions. This continues until the patient is stable, but is rapidly repeated if there is any significant change at any time.

The primary survey is carried out in the following sequence:

- Airway with cervical spine control
- Breathing and ventilation
- Circulation with haemorrhage control
- Disability (brief neurological assessment)
- Exposure with environmental control.

AIRWAY AND CERVICAL SPINE CONTROL

All trauma patients are assumed to have a cervical spine injury until proved otherwise. Cervical spine control must be established and maintained at all times, especially during airway management. This is achieved using a correctly fitting hard collar and sandbags at each side of the head, secured with strong adhesive tape across the forehead onto the stretcher frame. If it is necessary to remove the collar, e.g. to examine the neck, cervical spine and head alignment are maintained by manual in-line cervical spine immobilisation. The collar is replaced as soon as possible.

Airway obstruction may be sudden, complete, partial or insidious. Causes include prolapsed tongue and soft tissues, blood, secretions or vomit. Foreign bodies include teeth and bone from mandibular and facial fractures.

Initial airway management
The airway is opened using a chin lift and jaw thrust. Debris, foreign bodies and secretions are removed using a gloved finger, Magill's forceps and suction. The airway is maintained using an oral or nasal airway. Care must be taken with the patient who will tolerate an airway to ensure they have intact laryngeal reflexes to protect the lower airway. If in doubt the lower airway is protected by a cuffed endotracheal tube.

Intubation
Indicated if there is failure to maintain airway, if the lower airway is unprotected, or there is an existing or potential need for ventilation.

Oral endotracheal intubation is the method of choice in the UK. The nasal route (favoured in the USA) is useful when there is a

high possibility of cervical spine injury but may be associated with
significant epistaxis.

Before attempting intubation, the patient is preoxygenated with
100% oxygen. Prolonged attempts at intubation without
intermittent oxygenation must be avoided. Oxygen saturation
should be monitored using pulse oximetry. Once the tube is
placed, its position is checked by auscultation high up in both
axillae to avoid oesophageal or right bronchial intubation. End
tidal CO_2 monitoring confirms endotracheal placement. If in doubt,
remove and repeat.

Surgical airway

Indicated when other methods have failed, e.g. in severe glottic
oedema, foreign body or laryngeal fracture. Two methods are used
in the emergency department.

1. Needle cricothyroidotomy with jet insufflation of the airway.
   Indicated in children under 12 and in adults. A 12 or 14-gauge
   cannula is inserted through the cricothyroid membrane into the
   tracheal lumen. The cannula is attached to wall oxygen using
   plastic tubing at the end of which is either a side hole or a Y
   connector. The flow rate is set at 15 litres/min. Oxygen enters
   the lungs when the hole or Y piece is occluded for 1 second,
   it is released for 4 seconds to allow recoil of the chest for
   exhalation. Oxygenation can be maintained for up to
   40 minutes. However, there is a gradual build-up of CO_2 due to
   inadequate exhalation. This may be a problem in the case of
   head injury where hypercarbia should be avoided.
   Caution is required with total upper airway obstruction. If the
   obstructing body is not expelled, barotrauma may occur
   including tension pneumothorax. The flow rate should be
   reduced to 7–8 litres/min.
2. Surgical cricothyroidotomy
   Contraindicated in children under 12 as it causes trauma to the
   only circumferential support for the upper trachea in the child.
   A transverse skin incision is made over the cricothyroid
   membrane. The membrane is carefully opened under direct
   vision. A 5–7 mm cuffed tracheostomy or endotracheal tube is
   passed distally into the trachea and the cuff inflated.

BREATHING AND VENTILATION

The rate, depth and equality of respiratory movements are noted,
as well as use of accessory muscles or abdominal breathing. The
neck and chest are palpated for tracheal deviation, signs of
asymmetry, flail segments or surgical emphysema.

Oxygenation is monitored continually using pulse oximetry,
clinical observation and arterial blood gas measurement. Pulse
oximetry is the most useful non-invasive monitoring method, but

is unable to distinguish between oxyhaemoglobin, carboxyhaemoglobin and methaemoglobin. It is unreliable in profound anaemia (Hb < 5 g), marked peripheral vasoconstriction and in severe hypothermia.

All trauma patients receive supplemental oxygen delivered via a tight-fitting face mask with a reservoir bag with a flow rate of 10–12 litres/min. This provides an inspired oxygen concentration of up to 60%.

Effective assisted ventilation can be achieved using a bag and mask system, attached to wall oxygen, as long as the airway can be opened and a good seal maintained around the mask. This is used with or without endotracheal intubation. Caution is required with the non-intubated patient since assisted ventilation may lead to vomiting from gastric distension.

CIRCULATION WITH HAEMORRHAGE CONTROL

Circulatory failure leads to shock which is defined as: 'inadequate organ perfusion and tissue oxygenation'.

Five types of shock:

1. Hypovolaemic
2. Cardiogenic
3. Septic
4. Anaphylactic
5. Neurogenic.

Hypovolaemic shock

A high index of suspicion is essential in all trauma patients because of the effectiveness of physiological compensatory mechanisms in response to volume loss, particularly in the young, fit adult.

Blood pressure (BP) is not a reliable index of early shock. Look for:

• Tachycardia
• Peripheral vasoconstriction
• Pulse pressure
• Respiratory rate.

Physical signs associated with increasing blood loss may be used to describe four theoretical classes of haemorrhage (Table 3.1).

The volume of blood loss required to give a consistent drop in systemic BP is > 1500 ml, i.e. 30% blood volume. Therefore the patient who is obviously pale, clammy, tachycardic and hypotensive already has a significant deficit and needs urgent resuscitation. Good clinical management is aimed at detecting and resuscitating the patient showing subtle signs of volume loss.

Table 3.1 Classes of haemorrhage based on initial physical signs

	Class I	Class II	Class III	Class IV
% Blood loss	Up to 15%	15–30%	30–40%	> 40%
Blood loss (ml)	< 750	750–1500	1500–2000	> 2000
Pulse rate	under 100	100–120	> 120	> 140
Pulse pressure	Normal or increased	Decreased	Decreased	Decreased
Blood pressure	Normal	Normal	Decreased	Decreased
Respiratory rate	Normal	20–30	> 30	> 35
Mental state	Mild anxiety	Anxious	Confused	Lethargic
Urine output	Normal	Reduced	Oliguric	Negligible
	30 ml/hour	20–30 ml/hour	5–15 ml/hour	

Treatment

- Bleeding may be external or internal. Control obvious haemorrhage with firm pressure and consider sources of concealed haemorrhage: chest, abdomen, pelvis, retroperitoneum
- Site two intravenous cannulae (14-gauge) peripherally; antecubital fossa or femoral vein. The long saphenous vein at the ankle may be used percutaneously or as the site for a venous 'cut down'
- Rapidly infuse 2 litres of warmed fluids. Crystalloid or blood. Blood should be O-negative if very urgent, type-specific or fully X-matched if time allows. Fresh frozen plasma to supply clotting factors must be considered after 5 or 6 units
- Assess response.

Three patterns of response may be observed:

1. Responders
2. Transient responders
3. Non-responders.

Where the response to the initial fluid bolus of 2 litres is not sustained, a continuing source of fluid loss must be sought while continuing to fluid resuscitate. Non-responders usually need urgent surgical intervention to control catastrophic haemorrhage. Other causes to consider in non-responders:

- Pump failure: myocardial contusion, myocardial infarction
- Cardiac tamponade
- Tension pneumothorax
- Co-existing non-haemorrhagic shock.

Anaphylactic, septic and neurogenic shock
All cause impaired tissue perfusion by massive increases in the vascular space. Treatment is aimed at fluid replacement and

specific treatment of the cause, e.g. in anaphylaxis early treatment with intramuscular adrenaline. For septic shock – antibiotics and inotropes. Neurogenic shock is caused by interruption of sympathetic outflow from the spinal cord causing loss of vasomotor tone and sympathetic stimulation to the heart, resulting in vasodilatation, bradycardia and hypotension.

Problems in shock management

- The elderly have reduced compensation mechanisms
- Athletes may have a low resting pulse and increased blood volume by 15–20%
- Patients on β-blockers may not develop a tachycardia
- Pacemakers may not compensate for severe blood loss
- Pregnancy: venocaval compression by the gravid uterus causes decreased venous return making shock worse. Relieve by tilting patient to the left side
- Hypothermic patients do not respond to shock treatment fully until rewarmed
- Clotting deficiency after multiple trauma and massive transfusion.

DISABILITY (BRIEF NEUROLOGICAL ASSESSMENT)

A detailed neurological examination is carried out during the secondary survey. The primary survey involves a basic assessment of level of consciousness, pupillary responses, and an assessment of gross lateralizing signs. The Glasgow Coma Scale (see Table 3.2) is used to assess level of consciousness. It is vital to note *decreases in level of consciousness* and to consider causes:

Table 3.2   The Glasgow Coma Scale

Eye opening	Spontaneous	4
	To verbal command	3
	To pain	2
	None	1
Best verbal response	Fully orientated	5
	Confused conversation	4
	Inappropriate words	3
	Incomprehensible sounds	2
	No response	1
Best motor response	Obeys	6
	Localises pain	5
	Normal flexion from pain	4
	Abnormal flexion (decorticate)	3
	Extension (decerebrate)	2
	No response	1

Scores range from 3 to 15.

- Head injury
- Hypoxia – reassess airway, breathing and circulation
- Hypovolaemia
- Drugs and alcohol
- Hypoglycaemia.

EXPOSURE WITH ENVIRONMENTAL CONTROL

This is an integral part of the primary survey during which all the patient's clothing is removed, allowing accurate assessment of the whole patient. Hypothermia is avoided using warmed fluids and appropriate coverings.

SECONDARY SURVEY

As soon as possible a full history of the mechanism of injury is taken, from witnesses and ambulance crew. Past medical history including drugs and allergies is noted. The patient is examined from head to toe, including a log roll and internal examinations. Detailed investigations arranged as appropriate. A nasogastric tube is placed to decompress any post-traumatic gastric distension. The orogastric route is chosen if there is any suggestion of a cribriform plate fracture. Urinary catheterisation, after the rectal examination to exclude partial or complete urethral rupture, is carried out.

During the secondary survey, monitoring and clinical assessment continue to identify or anticipate changes that may require further resuscitation, especially when the patient is undergoing lengthy investigations. A detailed list of injuries and problems is made and a definitive plan of management made.

SPECIFIC TYPES OF TRAUMA

THORACIC TRAUMA

Approximately one in four patients with chest trauma die. Some of these deaths are preventable. The following conditions may be *immediately life-threatening* and must be rapidly excluded or treated during the primary survey. All may be treated by simple measures. They demonstrate par excellence the importance of the 'golden hour'.

- Airway obstruction
- Tension pneumothorax
- Open pneumothorax
- Massive haemothorax
- Flail chest
- Cardiac tamponade.

Airway obstruction
See Primary survey.

Tension pneumothorax
Caused by air in the pleural cavity that is unable to escape with expiration but which increases with inspiration. Increasing intrathoracic pressure causes collapse of the ipsilateral lung with mediastinal shift and eventually compression of the vena cava and heart, reducing venous return, leading to cardiovascular and respiratory compromise.

Diagnosis is clinical. Severe respiratory distress with signs of reduced cardiac output, tracheal deviation away from the tension, reduced breath sounds and hyper-resonance are classical findings.

Treatment is by needle thoracocentesis. A needle and cannula are inserted into the chest in the second intercostal space in the midclavicular line decompressing the tension. A formal chest drain is required to drain the now simple pneumothorax. Tension pneumothorax may develop during ventilation after chest injury.

Open pneumothorax
Also called a 'sucking' chest wound. If the opening in the chest wall is greater than two-thirds of the diameter of the trachea, air is sucked into the wound with each breath. Normal inspiration is impaired leading to hypoxia. Severe chest defects are associated with pulmonary contusion leading to further hypoxia.

Treatment is by covering the defect with a sterile occlusive dressing attached on three sides only. The open flap thus allows expulsion of trapped air with each expiration thus preventing the development of a tension pneumothorax. Surgical repair is usually required.

Massive haemothorax
Defined as the presence within the thoracic cavity of >1500 ml blood and/or the continued drainage of > 200 ml/hour blood.

Treatment is fluid resuscitation *before* drainage with a large caliber chest drain. Early thoracotomy is required. Penetrating wounds between the nipple lines and between the medial scapular borders suggest potential damage to the great vessels, hilar structures or the heart.

Flail chest
Multiple rib fractures causing a portion of the chest wall to move independently of the rest of the thoracic cage may produce paradoxical movement that can be detected clinically. Hypoxia is a result of both hypoventilation and, more importantly, underlying lung contusion, the effects of which can develop hours later and should be anticipated. The injured lung is susceptible to pulmonary oedema, therefore fluid replacement must be monitored. Treatment is analgesia, oxygen and often intubation and ventilation.

Cardiac tamponade

If blood accumulates in the fibrous and relatively unyielding pericardial sac, ventricular filling and contraction are rapidly impaired. Diagnosis is mainly by clinical suspicion, rather than by finding the classical Beck's triad of: raised venous pressure, falling arterial pressure and muffled heart sounds. Pulsus paradoxus, a decrease in systolic pressure of > 10 mmHg during inspiration, and Kussmaul's sign, a rise in venous pressure with inspiration, may be seen.

Electromechanical dissociation (the presence of a rhythm on the monitor that is normally associated with a cardiac output, but with no detectable output) may be caused by cardiac tamponade.

Treatment is by pericardial tap using a pericardial needle and 20 ml syringe. This is advanced into the pericardium using the subxiphoid route. An injury current may be observed on the ECG monitor, the needle is then withdrawn slightly and aspirated.

Aspiration of as little as 15 or 20 ml of blood may restore cardiac function. The cannula is left in situ with a tap to allow further aspiration if necessary. Thoracotomy is required to inspect the heart.

URGENT BUT NOT IMMEDIATELY LIFE-THREATENING CONDITIONS

Each of these frequently missed injuries may become life-threatening:

- Pulmonary contusion
- Aortic disruption
- Myocardial contusion
- Diaphragmatic rupture
- Oesophageal rupture
- Tracheal rupture.

Pulmonary contusion

Due to blunt trauma to the chest. May occur without a flail chest, especially in the young. Effects are often delayed. Causes hypoxia and can lead to pulmonary oedema. Treatment: maintain oxygenation, cautious intravenous fluids and ventilation if severe.

Aortic disruption

Rupture most frequently occurs at the level of the ligamentum arteriosum. Complete disruption is fatal. Partial rupture is tamponaded temporarily only to fatally rupture in the next few hours. Diagnosis is suggested by history of rapid deceleration injury.

Radiographic features

- Mediastinal widening (especially on PA chest X-ray)
- Tracheal deviation
- Oesophageal deviation to right

- Obliteration of aortic knuckle
- Fractures of 1st and 2nd ribs.

Most consistent finding is mediastinal widening which indicates the need for CT scanning or angiography. Treatment is surgical.

Myocardial contusion
Underdiagnosed. Due to blunt trauma to the heart. May cause impaired cardiac output and arrhythmias. ECG and cardiac enzymes are monitored.

Diaphragmatic rupture
Frequently missed. May present very late, including years later. More commonly diagnosed on the left because on the right the liver prevents herniation of abdominal contents into the chest. Presents with loops of bowel or the nasogastric tube in the left side of the chest. Treatment is surgical repair.

Oesophageal rupture
Causes extreme pain. Must be diagnosed to prevent the usually fatal mediastinitis. Pneumomediastinum may be seen on chest X-ray. Treatment is mediastinal drainage and repair.

Tracheal rupture
Presents with haemoptysis, stridor, surgical emphysema or pneumothorax. Treatment is surgical.

OTHER CHEST INJURIES

Rib fractures
Important because of associated injuries:

- Flail chest
- Sternal fracture and myocardial contusion
- Upper ribs 1–3: with great vessel damage, head, neck and spinal cord injury
- Middle ribs 4–9: if multiple with pulmonary contusion
- Lower ribs 10–12: with hepatosplenic, diaphragmatic or bowel injury.

Traumatic asphyxia
Due to strangulation or severe crush injury to the chest. Findings are plethora and petechial haemorrhages above the level of pressure due to venous compression. Massive swelling, cerebral oedema and retinal haemorrhages may also be found.

HEAD INJURY

Accounts for 50% of all trauma deaths. Mortality from severe head injury is 40%, with significant morbidity in the survivors.

Primary brain injury occurs at the time of trauma, resulting in untreatable neuronal and axonal injury.
Secondary brain injury occurs later due to:

- Intracranial haemorrhage
- Cerebral oedema
- Ischaemia and hypoxia
- Hypercarbia
- Raised intracranial pressure (ICP).

Head injury may be divided into diffuse and focal lesions.

DIFFUSE INJURY

- Concussion – transient loss of consciousness
- Prolonged traumatic coma – over 6 hours.

FOCAL LESIONS

- Skull fractures
- Contusions
- Intracranial haemorrhage
- Penetrating injury.

Skull fractures

1. Linear non-depressed fractures alone are usually not significant, it is the probability of underlying brain injury and haemorrhage that is important. Risk of intracranial haematoma:
   - Confused with skull fracture   1:4
   - Fully orientated with skull fracture 1:30
   - Confused but no fracture   1:120
   - Fully orientated with no fracture   1:6000
2. Depressed fractures are usually elevated if depressed more than the thickness of the skull
3. Basal skull fractures are usually not seen on X-ray; they are suggested by intracranial air. Features include:
   - Anterior fossa fractures: rhinorrhoea, scleral haematoma without a posterior limit, bilateral periorbital haematomas – racoon eyes
   - Middle fossa fractures: otorrhoea, haemotympanum
   - Posterior fossa fractures: Battle's sign – bruising in the mastoid region
4. Open skull fractures carry the risk of infection since the dura is open.

Contusion
May be directly under site of impact or on the contralateral side, i.e. a contracoup lesion.

Intracranial haemorrhage

Extradural (See Uncal herniation)   Occurs between the dura and bone. Usually from a dural artery, most commonly the middle meningeal artery. Usually associated with a linear skull fracture of the temporal or parietal bone that crosses the groove for the middle meningeal artery. A rare (< 1% of major head injuries), but important, injury. May be rapidly fatal but can be treated if diagnosed in the early stages.

History of loss of consciousness, then a lucid period usually with severe localised headache, followed by a secondary loss of consciousness with contralateral hemiparesis, signs of increasing ICP and an ipsilateral fixed dilated pupil. Treatment is urgent, surgical decompression. Burr holes may be indicated very occasionally as a holding measure – 'explore the side of the dilated pupil'.

Acute subdural   Caused by bleeding from bridging veins between cerebral cortex and the dura. Seen in 30% of severe head injuries, much more common than extradural. Morbidity of an acute subdural is partly from the mass effect but also from severe underlying brain injury. Mortality is 60%. Treatment is urgent decompression and supportive measures for underlying brain injury.

Subarachnoid   May be spontaneous, leading to the trauma or may be traumatic. Causes headache, meningeal irritation from blood in the cerebrospinal fluid (CSF), photophobia and vomiting.

Intracerebral   Haemorrhage within the brain substance. Varies in degree and may be delayed.

Penetrating injury
Damage depends on the site of penetration and energy of the projectile. Gunshot wounds causing damage far beyond their direct penetration because of the high energy expended.

Intracranial pressure (ICP)
Normal ICP is less than 15 mmHg. Cerebral blood flow depends on maintaining an adequate cerebral perfusion pressure (CPP). They are related by:

CPP = Mean arterial blood pressure – ICP

If ICP is elevated by an expanding lesion, compensatory mechanisms act to reduce intracranial volume, compensating for an increase in volume of 50–100 ml only. Above this, the ICP will elevate, causing an elevation in systemic blood pressure as seen in the Cushing reflex of progressive hypertension, bradycardia and decreased respiratory rate.

Herniation
Increased ICP can result in herniation at several locations.

1. Transtentorial or uncal herniation (Fig. 3.1)

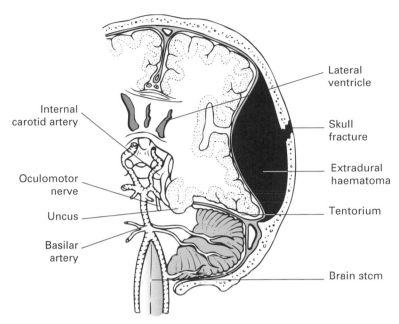

Internal
carotid artery

Oculomotor
nerve

Uncus

Basilar
artery

Lateral
ventricle

Skull
fracture

Extradural
haematoma

Tentorium

Brain stem

Fig. 3.1 Transtentorial uncal herniation.

Extradural or large subdural haematoma in the temporal lobe
area forces the ipsilateral uncus of the temporal lobe to herniate
through the tentorial hiatus, resulting in compression of the
oculomotor (IIIrd) nerve and parasympathetic paralysis of the
pupil on that side, causing it to become fixed and dilated.
Pressure on the cerebral peduncle may cause contralateral
hemiparesis and pressure on the brain stem causes decreasing
consciousness. Rarely the paralysis may be on the same side if
the opposite cerebral peduncle is compressed, causing a false
localising sign.
2. Cerebellar herniation through the foramen magnum may occur,
resulting in medullary compression causing bradycardia,
respiratory arrest and death.

Assessment and monitoring

History
Loss of consciousness and orientation. Mechanism of injury, drugs
or alcohol involvement.

Examination
ABC of trauma care is the first priority, with cervical spine
stabilisation. Neurological examination and monitoring using the

Glasgow Coma Scale (GCS) as devised by Teasdale and Jennett (Table 3.2).

Repeated examinations using the GCS are made to note if the patient is stable, improving or deteriorating. *The single most important factor is a deteriorating level of consciousness as a hallmark of secondary brain injury.*

Using the GCS

- Coma is defined as a GCS of 8 or less
- A deterioration of 2 or more points on the scale indicates significant elevation in ICP needing urgent investigation (CT scan) and treatment
- Severe head injury   GCS 8 or below
- Moderate   GCS 9–12
- Mild   GCS 13–15

Management of raised ICP

- ICP monitoring
- Paralyse and hyperventilate to produce controlled hypocarbia with $PaCO_2$ in the range of 3.5–3.7 kPa. This leads to cerebral vasoconstriction and a decrease of ICP
- Mannitol 1 g/kg may temporarily reduce ICP. Use remains controversial
- Control fits using intravenous diazepam, phenytoin or thiopentone
- Monitored intravenous fluids to prevent cerebral oedema
- Surgical removal of mass lesions.

Other manifestations of severe brain injury to consider are:

- Hyperpyrexia
- Hyperglycaemia
- Clotting abnormalities
- Neurogenic pulmonary oedema.

SPINAL INJURY

Management of a patient with a spinal injury is in three stages:

1. Ensure patient survival by following the ABCDEs of trauma care
2. Preserve residual spinal function by careful handling and immobilisation
3. Ensure the highest possible chance for the injured spinal cord to recover.

Any unconscious patient, head-injured patient or anyone with blunt trauma above the level of the clavicles must be strongly suspected of having a cervical spine injury. Spinal cord injury may occur with or without vertebral fracture.

Clinical findings associated with cord injury

- Sensory and motor level in the conscious patient
- Flaccid paralysis, flaccid areflexia (spinal shock)
- Loss of anal reflexes and anal tone
- Diaphragmatic breathing
- Neurogenic shock (hypotension with bradycardia)
- Priapism.

Clinical assessment

History
An unconscious patient admitted after a fall or road traffic accident
has a 5–10% chance of having a spinal injury.

Examination
Assume spinal injury. Manage with total spinal immobilisation on
a spine board. Log roll patient if movement required and when
assessing the back. A minimum of four people is required for a
safe log roll.
   Vertebrae are examined for bruising, muscle spasm, tenderness,
deformity. A 'step' may be felt or the spinous processes may be
abnormally prominent

Neurological examination
A complete spinal lesion causes total loss of motor and sensory
function distal to the lesion (Table 3.3). If the lesion is incomplete,

Table 3.3   Sensory and motor levels

Sensory level	Root	Motor function	Muscle
Occiput	C2		
	C3, C4	Shoulder elevation	Trapezius
Shoulder tops	C4	Respiration	Diaphragm
	C5, C6	Elbow flexion	Biceps
Thumb	C6		
Middle finger	C7	Elbow extension	Triceps
Little finger	C8	Finger flexion	Flexor digitorum
	T1	Finger abduction/adduction	Interossei
Nipple	T4		
Umbilicus	T10		
	T1–12	Respiration	Intercostals/abdominals
Inguinal crease	L1		
	L1–2	Hip flexion	Iliopsoas
Anterior thigh	L2–3		
	L3–4	Knee extension	Quadriceps
Medial calf	L4	Ankle dorsiflexion	Tibialis anterior
Lateral calf	L5	Big toe dorsiflexion	Extensor hallucis
Lateral foot	S1	Knee flexion	Biceps femoris
	S1–2	Foot plantar flexion	Soleus and gastrocnemius
Perineal	S2–4	Sphincter tone	Rectal sphincter

variable recovery may be possible. The only indication that a lesion is not complete may be the finding of 'sacral sparing', i.e. some sensation in the anal and perianal areas, or a flicker of movement in the big toe; however, it is not possible to diagnose an incomplete lesion during the period of spinal shock.

Spinal shock is a period of spinal cord 'concussion' during which cord-mediated reflexes are absent. It usually lasts for up to 24 hours but it may be prolonged for days or weeks. Return of reflex function is indicated by finding an intact bulbocavernosus or anal reflex, or priapism. The full extent of cord injury, and hence prognosis, cannot be determined until these reflexes return. Spinal shock should be distinguished from *neurogenic shock*, which is a loss of sympathetic tone to blood vessels and the heart resulting in vasodilatation, bradycardia and hypotension.

Respiratory function
Spinal lesions involving lower cervical and upper thoracic lesions cause impaired intercostal function. The diaphragm functions normally via the phrenic nerves (C3, 4, 5) resulting in abdominal breathing. High cervical lesions causing diaphragmatic paralysis are frequently fatal if complete.

Treatment

- ABC of trauma care
- Immobilisation and log rolling
- Treatment of neurogenic shock is with monitored fluids and atropine
- High-dose methylprednisolone may be beneficial if given within 8 hours of injury, although this remains controversial
- Pressure care. Denervated skin is especially susceptible to pressure necrosis during prolonged resuscitation on a rigid spine board. All paralysed patients must therefore be turned at least 2-hourly.

RADIOLOGY

Lateral cervical spine, look for presence of all seven vertebrae and the cervicothoracic junction. An increase in the prevertebral soft tissue shadow 5 mm or greater down to C3/4 level suggests haematoma secondary to fracture. Each vertebra is checked for fracture and the alignment of the normal lordotic curves. Full cervical spine series includes open mouth odontoid view, anteroposterior and oblique views.

ABDOMINAL TRAUMA

Identifying the need for early laparotomy rather than making an organ-specific diagnosis is the priority of management. Trauma may be blunt or penetrating, resulting in haemorrhage or perforation of a viscus in any of the three abdominal compartments:

- Peritoneal cavity
- Retroperitoneum
- Pelvis.

The upper part of the peritoneal cavity extends beneath the lower ribs and may be involved in thoracic trauma. The retroperitoneal space is difficult to examine and injuries are often missed.

BLEEDING

Splenic or hepatic rupture may present with catastrophic haemorrhage requiring urgent resuscitation and operation. Delayed, slower bleeding is also common. Bucket handle tear of the mesentery may occur during deceleration injury giving rise to subtle bleeding and devitalisation of bowel.

Diagnostic peritoneal lavage (DPL)

DPL is 98% sensitive for intraperitoneal bleeding. The open method is used using a 2–3 cm incision in the midline below the umbilicus (unless there is a pelvic fracture). The bladder and stomach are emptied first. The peritoneum is elevated and a peritoneal dialysis catheter inserted and advanced towards the pelvis. Warm saline up to 1 litre is instilled and gently agitated for 10 minutes. The fluid is then allowed to drain. Positive findings are:

- Gross blood *or*
- 100 000 RBC/mm^3 or more and greater than 500 WBC/mm^3.

The absolute contraindication for DPL is an existing indication for laparotomy. Relative contraindications include:

- Gross obesity
- Previous surgery and adhesions
- Clotting disorders.

False-positives may be caused by pelvic fracture or poor technique. False-negatives occur in up to 2%, usually due to trauma to the pancreas, duodenum, small bowel or bladder.

Other investigations

CT scanning is used to diagnose specific organ damage and to examine the retroperitoneum. Ultrasound in the resuscitation room is useful, especially for children.

Perforation

In the conscious patient this causes severe pain and tenderness with guarding. Prior to DPL an erect chest X-ray or a lateral decubitus may reveal subdiaphragmatic or extraluminal air.

Contrast studies using water-soluble contrast may confirm a perforation. Perforation should be considered in the days after trauma as it may be missed or develop late. Treatment is surgical with appropriate antibiotic cover.

Pelvic fracture
May lead to life-threatening haemorrhage or trauma to structures within the pelvic compartment of the abdomen. Disruption of the pelvic ring requires high energy trauma and is therefore associated with multiple other injuries. Heamorrhage is mainly from pelvic veins.

Examination should include pelvic 'springing' in longitudinal and lateral directions to look for obvious pelvic instability. Urethral injury may be seen. Anteroposterior X-ray of the pelvis is taken as part of the primary survey because of the potential for severe blood loss.

Initial treatment is to resuscitate the patient and to stabilise the pelvis by external fixation to reduce further vascular damage.

BURNS

May be:

- Thermal
- Electrical
- Chemical.

THERMAL BURNS

These are classified according to depth and percentage of body surface area involved:

- Partial thickness
- Full thickness.

Partial thickness burns may be superficial or deep. *Superficial partial thickness* (first-degree in USA) represented by moderate sunburn. The skin is red and painful, slightly oedematous but without blisters. There is minimal damage to the superficial layers of the epidermis. Healing is usually within 7 days with characteristic peeling of dead skin.

Deep partial thickness burns (second-degree) extend into the dermis but hair follicles and sweat glands are not destroyed. Characteristic blistering with painful redness, mottling and oedema are seen. Epithelial coverage takes 14–21 days. Healing is usually without scarring provided no infection develops.

Full thickness burns (third-degree) are charred, pearly white, translucent and leathery. All layers are destroyed. The surface is dry and pain-free. Healing is only possible by scarring with contractures or grafting.

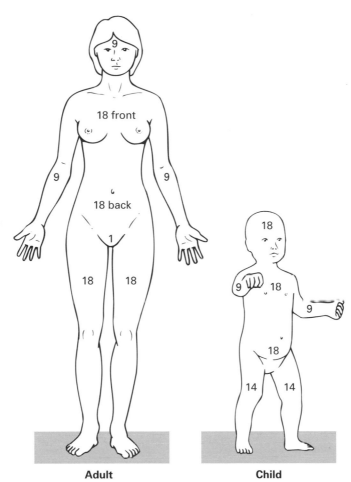

Fig. 3.2 'Rule of nines'.

Percentage of body surface area involved

Estimated using the 'rule of nines'. Used to calculate fluid replacement in severe burns (Fig. 3.2).

- 1% is approximately the palm of the patient's hand, excluding the fingers. Used to estimate the size of an irregular burn
- In children, the head is a greater percentage of surface area, the limbs are a smaller percentage area.

Clinical assessment of major burns

Three important elements to consider as well as the burn:

1. Acute inhalational injury with thermal damage to the airway
2. Carbon monoxide or other toxic gas poisoning
3. Associated other injuries, e.g. blunt trauma, falls or blast injury.

History

To include type of fire, enclosed space? Toxic chemicals involved? Other trauma likely, e.g. vehicle fires or falling masonry in house fires. Blast or electrical injury involved?

Examination and treatment

Airway, breathing and circulation are the priority. With facial and upper airway burns, early endotracheal intubation is necessary to avoid delayed airway obstruction. Finding singed facial or nasal hairs or carbonaceous sputum suggests inhalation injury with potential thermal damage to the airway. Tracheobronchial oedema, ulceration or bronchospasm, caused by inhalation of hot gases or chemical irritation, may present early or late with hypoxia, respiratory distress and wheezing. Pulmonary oedema results from damage to the alveolar capillary membrane from inhalation of chemicals in smoke and fumes. Chest X-ray and frequent arterial blood gasses are performed.

Circulation and fluid replacement must be maintained. Vasodilatation and capillary leakage from burned tissues leads to extensive fluid loss. Volume replacement due to burn losses is *in addition* to other fluid requirements and is calculated *from the time of the burn*, not from arrival in hospital.

A formula to estimate the replacement needed is:

2–4 ml/kg/% burn/24 hours

Half of this is given in the first 8 hours post burn and the other half in the next 16 hours. Amount is adjusted according to response. A urine output of 30–50 ml per hour should be maintained.

Other features of burns

- Rhabdomyolysis, the disintegration of striated muscle causing urinary excretion of myoglobin, may be seen in severe burns and electrical injury. Acute renal failure may result if adequate urine out put is not maintained
- Anaemia. In severe burns haemoglobin is lost, blood transfusion may be needed
- Hypothermia caused by loss of normal skin function
- Pain is treated with small doses of intravenous opiates
- Tetanus prophylaxis 0.5 ml tetanus toxoid booster is given to all burn patients or immunoglobulin if previous immunisation status in doubt

- Escharotomy may be necessary for circumferential burns of the chest or limbs where chest movement or distal pulses are compromised
- Antibiotics are not indicated prophylactically because of development of resistance.

CARBON MONOXIDE POISONING

Should be considered in all burns patients, especially when combustion was in a confined space. Causes headaches, confusion, coma and death. Carbon monoxide has an affinity for haemoglobin of at least 200 times greater than oxygen. It binds effectively irreversibly thus altering oxygen transport. It is also a mitochondrial toxin affecting cellular metabolism directly.

Treatment
High concentration oxygen or hyperbaric oxygen if clinically severe. This increases the elimination half-life from 250 minutes when breathing air, to 50 minutes on 100% oxygen, to 22 minutes on hyperbaric oxygen at 2.5 atmospheres. Carboxyhaemoglobin level may not correlate well with symptoms but is a good indicator of exposure. Levels of over 68% if untreated are usually fatal. The classical 'cherry red' appearance of carbon monoxide poisoning is only seen in severe or fatal cases.

FURTHER READING

American College of Surgeons Committee on Trauma 1993 Advanced Trauma Life Support Provider Manual. American College of Surgeons, Chicago

Tintinalli J E, Krome R L, Ruiz E (Eds) 1992 Emergency medicine: a comprehensive study guide, 3rd edn. American College of Emergency Physicians. McGraw-Hill, New York

Howarth P, Evans R 1994 Key topics in accident and emergency medicine. Bios Scientific, Oxford

Mendelow A D, Teasdale G, Jennett B, et al 1983 Risks of intracranial haematoma in head injured adults. British Medical Journal 187: 1173

Royal College of Surgeons of England 1988 Commission on the provision of surgical services. Report of the Working Party on the management of patients with major injuries. RCS, London

Skinner D V, Whimster F 1999 Trauma: a companion to Bailey and Love's short practice of surgery. Arnold, London

4. Anaesthetics

Sean Elliott, Stephen Eckersall

PREOPERATIVE ASSESSMENT

All patients should be assessed by an anaesthetist prior to anaesthesia in order to:

- Assess the risks involved
- Optimise preoperative condition
- Plan the anaesthetic technique and counsel patient.

Assessment of the airway

It is important to identify patients who may have a difficult airway so that appropriate personnel and equipment can be prepared

Risk factors

- Prominent upper teeth and premaxilla
- Receding lower jaw, high arched palate
- Obesity and pregnancy
- Reduced movement of cervical spine or mouth opening
- Congenital conditions, e.g. Pierre Robin and Treacher Collins syndrome
- Soft tissue abnormalities, e.g. previous radiotherapy, laryngeal carcinoma, epiglottitis.

A common assessment technique is the Mallampati classification of pharyngeal appearance with the mouth open and tongue protruded. This, however, has poor predictive power.

Investigations

To assess patient fitness for surgery, or to form a baseline recording for later comparison. In general, investigations are best guided by a good history and examination. There is a poor yield from preoperative screening investigations and thus any guidelines are controversial.

- ECG: age over 50. Cardiovascular or respiratory disease, or presence of risk factors
- CXR: Cardiovascular/respiratory disease without X-ray in last 6 months. New respiratory signs/symptoms. Possible metastases. High risk of TB, e.g. recent immigrant

- Haemoglobin: Age < 1 or > 50 years. Premenopausal women. Signs/symptoms of anaemia. Large blood loss expected
- Urea & electrolytes: age over 50. Metabolic disorders. Dehydration. Drugs such as diuretics, or those which are affected by electrolytes, e.g. digoxin
- Pulmonary function tests (PFT): Presence of functional respiratory impairment, e.g. COAD, kyphoscoliosis
- Arterial blood gases (ABG): if possible need for postoperative ventilation, significantly reduced PFT or severe exercise limitation
- Sickle cell testing: Patients from risk areas, e.g. Africa, Middle East and southern Mediterranean regions
NB. Positive Sickledex test occurs in hetero- and homozygous conditions, and requires serum electrophoresis to determine nature of haemoglobinopathy. Trait genotypes such as HbSC are at increased risk of sickling.

Scoring systems
The patient's physical condition is commonly summarised according to the American Society of Anesthesiologists (ASA) classification (Table 4.1). This system is validated as correlating with outcome.

Table 4.1   The ASA classification

Class	Physical status
1	Healthy
2	Mild systemic illness, not restricting activity
3	Disease restricting activity, but not incapacitating
4	Incapacitating, life-threatening disease
5	Not expected to survive 24 hours, e.g. ruptured aortic aneurysm

Another scoring system is the Goldman risk index. This multifactorial score assesses the risk of major perioperative cardiac complications in non-cardiac surgery. The two greatest risk factors are heart failure (third heart sound/elevated JVP) and myocardial infarction (MI) within the preceding 6 months. Perioperative MI has high mortality. Delay surgery 6 months if possible.

PREMEDICATION
Traditionally, patients received premedicant drugs before anaesthesia. However, with the smoothness and rapidity of action of modern drugs, the need for premedication is reduced (Table 4.2). Consider other drugs useful before surgery such as prokinetic agents, GTN patches and heparin thromboprophylaxis.

Table 4.2   The advantages and disadvantages of premedicant drugs

Indication	Benefits	Drugs	Problems
Sedation and anxiolysis	Patient preference, reduce dose of induction agent and incidence of complications at induction	Benzodiazepines, opiates, sedative anticholinergics, e.g. scopolamine	Respiratory depression and paradoxical preoperative excitation. Delayed recovery (hangover) postoperatively
Dry mouth	Reduce secretions during inhalational induction. Not required with non-irritant gases such as sevoflurane. Improve topical anaesthesia of airway	Anticholinergic, e.g. scopolamine	Unpleasant for patient, tachycardia, blurred vision, urinary retention
Analgesia	Reduce distress. 'Pre emptive analgesia' – blocking or treating pain prior to surgery reduces total postoperative pain (controversial)	Opiates	Respiratory depression, dysphoria, nausea

Fasting

A period of fasting is required to allow the stomach to empty and reduce the chance of gastric regurgitation and aspiration pneumonitis during anaesthesia (Mendelson's syndrome). However, there is often a substantial gastric residue especially if reduced gastric emptying due to pain, opiates or pregnancy beyond 20 weeks.

Recommended period of fasting:

- Clear fluids until 2 hours preoperatively
- Food until 6 hours preoperatively
- Breast milk until 4 hours preoperatively.

Medical therapy

In general, all medication should be continued, except:

- Anticoagulants
- Hypoglycaemic agents
- Monoamine oxidase inhibitors: traditionally stop 2–3 weeks preoperatively, hazardous interactions with sympathomimetic agents and opioids, e.g. pethidine
- Oral contraceptives: stop 1–3 months preoperatively, or use subcutaneous heparin prophylaxis to reduce risk of thromboembolism.

Management of a diabetic patient

Assess patient

- Quality of control: urinalysis, random serum glucose, serum HbA$_{1c}$ (reflects glucose control over previous 4–5 weeks)
- Presence of complications: ischaemic heart disease, peripheral vascular disease, nephropathy (often associated with retinopathy), neuropathy (autonomic neuropathy may lead to gastric stasis and vasomotor instability).

Plan management

- Minimise period of fasting, put early on list (see Fig. 4.1)
- Physiological stress response causes hyperglycaemia and disrupts diabetic control. Treat emergencies as soon as possible
- During the perioperative period, IDDM patients require a balanced amount of both insulin and carbohydrate to avoid ketosis. It is not sufficient to stop both insulin and carbohydrate and be content with normoglycaemia.

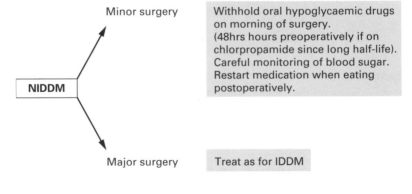

Minor surgery — Withhold oral hypoglycaemic drugs on morning of surgery. (48hrs hours preoperatively if on chlorpropamide since long half-life). Careful monitoring of blood sugar. Restart medication when eating postoperatively.

NIDDM

Major surgery — Treat as for IDDM

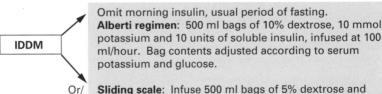

IDDM — Omit morning insulin, usual period of fasting. **Alberti regimen:** 500 ml bags of 10% dextrose, 10 mmol potassium and 10 units of soluble insulin, infused at 100 ml/hour. Bag contents adjusted according to serum potassium and glucose.

Or/ **Sliding scale:** Infuse 500 ml bags of 5% dextrose and 10 mmol potassium at 100 ml/hour,with a separate infusion of soluble insulin guided by hourly testing with reagent sticks.

Preoperative insulin regimens may be started once eating normally.

Fig. 4.1 Regimen for perioperative management of diabetic patients.

Plasma glucose should be maintained between 6 and 10 mmol/L. Hypoglycaemia is a possible cause of postoperative coma.

Management of anticoagulated patients
Assess need for and degree of anticoagulation (international normalised ratio (INR) for warfarin, activated partial thromboplastin time (APTT) for heparin).

If prosthetic heart valve: stop warfarin 3 days before surgery. Heparinise using intravenous (i.v.) bolus of 5000 IU, followed by infusion at rate of 1000–1500 IU/hour guided by daily measurement of APTT. Half-life of heparin (hepatic metabolism) is 90 minutes. Stop infusion 6 hours preoperatively. Most surgery can proceed with APTT ratio < 1.5. Heparin can be reversed using Protamine. Restart warfarin or heparin as soon as possible postoperatively.

Sickle cell disease
Patients with sickle cell disease should be assessed for possible pulmonary and renal impairment, and exchange transfusion may be required to achieve HbS concentrations of 30–40%.

Hypothermia, dehydration, hypoxia and infection may trigger crises and should be avoided in the perioperative period.

MONITORING
Minimum standard of monitoring
UK Association of Anaesthetists published a minimum standard of monitoring in 1988. This advises continuous monitoring from before induction of anaesthesia, through into recovery.

Invasive monitoring
In certain cases, more invasive monitoring is required (Table 4.3).

GENERAL ANAESTHESIA

No unified theory of action, possibly by activity on neuronal lipid membrane, or ion channels via receptors, e.g. GABA.

THE TRIAD OF ANAESTHESIA

A general anaesthetic is composed of elements of:

1. Hypnosis (unconsciousness)
2. Analgesia
3. Muscle relaxation.

Hypnosis
A reversible state of unresponsiveness.

Table 4.3   When to use invasive monitors

	Uses	Problems
Arterial line	Sampling blood gases Following rapid changes in BP Difficulty using cuff, e.g. obesity or poor access to limbs	Exsanguination if disconnected, emboli, risk of distal ischaemia
Central lines	Monitor right atrial pressure (~ 4 mmHg) to guide fluid replacement if large fluid shifts, or poor cardiac status For rapid fluid infusion or administration of irritant drugs	Pneumothorax, haematoma, line sepsis, air embolism Damage to: carotid artery, thoracic duct, phrenic nerve, brachial plexus, sympathetic chain
Pulmonary artery (PA) flotation catheter (Swan–Ganz)	Measures PA pressure (28/12 mmHg) When balloon wedged in pulmonary vessel, continuous column of blood between catheter tip and left atrium (LA) Wedge pressure ≃ LA pressure (8 mmHg) Useful for guiding fluid replacement if discrepancy suspected between LA and RA filling, e.g. in acute myocardial infarction Cardiac output: by thermodilution technique Measuring oxygen tensions and pressures in various chambers to assess shunt	Above, plus arrhythmias, valve disruption or endocarditis, catheter knotting within heart, pulmonary artery rupture, pulmonary infarction

Induction

Either by i.v. injection of anaesthetic drug (rapidly attains deep level of anaesthesia) or by inhalation of volatile agents, e.g. sevoflurane (ideal in airway obstruction, needle phobia and children).

Rapid sequence induction

Used in emergency surgery to minimise risk of gastric aspiration. Patient is 'preoxygenated' by breathing 100% oxygen. An i.v. induction is followed by suxamethonium muscle relaxant. This provides optimal intubating conditions within 30 seconds, yet in event of failed intubation muscle power and spontaneous ventilation returns in 2–5 minutes. The preoxygenation of functional lung capacity means that ventilation by mask with attendant risks of gastric insufflation and distension is not required. Cricoid pressure (Sellick's manoeuvre) is applied until the airway is secured. This uses anterior pressure on the cricoid ring to compress the oesophagus and prevent passive gastric regurgitation.

Maintenance

The hypnotic effect of an i.v. anaesthetic drug lasts only a few minutes. To maintain anaesthesia, may use volatile anaesthetic agents, or total intravenous anaesthesia (TIVA). This uses i.v. infusion of anaesthetic agent (usually propofol), which allows rapid recovery, and may have anti-emetic effects.

Intravenous anaesthetic drugs

Rapid onset in single 'arm–brain circulation time'. Mostly cerebral depressants, e.g. propofol, etomidate, thiopentone. (Ketamine is unique, it is a stimulant, yet it induces a state of profound 'dissociation').

Problems Cardiovascular and respiratory depressants with risk of apnoea, and cardiovascular collapse (especially if hypovolaemic). Contraindicated in airway obstruction and porphyria (thiopentone).

Volatile anaesthetic agents

- Isoflurane
- Enflurane
- Halothane
- Sevoflurane
- Desflurane.

Liquids which vaporise in sophisticated vaporisers to produce accurately controlled concentrations. At the minimum alveolar concentration (MAC), 50% of patients will not move to a surgical stimulus.

Side-effects Respiratory and cardiovascular depression, increased cerebral blood flow, relaxation of skeletal and uterine muscle. Halothane has been associated with an acute fulminant hepatic failure.

Analgesia

Reduces autonomic responses to pain, e.g. tachycardia, hypertension, tachypnoea, sweating and lacrimation.

Usually use opiates, e.g. morphine. Newer synthetic opioids, e.g. fentanyl and remifentanil, have more rapid onset and offset allowing quicker recovery. Still have side-effects of respiratory depression, nausea, itching, etc.

Non-steroidal anti-inflammatory drugs (NSAIDs) are effective alone, but also have 'opioid sparing' effect, i.e. require less opioids for same analgesia. Side-effects include peptic ulceration, bronchospasm, renal failure and bleeding from impaired platelet function. Analgesia is also provided by local anaesthetic techniques.

Muscle relaxation

Non-depolarising muscle relaxants (e.g. atracurium, vecuronium) competitively bind with acetylcholine receptors at the neuromuscular junction, and are effective for approximately 30–45 minutes. Their effects can be reversed by the use of neostigmine, an anticholinesterase which increases the availability of acetylcholine. Monitored using peripheral nerve stimulator. Suxamethonium is a depolarising muscle relaxant, which non-competitively depolarises the muscle end plate causing fasciculation and a rapid onset paralysis. The drug is rapidly metabolised by plasma cholinesterase enzymes.

Indications for muscle relaxation

- Facilitate surgery, e.g. retraction of abdominal wall
- Facilitate intubation and ventilation
- Prevent reflex movements under light anaesthesia, e.g. for Caesarean section or cardiac bypass, but introduces the potential for 'awareness' – explicit or subconscious recall of procedure.

Airway maintenance

Once unconscious, the usual muscle tone maintaining a patent airway is lost. Respiratory obstruction leads to hypoventilation with hypoxia, hypercapnia and lightening of anaesthesia, and increases the risk of gastric regurgitation. The simplest method is to hold the patient in the 'sniffing the morning air' position, with flexion of the neck, extension of head on neck, and jaw thrust. If inadequate, a Guedel or nasal airway may be used to bypass the tongue.

Laryngeal mask airway

Tube conducts gases to a small mask with an inflatable cuff. Designed so that when cuff is inflated, the tip of the mask lies in the oesophagus, while the mask sits over the laryngeal inlet.

Advantages Easily and blindly inserted. Maintains airway while leaving hands free. Less stimulating to patient than intubation. Provides good seal preventing contamination of airway from oral debris. Allows positive pressure ventilation.

Disadvantages During positive pressure ventilation, there is a risk of inflating stomach, and there is no protection from aspirating gastric contents.

Endotracheal tubes: indications for intubation

- Inflatable cuff protects airway from soiling
- Allows use of positive airway pressure for ventilation, or CPAP in the ITU

- Secures airway when access difficult, e.g. ENT surgery
- Access to airway for effective suctioning of secretions.

Difficult intubation

1. Incidence of difficult intubation, 1%. Defined as inability to see the glottis on laryngoscopy.
2. Incidence of failed intubation: 1 in 3000 (1 in 300 in obstetric anaesthesia).

   If predicted, options available are:

- Inhalational induction, with spontaneous ventilation maintained. If able to ventilate patient by mask then dose of suxamethonium given
- Retrograde intubation: Endotracheal tube railroaded over guidewire passed in cephalad direction via cricothyroid puncture
- Fibreoptic intubation with endotracheal tube railroaded over bronchoscope
- Blind nasal intubation
- Tracheostomy.

   The latter four may be performed under general or local anaesthetic.

GENERAL CARE OF PATIENT UNDER ANAESTHESIA

TEMPERATURE REGULATION

On induction of anaesthesia, there is vasodilatation and redistribution of heat from core to the peripheries, resulting in unavoidable heat loss. Thenceforth there is a steady heat loss from patient to surroundings mainly by radiation and convection. Homeothermic mechanisms absent. Children are far more prone to hypothermia due to their increased surface area to volume ratio and low heat capacity.

While the protective effects of hypothermia against tissue hypoxia are useful in certain neuro- and cardiothoracic operations, in general the effects are deleterious:

- Shivering postoperatively increases oxygen consumption up to 10 times and may lead to hypoxia and cardiac ischaemia
- Impaired coagulation
- Increased duration of action of anaesthetic drugs, e.g. muscle relaxants
- Reduced conscious level.

To avoid hypothermia

1. At risk patients are identified, e.g. elderly, babies, long cases
2. Temperature is monitored: centrally via nasopharynx and also skin of peripheries

3. Heat conservation devices used:
   - Maintain temperature of theatre at 22–24° Celsius and 50% humidity (higher in neonatal cases)
   - Heat and humidify anaesthetic gases
   - Warm blood and other fluids being infused, e.g. bladder irrigation, peritoneal lavage
   - Keep patient covered as much as possible and use metallised sheets
   - Actively heat the patient using heated mattresses or hot air blankets.

FLUID MANAGEMENT

Deficits

Pre-existing dehydration/hypovolaemia, e.g. preoperative fasting overnight in adult results in approximately 1 litre deficit. Children are more prone to dehydration.

Maintenance fluids

- In adults: 2 ml/kg/hour
- In children:
  for first 10 kg of weight   4 ml/kg/hour
  for second 10 kg of weight 2 ml/kg/hour
  for remaining weight   1 ml/kg/hour

  e.g. child weighing 28 kg requires

  $(10 \times 4) + (10 \times 2) + (8 \times 1) = 68$ ml/hour

Rate increased peroperatively due to evaporative losses from exposed viscera, e.g. up to 10 ml/kg/hour during laparotomy.

Losses

General guidelines for blood transfusion relate to patient blood volume, which is 60–70 ml/kg in adults, 80–90 ml/kg in children.

Transfuse when lost 15% of blood volume in adults, 10% in children.

Obviously also depends on starting Hb, physical status of patient, predicted ongoing losses.

PATIENT POSITIONING

Anaesthetised patients are at risk of prolonged pressure and damage to tissues, e.g. retinal infarction from pressure on the eye, ulnar nerve palsy at the elbow. Thus padding of at risk areas is vital. Eyes are vulnerable to corneal ulceration due to drying, and lids are often taped shut.

ANAESTHETIC CONDITIONS

Malignant hyperpyrexia

- Autosomal dominant inherited abnormality of skeletal muscle calcium metabolism. Trigger agents, especially suxamethonium and volatile anaesthetic agents, cause muscle contraction. Leads to: rigidity, rapid and severe hyperpyrexia, hypoxia, hypercapnia, acidosis, hyperkalaemia, arrhythmias
- Incidence: 1 per 200 000
- Treatment: dantrolene up to 10 mg/kg reduces mortality from 80 to 2% otherwise supportive measures and discontinue trigger substance
- Diagnosis: requires muscle biopsy and contractility tests in response to trigger agents. Relatives should also be tested.

Suxamethonium apnoea

- Inherited deficiency of plasma cholinesterase causes prolonged activity of suxamethonium, leading to 2–4 hours of paralysis
- Management requires postoperative ventilation until return of muscle power
- Diagnosis of patient and relatives requires analysis of serum cholinesterase activity.

LOCAL AND REGIONAL ANAESTHESIA

LOCAL ANAESTHETIC DRUGS

Classified: as esters (cocaine) or amides (lignocaine, bupivacaine, ropivacaine) depending on chain-linking hydrophobic aromatic group to a hydrophilic amine group. Amides are metabolised in the liver (esters by plasma cholinesterase) and cause fewer allergic reactions.

Work by entering nerve cell and plugging Na^+ channels, thus preventing depolarisation. pKa of drug determines onset of block since drug enters nerve in un-ionised form and enters ion channel in ionised form.

SAFE AND TOXIC DOSES

Toxic effects of local anaesthetics depend on their intrinsic toxicity and the serum level achieved which depends on:

1. Dose given and speed of injection
2. Condition of patient: reduce dose in frail or those with liver disease
3. Rate of absorption, which depends on
   a. addition of vasoconstrictors: except cocaine, local anaesthetics cause vasodilatation, therefore adrenaline is

added to reduce rate of absorption thus extending duration of action and reducing plasma levels; should not be used near end arteries, and may cause tachyarrhythmias especially in presence of halothane
b. vascularity of site of injection. For rate of absorption, intercostal > brachial plexus > infiltration.

'Maximum' dose guide therefore dependent on individual case:

- Lignocaine: 3 mg/kg (7 mg/kg with adrenaline)
- Bupivacaine, 2 mg/kg
- Prilocaine, 5 mg/kg.

Concentration of local anaesthetic expressed as 'percent' means the number of grams of drug within 100 millilitres. A 1% solution contains 10 mg/ml.

Symptoms of toxic complications
With increasing serum levels:

- Dizziness
- Tinnitus
- Circumoral numbness
- Twitching
- Convulsions
- Unconsciousness
- Respiratory arrest
- Cardiovascular collapse

Treatment: treat fits (diazepam or thiopentone), cardiorespiratory support until drug cleared.

PREPARATION OF PATIENT

There is always the danger of drug toxicity or technique failure. Therefore, the patient should be prepared as for a GA, i.e. general condition optimised, starved, i.v. access, monitoring, resuscitation equipment available.

LOCAL ANAESTHETIC TECHNIQUES

Infiltration
Simple, with few hazards. Provides postoperative analgesia as effective and possibly longer lasting than regional block, e.g. hernia surgery. Preincisional infiltration more effective than at end of operation (?pre-emptive analgesia). Possibly a local anti-inflammatory effect of bupivacaine.

Field blocks, e.g. for hernia repair
Combination of nerve block and infiltration.

Nerve blocks, e.g. femoral, brachial plexus

Rely on accurate placement of local anaesthetic adjacent to nerve. Achieved by using nerve stimulator (electrical impulses applied to needle tip cause muscle twitch due to stimulation of motor neurones) or eliciting paraesthesia. May have prolonged effect, e.g. 20 hours for interscalene block using bupivacaine.

Intravenous blocks (Biers)

Limb is exsanguinated, tourniquet is applied at double systolic arterial pressure. Prilocaine (3 mg/kg) is given intravenously, it is considerably less cardiotoxic than bupivacaine. Local anaesthetic binds to nerve and other tissue. Tourniquet may be released after half an hour. Local anaesthetic gradually leaches out of the limb tissues into the systemic circulation to be metabolised in the liver. Key point is that the *peak* serum concentration never approaches toxic levels. Main danger is accidental early cuff deflation.

SPINALS AND EPIDURALS (Table 4.4)

Action of local anaesthetic on spinal nerves and cord causes:

- Sensory block
- Motor block: weak legs, intercostal and abdominal muscles
- Autonomic block: sympathectomy with vasodilatation. Treated with i.v. fluids and ephedrine.

Complications of spinals and epidurals

- Due to block: hypotension, heavy numb legs, urinary retention
- Dural puncture headache: severe, postural, occipito-frontal headache usually occurs next day. Incidence related to size of

Table 4.4   Differences between spinals and epidurals

	Spinals	Epidurals
Needle type	Atraumatic tip, e.g. Whitacre	Tuohy (curved blunt tip)
Needle size	Small, e.g. 25 G	Large, e.g. 16 G
Anatomical end point	Puncture dura	Peridural (between ligamentum flavum and dura)
Functional end point of injection	CSF aspirated	Loss of resistance to air or saline injection entering loosely fat-filled peri-dural space from dense ligament
Onset of block	Rapid (< 5 minutes)	Slow, 15–30 minutes
Duration	1–2 hours	Longer (2–3 hours)
Insertion of catheter	No	Yes – allows top-ups
Dose of local anaesthetic	Small, e.g. 2–3 ml	Large, e.g. 20 ml

needle. Incidence approximately 1% for spinal or epidural.
Treated with epidural 'blood patch'
- Misplaced epidural injection:
  a) Into CSF causing 'total spinal' with unconsciousness, apnoea, and cardiovascular collapse
  b) intravenous injection
- Infections: meningitis, epidural abscess
- Neuropraxia
- Extradural haematoma and cord compression.

Epidural/spinal opioids

Opioids, e.g. fentanyl 2 µg/ml, have a synergistic effect when used with local anaesthetics. There are opioid receptors in the spinal cord. Thus weaker solutions of, e.g. 0.1% bupivacaine, can be used in infusions postoperatively. This reduces the degree of motor block and hypotension (allowing 'walking epidurals').

Complications of epidural/spinal opioids

- Nausea
- Urinary retention
- Itching
- Respiratory depression: may be severe and delayed up to 24 hours.

SEDATION

A reduced level of consciousness, while retaining verbal contact with the patient. Facilitates uncomfortable procedures. Use single agent only, to avoid drug interactions. Drug of choice is midazolam: short-acting i.v. benzodiazepine providing sedation and amnesia. May cause respiratory depression and loss of consciousness.

Therefore patient needs preoperative assessment, i.v. cannula, monitoring, trained person observing patient, full resuscitation facilities. Flumazenil is specific antagonist, routine use inadvisable since shorter action than benzodiazepines with potential for resedation, may cause fitting and expensive. Newer ideas: propofol in subanaesthetic boluses: 'patient-controlled sedation', for quicker recovery and better patient control.

POSTOPERATIVE CARE

PROBLEMS IN RECOVERY

- Cardiovascular: hyper/hypotension, arrhythmias
- Respiratory: laryngospasm, hypoventilation, aspiration
- Gastrointestinal: nausea and vomiting
- Neurological: inadequate reversal of muscle relaxant, agitation, oversedation
- Others: hypothermia, surgical (e.g. bleeding).

Consider requirements for pain relief, fluid management, oxygen therapy, level of observation and monitoring, e.g. ward, HDU or ITU.

PAIN RELIEF

Inadequate management of postoperative pain identified by Joint College Report in 1990. In response, acute pain teams set up.
Functions of acute pain teams:

- Education
- Monitoring and audit
- Introduction of effective methods of pain relief.

Patient-controlled analgesia (PCA)

Computer-controlled pump, usually containing opioids. Patient control device triggers administration of small bolus. Then follows lockout period during which pump will not function. May also set a continuous background infusion.

Advantages

- Caters for the large and unpredictable inter-individual variations in opiate requirements, allowing optimum dosing. Provides more constant plasma levels
- Inherent safety mechanism whereby patient falls asleep before seriously overdosing themselves
- Avoids need for nurses to sign out and administer intramuscular drugs
- Adds psychological aspect of improved patient control.

Disadvantages

- Frequent monitoring of pump function by nursing staff
- Danger of pump malfunction and opiate overdose
- Under-use of pump due to patient fears regarding addiction or overdose, or problems with nausea and vomiting. Patients tend not to dose themselves to complete analgesia
- Problems operating control button, e.g. arthritic hands. Patients need to be selected and educated in use of pump preoperatively. Generally considered as option for use in children over the age of 5 years.

Epidurals

A catheter may be left in the epidural space for several days. Local anaesthetic drugs (e.g. bupivacaine) or opioids (e.g. fentanyl) or combinations are then given either as a continuous infusion, or boluses given either by nurses or using a PCA pump. There is a dermatomal distribution of epidural analgesia, and so thoracic epidurals are most effective for upper abdominal incisions, whereas a lumbar epidural is best for hip/knee surgery.

BENEFITS OF GOOD ANALGESIA

● Humane
● Improves pulmonary function by facilitating chest physiotherapy and avoiding respiratory depression of systemic opioids.

However, little evidence that has any impact on overall recovery and time to discharge. Pain is often measured using a visual analogue scale.

INDICATIONS FOR POSTOPERATIVE VENTILATION

● Pre-existing respiratory impairment, e.g. pulmonary disease, obesity
● Iatrogenic, e.g. after high-dose opioid technique used for cardiac stability
● Stabilisation, e.g. to allow patient time to warm up, correct coagulation, acid-base, etc.
● Physiological control, e.g. for hyperventilation to decrease raised intracranial pressure, or heavy sedation to ensure BP control, e.g. aortic surgery
● Predictable deterioration, e.g. after faecal peritonitis, prolonged shock, gastric acid aspiration.

FURTHER READING

Smith G, Aitkenhead A R (eds) 1996 Textbook of anaesthesia. Churchill Livingstone, London
Yentis S M, Hirsch N P, Smith G B 1993 Anaesthesia A to Z. An encyclopaedia of principles and practice. Butterworth-Heinemann, Oxford

5. Vascular surgery

Louis Fligelstone, Alun H. Davies

ARTERIAL ASSESSMENT

Assessment of the vascular patient relies on obtaining an accurate history and examination and the results of complementary investigations both non-invasive and invasive. The decision to perform invasive assessment should **only** be made in a patient being considered for vascular intervention.

HISTORY – GENERAL

Assessment relies on careful history and examination directed at the presenting complaint and attention to risk factors for vascular disease, especially smoking hypertension, hyperlipidaemia and diabetes mellitus.

Lower limb assessment
The distinction between intermittent claudication and spinal claudication (due to spinal canal stenosis) is important (Table 5.1).

Table 5.1 **Distinction between intermittent and spinal claudication**

	Intermittent claudication	Spinal claudication
Cause	Vascular insufficiency unmasked by increased metabolic demands of exercising tissue	Paraestheslae due to compression of cauda equina by osteoarthritic abnormality of the lumbar spine, spinal canal narrowed further by lumbar lordosis induced by standing erect
Nature	Aching discomfort, mostly affecting the calf, but may affect the buttocks and thighs in iliofemoral disease	Aching numbness of hips, thighs, shin, calf, heel and foot. Often affects dermatome distribution L4,5, S1
Pain		
Onset	Gradual, same degree of exercise	Rapid on exercising in the erect posture Onset may occur whilst standing still
Offset	Prompt on rest	Rarely relieved on stopping exercise if remain upright but passes off rapidly on sitting
Pulses	Reduced or absent	Usually present
Straight leg raising	Within normal limits	Reduced, often reproduces symptoms

Investigation of possible spinal stenosis includes plain X-rays of lumbosacral spine and MRI.

Osteoarthritis may cause pain but it occurs with movement, often present at rest and is not relieved by rest. Typical features of arthritis are evident on plain radiographs.

The current definition of critical leg ischaemia has been devised by the European Working Group on Critical Leg Ischaemia: 'Chronic critical leg ischaemia, in both diabetic and non-diabetic patients, is defined by either of the following criteria: persistently recurring rest pain requiring regular analgesia for > 2 weeks and/or a toe systolic pressure of ≤ 30 mmHg; or ulceration or gangrene of the foot or toes with an ankle systolic pressure ≤ 50 mmHg or a toe systolic pressure of ≤ 30 mmHg.' A new definition and management structure is due to be published by a new working group consisting of European and American participants that should provide a more universally applicable management plan.

Rest pain usually presents as severe forefoot pain and may be relieved temporarily by dependency. Rest pain is an indication for intervention as it signifies impending tissue necrosis.

Examination

General
Cardiovascular, respiratory to assess fitness for surgery.

Specific
Trophic changes of skin and adnexae, peripheral circulation, pulse status (including radiofemoral delay and arm pressures), areas of ischaemic necrosis especially over pressure points and between the toes, presence of vascular bruits, palpation for aneurysmal disease.

Pulses should be recorded as:

0 Absent
1 Reduced volume
2 Normal volume
3 Ectatic (enlarged, but not truly aneurysmal)
4 Aneurysmal.

NON-INVASIVE ASSESSMENT

Ankle brachial pressure index (ABPI)

- Systolic pressure measurement using handheld Doppler probe. Ankle pressure divided by brachial pressure provides the ABPI
- Normal > 0.8
- Claudication 0.6–0.8
- Rest pain, critical ischaemia < 0.5 (or pressure < 50 mmHg)
- Diabetic patients suffer vascular calcification of medium-sized vessels, which gives falsely high ABPI; also in claudicants,

stenoses may give normal ABPI at rest but repeat readings postexercise will produce a significant fall in ABPI
• The audible waveform is also important and is recorded as:
Triphasic – normal
Biphasic – demonstrating some loss of elasticity of the arterial wall
Monophasic – poor waveform
'Whooshy' monophasic – nearly inaudible (in this situation repeating the assessment with the leg dependent is advisable).

Colour duplex
Combination of real time B-mode imaging with the Doppler shift pattern has been enhanced by colour coding the pixels of a television screen image according to the velocity of flow of the blood within the vessel. The faster the flow the brighter the colour; flow in the forward direction is traditionally coded red and reverse flow blue. This assesses vessel wall abnormalities and effect on flow by lesions. An increase in the ratio of velocity at the stenosis to velocity proximal to the stenosis > 2 is significant.

Colour duplex imaging is quick, does not expose the patient to radiation and can be repeated safely. It is ideal for initial assessment of patients with symptoms of occlusive vascular disease, including carotid stenosis, limb claudication, aneurysmal disease and for surveillance of vascular bypass grafts. Many surgeons are now willing to operate on the basis of the results of colour duplex alone for carotid artery disease.

Magnetic resonance angiography (MRA)
The application of a strong magnetic field results in repolarisation of hydrogen nucleus, this results in the emission of the transferred energy as radio waves that are detected by a short wave antenna and converted to a digital image. The movement of blood in the circulation results in a flow void an image of the vascular system without the need for contrast. The digital images obtained can be manipulated to provide a 3-dimensional (3D) image that can be viewed from any perspective desired. At present it is time-consuming and expensive.

Pulse-generated run-off
Angiographic assessment of severely diseased lower limb vessels fails to demonstrate the run-off vessels in a small percentage, in addition Doppler insonation may be unhelpful. Planning reconstruction to the crural or pedal vessels is very difficult. Using a Doppler probe to insonate over the anatomical site of the leg arteries whilst a cuff is inflated rapidly causes an acceleration of blood within the artery resulting in a flow signal. The patency of the vessel and flow signal indicates suitability for use as a run-off vessel.

Management of patients with intermittent claudication

Management of patients with intermittent claudication due to occlusive peripheral vascular disease varies; however, the degree of individual disability and risk–benefit analysis is required for all patients. An algorithm of current management of patients with intermittent claudication is provided (Fig. 5.1). The phrase 'stop smoking, keep walking' holds true and the addition of 75 mg of aspirin daily to this advice is associated with a reduction in stroke and myocardial infarction, the major causes of disability and death in patients with peripheral vascular disease.

INVASIVE ASSESSMENT

Angiography
Assessment of in-flow and run-off is important to determine the procedure best suited for the patient. Recognition of named arteries and anatomical terminology is important:

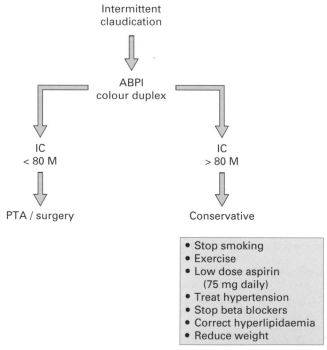

Fig. 5.1 Algorithm for management of intermittent claudication. A general protocol is given; however, each patient should be evaluated for actual disability from their disease and the decision to treat should take account of this. Angioplasty has no advantage over a structured exercise programme for intermittent claudication at 2 years.

- Common iliac
- External iliac
- Common femoral
- Profunda femoris
- Superficial femoral artery

- Popliteal artery
- Anterior tibial
- Tibio-peroneal trunk
- Posterior tibial
- Peroneal vessels.

Contrast

Arterial cannulation using the Seldinger technique, with timed injection of set volumes of contrast using an automated power syringe driver, with conventional film radiographs.

Arterial digital subtraction angiography (DSA)
This technique involves cannulation and injection of contrast as above; however, an initial digitised X-ray image of the area being assessed is taken first and subtracted from subsequent images. This provides a clearer image of the vessels being assessed and a reduction in the contrast load.

Intravenous DSA
The same technique can be applied following an injection of intravenous contrast but the quality of the image obtained is inferior to that of intra-arterial injection and requires a larger volume of contrast to be delivered due to rapid dilution of the media as it passes from the venous to arterial circulation.

Allergy

Allergy to contrast media can result in anaphylactic reaction with possible loss of life. This is less common since the introduction of non-ionic contrast media. In the presence of an allergy, if MRA is not available, medical-grade carbon dioxide can be used as a contrast agent in combination with digital subtraction imaging.

Angioscopy

Direct inspection of the lumen of a vessel. This technique may be successfully applied in the assessment of carotid endarterectomy to exclude the presence of intimal flaps and thrombus, and may be used to direct destruction of venous valves for the technique of in situ venous bypass.

Therapy

Catheter-based therapeutic modalities are becoming increasingly effective and have results approaching that of surgery in selected situations, with a lower initial morbidity and mortality.

Percutaneous transluminal angioplasty (PTA)

Transluminal angioplasty is used to dilate arterial stenoses and recanalise short segments of occluded arteries (up to 10–15 cm). Modification of the technique, termed sub-intimal angioplasty, where the intima is punctured by a guidewire and re-enters the vessel lumen in the distal vessel, has been used successfully to treat longer occlusions in some centres. This technique was developed by Dotter and Judkins in 1964 and subsequently modified by Grüntzig and Hopff in 1974 who developed a special double lumen balloon catheter.

Arterial puncture is carried out under local anaesthesia using the Seldinger technique, usually via the common femoral artery. The puncture site is dilated to accommodate a sheath through which is passed an angioplasty catheter. The flexible polyvinyl catheter with a double lumen has a radio-opaque balloon at its end and is inserted into the arterial lumen either percutaneously or peroperatively via an arteriotomy. The balloon can be distended at high pressure whilst maintaining its profile. A guidewire is used to negotiate the stenosis of occlusion and the catheter is passed over the guidewire such that the balloon is placed across the stenosis or short occlusion; 5000 units of heparin are injected intra-arterially before inflation of the balloon to a pressure of 4–8 atmospheres, for 20–30 seconds. This ruptures the atherosclerotic plaque, creating a longitudinal split in the vessel wall, thus increasing the cross-sectional diameter of the vessel, restoring flow. Platelet and fibrin deposition followed by fibrosis later remodels the irregular area, restoring laminar flow.

The immediate effect of angioplasty can be assessed clinically and by comparison of pre- and post-dilatation angiograms or the pressure gradient across the lesion before and after its dilatation.

Aspirin 75–300 mg daily is prescribed for a minimum of 3 months following successful angioplasty to prevent re-occlusion, reduce disease progression and mainly for its cardiovascular protective action.

PTA may be used as an adjunct or alternative to conventional reconstructive vascular surgery, e.g. external iliac angioplasty prior to femoro-popliteal bypass grafting, or in addition to percutaneous intra-arterial thrombolysis.

Case selection is very important in order to achieve good results.

Applications for PTA

- Isolated stenoses and occlusions of the common and external iliac arteries
- Stenoses and short occlusions (< 10 cm) of the superficial femoral and popliteal arteries
- Renal artery stenosis
- Coronary artery disease
- Localised strictures of the proximal part of a main coronary artery may be suitable for percutaneous angioplasty
- Other lesions, especially those situated more distally, may be suitable for dilatation at the time of coronary artery bypass grafting
- Under evaluation for the treatment of symptomatic carotid stenoses and visceral artery stenoses

- Sub-intimal dissection techniques are under evaluation for longer and more distal stenoses
- Occlusion of the distal aorta and common iliac occlusions
- Iliac occlusions benefit from thrombolysis-assisted angioplasty
- Treatment of ostial lesions is more difficult but results are improved by the use of stents
- Proximal iliac stenoses close to or flush to the bifurcation are at risk of creating a dissection of the vessel wall but use of the 'kissing balloon technique' prevents this.

Contraindications

- No arterial lumen visualised distal to the obstruction
- Complete occlusion of superficial femoral artery.

Complications

At the site of arterial puncture

- Haemorrhage
- Haematoma
- False aneurysm
- These complications can be reduced by application of adequate pressure for a minimum of 15 minutes after removal of the balloon catheter at the end of the procedure.

At the site of angioplasty

- Sub-intimal arterial dissection
- Arterial perforation by guidewire
- Arterial rupture
- False aneurysm formation.

Within the distal vasculature

- Embolisation occurs in 3–5% of cases but is rarely of clinical significance
- Arterial spasm
- Thrombosis.

Advantages

- Minimal in-patient hospital stay of only 24 hours, with low overall morbidity and mortality of PTA comparing favourably with those of conventional vascular surgical procedures
- This technique can be used selectively in elderly patients who present an unacceptably high risk for vascular reconstruction
- Repeated angioplasty is an option with stent placement for resistant stenoses
- In patients fit for surgery, reconstructive arterial surgery can be performed at a later date if necessary.

Table 5.2 Cumulative patency (%)

Segment	1-year	3-year	5-year
Aortic	98	87	80
Iliac	91	80	72
Femoro-popliteal	63–82	51–61	38–58

Disadvantages

* A study comparing the outcome of claudicants treated by angioplasty or by strict exercise programme failed to show a significant difference in pain-free walking distance at 24 months.

Patency rates for angioplasty (Table 5.2)

* Late re-occlusion depends on the site and nature of the lesion
* Antiplatelet agents can improve long-term patency results
* Improved patient assessment, selection and newer techniques are expected to improve this significantly.

Stent
The development of expandable metal stents has led to a rapid advance of endovascular techniques. Patients with recurrent stenosis following PTA or lesions resistant to dilatation may be supported internally by the placement of a stent. Current work suggests that, in lesions that have eccentric calcification, or significant recoil after angioplasty, primary stenting has a role. Stents are currently in use in the aortic, renal, iliac, coronary circulation, long-term results are awaited.

Stents have also been used to secure intimal flaps causing haemodynamic abnormality or occlusion following angioplasty.

Stent graft combinations
A natural progression from the placement of stents within the arterial tree is the combination of stents with vascular grafts. Endoluminal placement of such combinations is becoming commonplace, over 9000 have been placed to date. The variety of applications is expanding rapidly. A covered stent may be used to isolate and seal arteriovenous fistulae, false aneurysms, or dissection of a vessel wall. A graft may be held in situ with stents proximally and distally, this has been carried out successfully in the treatment of aorto-iliac aneurysm disease and is currently under prospective evaluation.

Transfemoral placement of these devices at present requires open arteriotomy of the common femoral vessels under general anaesthetic but as technology advances percutaneous techniques may be developed. Most new aortic stent graft devices have stents supporting all of the graft.

Endoluminal replacement of abdominal and thoracic aortic aneurysms can be complicated by an ENDOLEAK in up to 24% of cases. Endoleaks are classified as:

Type I   Perigraft endoleak
Type II   Retrograde endoleak
Types I & II are further subdivided into:
             A – Inflow **but no** outflow from aneurysm sac
             B – Inflow **and** outflow from aneurysm sac
Type III   Leak through fabric tears, disconnection of the graft, or
             due to disintegration of the graft fabric
Type IV   Leak due to porosity of the fabric.

THROMBOSIS

With the reduction of rheumatic heart disease the incidence of acute arterial occlusion due to distal embolisation is falling. An increasingly aged population with atherosclerotic disease has resulted in the major cause of acute lower limb ischaemia being thrombosis. Correct diagnosis is essential and may require angiography; if thrombosis is confirmed the angiography catheter is replaced by an infusion catheter to administer thrombolytic agents into the thrombus. Most experience has been with continuous infusion of the thrombolytic agent with repeat angiograms and advancement of catheters. This takes up to 72 hours in some cases. The technique of pulse spray thrombolysis has been advocated by some groups as this has been shown to achieve more rapid thrombolysis with an equal complication rate.

Intra-arterial thrombolysis
Systemic thrombolysis similar to that used for patients with myocardial infarction has been attempted; however, local low-dose intra-arterial thrombolysis is the treatment of choice. The first reported use of intra-arterial administration of thrombolytic agents was by Cotton in 1962, subsequently adopted, improved and popularised by Dotter. Intra-arterial low-dose regimens can result in a limb salvage rate of 69%, and low-dose thrombolysis for occluded bypass grafts has achieved complete clot lysis in up to 88% and a limb salvage rate of 74%.

Indications for thrombolysis have yet to be clearly defined. The lag time between onset of treatment to the restoration of flow has been a limiting factor as for many patients the ischaemic process will have progressed, rendering the limb beyond salvage, prior to recanalisation. Revascularisation of limbs with irreversible changes of ischaemia can result in renal failure secondary to myoglobinuria.

Careful assessment and patient selection is necessary. Thrombolysis is suitable for patients that present with a history consistent with acute or chronic ischaemia, embolism post-myocardial infarction, late distal graft thrombosis, or popliteal aneurysm thrombosis.

Arteriographic findings associated with higher success rates are occlusion of the iliac vessels, an occlusion < 10 cm long, findings consistent with an embolus. The presence of good distal run-off is a favourable finding, but may only become evident following thrombolytic therapy.

Arteriographic assessment and X-ray-guided placement of the arterial cannula is followed by intrathrombus infusion of the thrombolytic agent. Repeat angiography with catheter advancement is continued until thrombolysis is complete.

Local complications

- Haematoma at the site of the arterial cannula and pericatheter thrombosis. The use of finer cannulae and local pressure at the time of removal can reduce the former, and the addition of 200 units of heparin in the infusion can reduce the latter
- Generalised fibrinolytic state can result in major haemorrhage in up to 5% of cases. The risk of this occurring is significantly reduced if the fibrinogen level is maintained at > 1 g/l, but surprisingly this complication is not reduced by monitoring with regular coagulation screening
- 1% incidence of death during thrombolytic therapy due to major stroke or concealed haemorrhage.

Revised absolute contraindications to thrombolysis

- Recent stroke (within the previous 2 months)
- Uncontrolled hypertension
- Presence of a bleeding diathesis.

Revised relative contraindications

- Recent major surgery
- Active peptic ulceration
- Renal failure
- Hepatic failure.

The presence of left heart thrombus is no longer considered a contraindication. There is considerable debate concerning the mode of action, cost and side-effects of the currently available thrombolytic agents and continuing research is being undertaken to achieve improved agents.

Streptokinase
Streptokinase is a non-enzyme protein that activates endogenous plasminogen by inducing a conformational change on binding to it, exposing an active site of the plasminogen molecule. The streptokinase–plasminogen complex is a potent plasminogen activator and therefore results in the production of plasmin and therefore fibrinolysis. Streptokinase is a foreign protein and

antibodies to it are formed following administration, anaphylaxis may result on repeated therapy if a 3-month period has not elapsed between first and second treatments. Previous streptococcal infection can lead to a reduction of response for a given dose. Some patients may suffer pyrexia during the infusion. Low-dose intra-arterial thrombolysis: 5000 units per hour

Urokinase
Urokinase is a serine protease similar to trypsin. It acts directly on plasminogen, to form active plasmin by cleavage of several amino acid bonds. Urokinase is non-antigenic and may therefore be used on more than one occasion without the risk of reduced efficacy or anaphylaxis. Despite costing up to six times more than streptokinase it is the agent most commonly used in the USA on the basis that it is a more potent thrombolytic agent than streptokinase and has fewer side-effects, thus leading to an overall cost advantage from early discharge from hospital. Intra-arterial thrombolysis: 30 000–50 000 units per hour, initially given at a rate of 2000–4000 units per minute for the first 2 hours, and subsequently 1000–2000 units per hour.

Tissue plasminogen activator (t-PA)
This is a naturally occurring substance produced by vascular endothelium, it is a serine protease and is the initiator of the fibrinolytic system in vivo. It is poorly active in the circulation; however, its activity increases several thousand percent on binding to fibrin, therefore it has a preferential activity upon plasminogen bound within and on the surface of a clot. It has been produced from melanoma cell lines but currently production utilises recombinant DNA technology. Recombinant tissue plasminogen activator (rTPA), has been associated with lower dosage administration and lower complication rates. It is also non-antigenic and repeat administrations are therefore permissible. Intra-arterial thrombolysis: 0.1 unit/kg/hour until lysis occurs.

Other newer agents undergoing evaluation include:

- Anisoylated plasminogen streptokinase activator complex (APSAC)
- Single-chain Urokinase-type plasminogen activator (Scu-PA or Pro-Urokinase)
- K1K2PU.

ACUTE LIMB ISCHAEMIA

Management
The management of acute limb ischaemia has changed over the past two decades. Previously the majority of patients developed an acutely ischaemic limb due to embolic disease, often as a

complication of rheumatic heart disease. Currently the vast majority of patients develop acute limb ischaemia due to thrombosis in vessels affected by atherosclerosis, an inappropriate embolectomy can result in significant damage to the native vessel and destroy vital collateral circulation, which may result in limb loss. An algorithm for the management of acutely ischaemic limbs is given in Figure 5.2.

Preoperative checklist for all vascular cases

1. Identify patient
2. Mark side (if appropriate)
3. Group and save or cross-match blood
4. Radiological films available for reference in theatre
5. Image intensifier, radiographer, still films if required
6. Antibiotic prophylaxis
7. Anticoagulant therapy (if appropriate).

Bypass grafts

Indications for operative intervention include critical ischaemia (see above for definition), peripheral gangrene due to a surgically correctable lesion, incapacitating intermittent claudication (< 80 yards), or trauma. The natural history of patients with intermittent claudication, who 'stop smoking and keep walking', with correction of hyperlipidaemia and hypertension, is that over 5 years a third will have improved symptoms, a third will remain stable and the remainder will progress to a point that requires intervention. Overall, 10% of patients with intermittent claudication develop rest pain.

Operative intervention for intermittent claudication may result in worsening of symptoms or limb loss. These patients have widespread vascular disease and the same group of patients will have a 25% 5-year mortality, from other causes including myocardial infarction, ruptured aortic aneurysms and stroke.

The decision to carry out a reconstructive procedure is based on a risk–benefit analysis.

Technique
The arterial graft bypasses the occlusion utilising a route different to the native vessel, examples include axillo-bifemoral, femoro-femoral cross-over grafts, obturator bypass and sub-scrotal bypass.

General factors affecting graft failure

- The vessel of supply should provide sufficient in-flow (both pressure and volume), if inadequate this should be corrected
- There should be adequate run-off, i.e. the vascular tree beyond the occlusion should allow sufficient flow to maintain patency
- Careful surgical technique to create a widely patent anastomosis, avoiding kinking or compression of graft. Correct

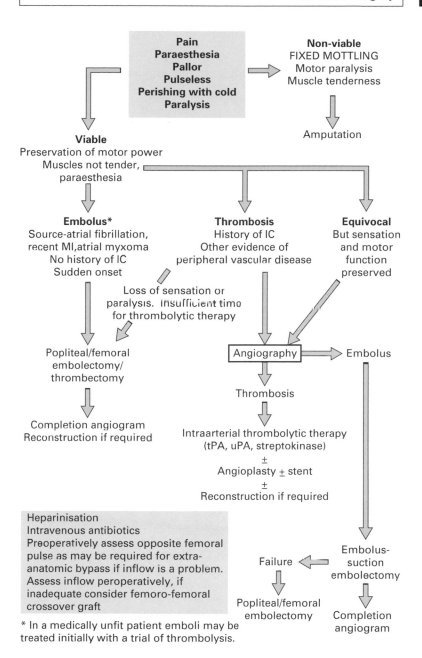

Fig. 5.2 Acute limb ischaemia

suturing technique will prevent intimal flap formation and dissection
- Choice of bypass conduit
  - Autogenous vein (saphenous vein, arm veins)
  - Synthetic grafts: PTFE, Dacron
  - Human umbilical vein grafts
  - Tanned heterografts.

Graft material
The ideal vascular bypass graft would have the following properties:

- Non-thrombogenic flow surface
- Resistance to infection and biodegradation
- Predictable host tissue response
- Ease of handling and suturing
- Elastic properties similar to those of host artery
- Available in a wide range of lengths and diameters
- Ease of storage with long shelf life
- Minimum preparation prior to use.

Reversed autogenous long saphenous vein graft

- Easily accessible and inexpensive but harvesting may be time-consuming
- The graft of choice for femoro-popliteal and coronary artery bypass procedures
- External diameter should exceed 4 mm
- There should be no pre-existing disease of the vein to be used (e.g. thrombophlebitis or varicose veins)
- During harvesting the vein must be handled gently and kept moist with heparinised Hartmann's or saline (5 units per millilitre)
- The patency of femoro-popliteal bypass grafts is related to the indication for the graft, the in-flow, graft length and the quality of the run-off circulation.

In situ non-reversed long saphenous vein graft
This is the graft of choice for femoro-popliteal and femoro-distal bypass procedures (Table 5.3). Preoperatively the vein is assessed for suitability as a conduit by colour duplex, noting patency, diameter, wall characteristics and presence of endoluminal echoes. The vein and all tributaries are mapped (marked on the skin) to guide the incision to prevent excessive tissue dissection, reducing wound-associated morbidity. The long saphenous vein is exposed throughout the length required for the bypass, several incisions may be used, creating skin bridges that reduce the risk of scar contracture and poor healing. Valves are destroyed using special valve strippers, valvulotomes or micro-scissors inserted through transverse venotomies. All tributaries are ligated to prevent development of arteriovenous fistulae. Vasa vasorum of the vein remain intact and hence its nutrition is preserved. The theoretical

Table 5.3 Patency of autogenous saphenous vein femoro-popliteal bypass grafts (%)

	5 years	10 years
Indication		
Intermittent claudication	72–75	45
Limb salvage	58–63	20
Distal run-off		
Good	70	40
Poor	40	30
Length of graft		
Above-knee	59–76	40
Below-knee	66–76	25

Table 5.4 Patency of tibial and peroneal bypass grafts (%)

Indication	1 year	5 years
Autologous saphenous vein		
Limb salvage and Intermittent claudication	64–85	31–68
Limb salvage	47–88	47–71 (4 years)
Human umbilical vein		
Limb salvage and intermittent claudication	18–84	14–32
Limb salvage	20 30	27 (4 years)
PTFE		
Limb salvage and intermittent claudication	40–68	14–28
Limb salvage	35–75	35–61 (4 years)

benefit of in situ grafts is that as the graft narrows distally the velocity of blood flow increases and is maximal at the distal anastomosis thus tending to maintain its patency.

Multiple anastomoses to the distal calf arteries using tributaries of the saphenous vein are often feasible. Saphenous vein with a diameter of only 2.5–3 mm may be used. Provided cases are well selected, an 80% 1-year patency rate for femoro-tibial bypass procedures is obtainable (Table 5.4). No benefit of in situ over reversed vein has been demonstrated.

The skin incision over the vein can be reduced by angioscopic-controlled valve destruction with angioscopic-guided ligation of tributaries, where small incisions can be made near the illuminated light source of the angioscope directly over the tributary. Angioscopy can identify lesions within the vein not detected by colour duplex or venography.

Synthetic grafts

Expanded polytetrafluoroethylene (PTFE), e.g. Gore-Tex, Impragraft Expanded PTFE is a hydrophobic polymer with high strength, microporous, non-elastic material, with a high electro-negative surface charge. Its inert smooth surface prevents platelet deposition, giving a low thrombogenic potential. PTFE allows tissue ingrowth and neointima formation. Preclotting is not required.

PTFE grafts may kink, especially when passing over a joint, this is prevented by external reinforcement with a spiral of polyethylene. This spiral can be removed from the graft over variable lengths to facilitate formation of anastomoses.

It may be used for above-knee and below-knee femoro-popliteal and extra-anatomic bypasses, e.g. axillo-femoral and femoro-femoral bypasses. If used for femoro-distal reconstruction patency is improved by interposing a 'Miller cuff' or 'Taylor patch' of saphenous vein to improve haemodynamics between the relatively stiff PTFE and the native vessel. Newer grafts are utilising a pre-dilated distal end of the PTFE graft to create a haemodynamically favourable cuff, which may improve patency rates in grafting to tibial vessels (Table 5.5).

Haemorrhage from suture holes at the anastomoses has proven problematic especially in patients with coagulation defects; however, with the newer suageless PTFE sutures this is reduced because the size of the puncture made by the needle is the same diameter as the suture.

There is a high risk of pseudoaneurysm formation with repeated puncture, thus limiting its use for direct puncture vascular access. PTFE is used for creation of arteriovenous fistulae, allowing repeated puncture of the arterialised vein.

Dacron A synthetic fibre made from the polymerisation of polyethylene terephthalate.

1. Woven dacron
   - Fibres are packed tightly together to produce a material with low porosity
   - Only slight haemorrhage through graft wall occurs following implantation and preclotting is not essential
   - Minimal ingrowth by fibrous tissue
   - Prosthetic material of choice for repair of ruptured abdominal aortic aneurysms
2. Knitted dacron
   - High porosity allows penetration by granulation tissue and fixation of endothelium
   - Previously marked leakage of blood through the graft wall would occur after implantation if the graft was not pre-clotted (filled with blood drawn from the patient prior to

Table 5.5 Patency of expanded PTFE femoro-popliteal bypass grafts

	1 year	3 years	5 years
Length of graft			
Above-knee	64–95	44–73	42–62
Below-knee	55–88	45–80	32–43
Indication			
Intermittent claudication	68–95	75	65
Rest pain	75	60	35

heparinisation and allowed to clot). This is no longer required as the grafts are impregnated with albumin or collagen
- Easier to handle, more conformable and less likely to fray than woven dacron
- Suitable for replacement or bypass of the aorta and the visceral and proximal limb arteries

3. Dacron velour
- Highly porous graft which must always be pre-clotted prior to use
- Should not be used in the presence of coagulation defects
- Internal velour promotes formation of pseudointima and endothelium
- External velour encourages adherence of fibrous tissues.

Impregnated grafts The porosity of a graft can be reduced by precoating with collagen or albumin. In 're-do' surgery use of a graft impregnated with an antibiotic, e.g. rifampicin, has the potential benefit of increased resistance to infection. A new variant that has promise is collagen-coated grafts impregnated with silver nitrate.

Complications of synthetic arterial grafts

- **Haemorrhage** through the graft wall is a potential problem with all synthetic grafts, especially those of high porosity
- **Graft sepsis** is associated with a high mortality and morbidity, with high amputation rate. Manifestations include fever, purulent wound discharge, false aneurysm formation, septic infarcts and septicaemia. Abdominal aortic graft infection may lead to aorto-enteric fistulation presenting with massive gastrointestinal haemorrhage, with a high mortality. Often mixed flora are responsible, staphylococci usually infect grafts placed in the inguinal region; coliform and other aerobic Gram-negative organisms are often cultured from infected aorto-iliac grafts. Reduction of graft infection is obtained by attention to detail: skin preparation, operative technique, broad-spectrum antibiotic prophylaxis. Once infected a synthetic graft must usually be removed; however, local groin infections have been successfully treated by debridement, placement of gentamicin-impregnated beads and intravenous antibiotics. In high-risk situations use of grafts impregnated with rifampicin may reduce subsequent infection rates
- **False aneurysms** occur at the suture line as a late complication. Attention to anastomotic technique and inert suture material, such as prolene, reduces this risk. Despite these measures the diseased vessel wall may allow the stitch to cut out, leading to loss of tension in the anastomosis
- **Early graft failure within 30 days** is usually related to technical errors. Graft thrombosis is a common cause of early graft failure; graft thrombectomy with exploration, on-table angiography and correction of the error is required

- **Intermediate graft failure – 30 days to 1 year –** may be due to progressive pseudointimal fibrous hyperplasia occurring at the site of arterial-graft anastomoses, or within the autologous vein graft. This is more common if prosthetic materials are used. Intra-arterial thrombolysis may restore patency in late graft failure, and the reason for failure identified. Patch angioplasty is used when revising the graft, some centres prefer PTA; however, the long-term results are inferior
- **Long-term graft patency – greater than one year –** can be improved by administering low-dose aspirin.

Healing of synthetic arterial grafts   Endothelialisation from the adjacent host artery across the anastomotic line occurs to a maximum distance of 10 mm. Haematoma around the graft is organised by fibroblasts to form a surrounding capsule. Fibroblasts also grow through the interstices of the graft material to reach its luminal surface; grafts of high porosity allow greater ingrowth of fibroblasts. The luminal surface of the graft eventually consists of collagen fibres which are incompletely covered by endothelial cells. Seeding synthetic grafts with endothelial or mesothelial cells aims to reduce the thrombogenic potential of their luminal surface.

Allografts, e.g. human umbilical cord vein allograft (HUCVAG)

- Lined by intima and has no branches or valves
- Available in large quantities but usually in limited lengths; a longer graft can be made by joining two or more grafts by end-to-end anastomosis
- Chemical processing involves tanning with glutaraldehyde which renders the graft non-antigenic and increases its tensile strength
- Dardik biograft is strengthened by an outer polyester mesh wrap to prevent aneurysmal dilatation
- Used for below-knee femoro-popliteal and femoro-distal bypasses when saphenous vein is not available.

Heterografts, e.g. bovine carotid arterial grafts

- Prepared by digestion of bovine carotid artery in protease enzymes then tanned with dialdehyde starch or glutaraldehyde to produce a tube of non-antigenic collagen
- High incidence of calcification and aneurysmal dilatation when used for arterial bypass but still used for vascular access.

Follow-up of bypass grafts

- Lower limb bypass grafts may fail as described above
- Graft surveillance (Fig. 5.3) is commonly employed to detect features predicting graft failure that may be treatable
- Graft surveillance is frequently used but has yet to be convincingly shown to prolong limb survival.

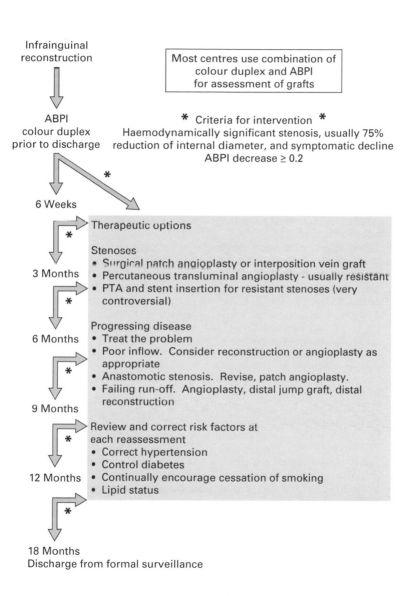

Infrainguinal
reconstruction

Most centres use combination of
colour duplex and ABPI
for assessment of grafts

ABPI
colour duplex
prior to discharge

* Criteria for intervention *
Haemodynamically significant stenosis, usually 75%
reduction of internal diameter, and symptomatic decline
ABPI decrease ≥ 0.2

6 Weeks

Therapeutic options

Stenoses
• Surgical patch angioplasty or interposition vein graft
• Percutaneous transluminal angioplasty - usually resistant
• PTA and stent insertion for resistant stenoses (very
  controversial)

3 Months

6 Months

Progressing disease
• Treat the problem
• Poor inflow. Consider reconstruction or angioplasty as
  appropriate
• Anastomotic stenosis. Revise, patch angioplasty.
• Failing run-off. Angioplasty, distal jump graft, distal
  reconstruction

9 Months

Review and correct risk factors at
each reassessment
• Correct hypertension
• Control diabetes
• Continually encourage cessation of smoking
• Lipid status

12 Months

18 Months
Discharge from formal surveillance

Fig. 5.3 Graft surveillance protocol. (Results of multicentre randomised control trials
of ABPI and clinical assessment versus ABPI, clinical assessment with colour duplex
scanning are awaited.)

CAROTID ENDARTERECTOMY

At present, endarterectomy is used for disease of the following vessels:

- Carotid bifurcation
- Common femoral artery
- Renal arteries.

The use of endarterectomy at other sites is controversial and is being re-evaluated, especially in the iliofemoral circulation.

Differential diagnosis of stroke

- 85% of all strokes result from cerebral infarction, the majority are due to embolisation, but some are due to thrombosis
- 15% of strokes are haemorrhagic in origin, most due to intracerebral haemorrhage, but some due to subarachnoid haemorrhage
- The majority of emboli originate from plaques that develop at the carotid bifurcation. Emboli comprise platelet aggregates, cholesterol crystals, or other atheromatous debris. Emboli may also originate from the heart (mural thrombus secondary to subendocardial infarct, atrial myxoma), and the arch of the aorta
- The neurological deficit may be permanent or transient. A transient ischaemic attack (TIA) is a neurological deficit resolving within 24 hours. Strokes may be classified as:
  — Transient: resolve within 21 days
  — Established: persist beyond 21 days
- Further classification according to residual function is beneficial in deciding appropriateness of carotid endarterectomy
- A carotid stenosis of > 70% is associated with a risk of stroke of 6–15% per annum
- Emboli from a carotid plaque will cause ipsilateral visual disturbance, including blurring of vision and temporary visual field loss (amaurosis fugax), a contralateral motor or sensory impairment, and dysphasia if dominant hemisphere affected
- Vertebro-basilar arteries may also be a source of emboli causing TIA and stroke. Classically they cause visual disturbances including diplopia and homonymous hemianopia, ataxia and syncope (drop) attacks.

Diagnosis

- Clinical history of TIA or occlusive stroke
- Presence of an arterial bruit on auscultation; however, this disappears with high-grade stenosis
- Colour duplex assessment is now used alone in the assessment of patients to identify the degree of stenosis, morphology of plaque, and presence of ulceration of the plaque

- Carotid duplex may fail to demonstrate the presence of flow in a high-grade stenosis and carotid angiography should be performed to confirm occlusion, as this is a contraindication to surgery
- Exclusion of cardiac arrhythmia by ECG and Holter monitoring is useful in equivocal cases.

Treatment

Surgery

- Indicated in high-grade stenoses (70%) and symptomatic stenoses not controlled on medical therapy (aspirin/warfarin)
- Many believe that patients with asymptomatic stenosis should receive aspirin therapy; however, the results of controlled trials of surgery versus medical management of asymptomatic stenoses are awaited
- Rarely a slowly evolving ('stuttering') stroke may be an indication for surgery
- Previously when extracranial surgery has not been possible, usually because of occlusion of the internal carotid artery, the patient may have been considered for extracranial–intracranial bypass. This was abandoned following poor results of a multicentre trial of this therapy.

Conservative medical therapy

- First-line therapy is 75 mg of aspirin, if this fails to control the symptoms surgery is indicated
- Warfarinisation is indicated if emboli arise from the heart.

Contraindications to surgical treatment

- Dense acute completed stroke
- Rapidly progressing or rapidly improving strokes
- Advanced biological age
- Severe coronary arterial disease
- Marked hypertension
- Generalised intracranial and extracranial arterial disease.

Despite improved techniques, invasive arteriography is still associated with a small risk of stroke.

Surgical treatment

Carotid endarterectomy
Indicated in the presence of an ulcerating non-stenosing atheromatous plaque or stenosis of the internal carotid artery reducing its luminal diameter by $\geq$ 70%. The risk–benefit analysis for carotid endarterectomy is important, and a benefit is derived if the stroke rate of the surgeon is low (acceptable results < 5% overall). Further information regarding risk and benefit has been

reported in the North American Symptomatic Carotid Endarterectomy Trial and European Carotid Surgery Trials.

1. Usually performed under general anaesthesia although local anaesthetic techniques may be used
2. The common carotid, external and internal carotid arteries are clearly displayed and clamped after heparinisation
3. Manipulation of the vessels is minimised to prevent:
   a. distal embolisation
   b. stimulation of the carotid sinus nerve, as this can produce profound hypotension. This may be prevented by local anaesthetic blockade of the carotid sinus nerve
4. A longitudinal arteriotomy in the common carotid artery is extended into the internal carotid artery
5. A shunt may be used to preserve cerebral blood flow and is placed between the proximal common carotid artery and the internal carotid artery distal to the stenosis
6. Some surgeons shunt routinely, others only on a selective basis, i.e. if the stump systolic pressure is less than 50 mmHg, or in the presence of vertebral or contralateral carotid arterial disease. Transcranial Doppler and perioperative EEG changes on cross-clamping may also be used to determine the requirement of a shunt
7. Shunts may be of the inlay type (Harvey shunt) or outlay shunt (Javid shunt – held in place by special external vascular clamps, or the Pruitt Innahara shunt – held in place by intravascular balloons)
8. The plain of cleavage is between the adventitia and the media
9. After endarterectomy is completed the distal intima may need to be fixed with fine axial sutures to prevent dissection. Closure of the arteriotomy is usually performed using fine prolene sutures, and the use of a patch angioplasty may be included in small arteries and to prevent kinking. If used, PTFE or Dacron patches are preferable to saphenous vein patches as the latter are prone to rupture. The operative mortality should be less than 2%; approximately 1–2% of patients will develop a stroke following carotid endarterectomy
10. There is risk of damaging cranial nerves X and XII during the dissection
11. About 1% of patients suffering TIAs and undergoing carotid endarterectomy can be expected to develop a significant stroke in each of the following years; in contrast, 6–15% of similar patients not treated surgically will develop a stroke each year.

Surgical treatment of lesions of other extracranial arteries

- Single occlusions of the proximal part of the subclavian artery causing subclavian steal syndrome. This can be successfully treated **surgically** by using axillo–axillary,

subclavian–subclavian or carotid–subclavian grafts, provided the other major vessels are relatively free of disease, or by percutaneous transluminal balloon angioplasty. This obviates the need for thoracic reconstruction
- Multiple stenotic lesions of the origins of the innominate, left common carotid and left subclavian arteries require extensive reconstruction of the aortic arch and its major branches
- Vertebral endarterectomy can be performed via a medial supraclavicular approach; access to the origin of the vertebral artery is through a short subclavian arteriotomy
- Extracranial intracranial revascularisation. This was indicated when distal internal carotid artery occlusion precluded carotid bifurcation endarterectomy and other forms of vascular reconstruction were not feasible. This is very rarely carried out today.

RENAL ARTERY STENOSIS

Post-mortem studies have shown that renal artery stenosis (RAS) is more common than current teaching suggests. Many cases are not identified. Patients over 50 years of age with end-stage renal failure have a 14% incidence of RAS, which has failed to be diagnosed prior to the onset of renal failure. A stenosis of 60% is considered to be significant as it is associated with imminent renal damage and progression to occlusion in up to 10% at 2 years. Stenosis is most often due to atherosclerosis, but fibromuscular dysplasia is encountered in younger patients.

Investigation
Renal angiography is at present the gold standard.
  Options include:

1. Colour duplex examination is of variable usefulness due to overlaying bowel gas and operator dependence. Quality of evaluation is improved if overlying bowel gas is avoided. This may be achieved by patients fasting for a minimum of 12 hours pre-investigation and the scan performed early in the morning to prevent accumulation of gas from swallowing. Sensitivity of colour duplex is improved by:
   a. assessing the peak velocity of flow in the renal artery and aorta. If the renal/aortic ratio is ≥ 3.5 there is a significant stenosis
   b. In view of the above-mentioned difficulties of visualising renal arteries directly, attempts have been made to quantify renal cortical flow to provide an indirect indicator of renal artery disease
2. Magnetic resonance angiography (MRA) using time of flight (TOF) to display the vessel and phase contrast MRA to impart information on velocity of flow. MRA provides 3D imaging and can be used to plan endovascular intervention.

Treatment

1. Conservative
2. Percutaneous transluminal angioplasty
   - Indicated in patients with > 50% stenosis, with associated hypertension or renal impairment
   - Associated with a high incidence of re-stenosis and is not suitable for ostial lesions
   - Recent work using PTA combined with stent placement may offer satisfactory results and is currently under evaluation
   - Re-stenosis after PTA alone is in the region of 30%
   - Complications, including intimal dissection, thrombosis and renal puncture, occur in up to 10%
3. Surgical bypass
4. Bench endarterectomy and autotransplantation.

MESENTERIC ISCHAEMIA

Mesenteric ischaemia may be the result of:

- Arterial embolism
- Arterial thrombosis
- Mesenteric vein thrombosis
- Non-occlusive mesenteric ischaemia (NOMI). NOMI is the result of vasoconstriction of the mesenteric vessels as a part of the physiological response to trauma. NOMI is an exaggerated response leading to significant bowel ischaemia and in extreme circumstances may result in bowel infarction.

CHRONIC MESENTERIC ISCHAEMIA

- Chronic mesenteric ischaemia is infrequently diagnosed
- History is variable and classical presentation of mesenteric angina is rare
- Diagnosis can only be made when a high index of suspicion is maintained
- Colour duplex and angiography are used in combination to confirm the diagnosis
- Mesenteric angina is described by patients as severe pain which has an onset immediately after eating. They are often emaciated and have difficulty eating at all. Usually two of the three visceral vessels are occluded, with stenosis in the third. It is unusual to have symptoms even in the presence of three tight stenoses, and it is usual for at least one vessel to be occluded and two others to be stenosed greater than 95%.

Treatment

- Angioplasty is currently the treatment of choice for non-ostial lesions. Failure usually does not produce significant worsening of the patient's condition

- Surgical options include in-flow from the supracoeliac aorta utilising Dacron grafting either to a single vessel or to the coeliac and superior mesenteric arteries. Long saphenous vein interposition or aorto-mesenteric jump graft is more suited for use where the iliac vessels are the source of in-flow. It is rare to have to revascularise the inferior mesenteric artery
- Success rates of surgical bypass vary according to the site affected
- Surgery is relatively high risk.

ACUTE MESENTERIC ISCHAEMIA

- Despite all advances this condition still has a mortality of 50%
- Acute mesenteric ischaemia may be the result of a thrombosis in a diseased artery, embolism, or venous thrombosis. Angiography may be employed to confirm the diagnosis and the catheter used to administer thrombolytic agents in cases of venous thrombosis
- Superior mesenteric artery thrombosis can result in infarction from the duodeno–jejunal junction to the junction of the middle and distal third of the transverse colon
- Massive bowel infarction may occur secondary to thrombosis of a diseased superior mesenteric artery or infrequently due to venous thrombosis in a patient with a hypercoagulable state (Antithrombin III deficiency, protein C or S deficiency, etc.)
- Commonest form of mesenteric ischaemia is ischaemic colitis that may follow major vascular reconstructions, secondary to thrombosis of the left colic artery. Usually a self-limiting condition and can be managed conservatively with intravenous fluids and antibiotic therapy. The long-term complication of colonic stricture may require endoscopic intervention or resection
- Embolectomy should be attempted in cases requiring revascularisation
- Bypass of the stenosis is often disappointing
- The mainstay of treatment is resection of infarcted bowel, exteriorisation and early reassessment with further resection as required.

ANEURYSMAL DISEASE

An aneurysm is an abnormal dilatation of a blood vessel. A vessel is considered to be aneurysmal if the diameter exceeds twice that of the normal artery.

Presentation of aneurysmal disease includes localised pulsatile swelling, symptoms from local compression, haemorrhage from rupture, distal ischaemia secondary to thrombosis and distal embolisation. The functional abnormality varies according to the anatomical site, e.g. cerebrovascular accident and subarachnoid haemorrhage for intracranial aneurysms.

Aetiology of aneurysms

- Atherosclerotic – commonest
- Inflammatory
- Mycotic, i.e. infective – rare
- Trauma
- Metabolic e.g. Marfan's and Ehlers Danlos
- False aneurysms – arterial puncture, suture line failure.

Abdominal aortic aneurysm (AAA) is common, with a prevalence of 5.4% in men aged 65–74. AAA is diagnosed when the anteroposterior diameter of the infrarenal aorta exceeds 4 cm. Ninety five percent arise below the origin of the renal vessels, 5% involve the suprarenal aorta. The aetiology of most aneurysms is atherosclerotic degeneration.

Assessment

- Ultrasound: confirms diagnosis, may be used as a screening tool in the future. Diameter dependent on correct orientation of the ultrasound probe. Accurate to within 5 mm over time. May be difficult to determine proximal extent and origin of renal arteries
- CT, spiral CT: this modality is very useful to assess renal artery origin and in 3D modelling for assessment for endovascular stent graft repair of aneurysm. With conventional CT scanning the renal artery origin may still be unclear
- Intravenous intra-arterial subtraction angiography: may be used as an adjunct to the above methods to determine the origin of the renal arteries
- MRI/MRA: may be the diagnostic tool of choice for the future as it provides 3D modelling and angiographic detail without recourse to X irradiation and contrast agents.

Treatment

The problems associated with AAA are distal embolisation and rupture. The risk of rupture increases with size of the aneurysm and most aneurysms increase by 0.4 cm per annum. If the rate of increase exceeds this, surgical intervention would be wise. The rupture rate over 5 years is:

< 4.5 cm	9%
4.5–7 cm	35%
> 7 cm	75%

The UK Small Aneurysm Trial has reported that operating on aneurysms < 5.5 cm does not confer any clinical benefit. It is reasonable to operate on smaller aneurysms if they are symptomatic or rapidly expanding (> 1 cm per annum).

Conservative

Abdominal aortic aneurysms < 5.5 cm monitor with regular USS estimation, control hypertension and other risk factors.

Beta-blocker administration has reportedly been associated with reduced expansion rates, controlled clinical trials are not available to support this. If considered for surgery, preoperative cardiac evaluation is required as cross-clamping the aorta places very severe stress on the heart. If significant coronary artery disease is discovered, coronary angioplasty or coronary artery bypass grafting takes precedence as complication of myocardial infarct or death from cardiac disease is otherwise common.

Surgical

Open repair Abdominal inlay graft with a straight or bifurcated prosthesis.

Endovascular repair Transfemoral placement of an aortic graft is now feasible and undergoing evaluation in clinical trials. It has initially been associated with a faster postoperative recovery and a reduced metabolic response to trauma. Patient selection is paramount. The neck of the aneurysm, that is the area between the origin of the renal arteries and the onset of aneurysmal dilatation, must be of sufficient length to enable the stent to secure the graft without occlusion of the renal arteries. Factors suggesting that an aneurysm is unsuitable include excessive angulation between the neck and the aneurysm, calcified plaques within the wall of the neck and a neck diameter > 30 mm. Initial work with straight tube grafts was disappointing as percentage of aneurysms had a sufficiently long distal neck for stent placement. Bifurcate grafts to the iliac vessels are currently favoured.

Complications of this technique include displacement of graft, continuing expansion of the aneurysm wall due to back flow from patent lumbar and inferior mesenteric vessels and possible rupture. This is covered earlier in the chapter. Complications secondary to groin dissection and damage at the site of arterial insertion have been reported.

Massive blood transfusion may be required in ruptured AAA and thoraco-abdominal aneurysms. Cell-saving equipment recycles blood lost during the procedure and processes it in a form suitable for auto-transfusion. This can significantly reduce the need for large donor supplied blood.

ANEURYSMAL DISEASE SPECIAL CASES
POPLITEAL ANEURYSMS

- Usually treated by exclusion femoro-popliteal bypass, rarely excision and bypass
- If thrombosis has occurred, thrombolysis may be necessary to clear the distal run-off at the time of surgery, this has improved the outcome of surgery for popliteal aneurysms

- Popliteal aneurysms are often bilateral, in the acute situation the occluded vessel should be treated and the other side dealt with electively
- There is considerable variation with respect as to when to operate; however, in the presence of distal embolisation, occlusion, onset of symptoms of claudication intervention is required. The diameter at which intervention is advisable is ≥ 2 cm as other complications occur more frequently.

VISCERAL ARTERY ANEURYSMS

- Are very uncommon
- **Hepatic artery aneurysm** is the most frequent visceral artery aneurysm followed by splenic artery aneurysm
- **Splenic artery aneurysms** classically present in pregnant women, with an episode of severe upper abdominal pain and collapse. Haemorrhage is initially into the lesser sac and therefore abdominal signs are limited. This is followed by temporary haemodynamic compensation. Several hours later, free intraperitoneal haemorrhage occurs and is associated with significant mortality. Diagnosis relies on high index of suspicion, plain abdominal X-ray will show eggshell calcification in the wall of the aneurysm in the left upper quadrant
- Treatment is by excision of the aneurysm with end-to-end anastomosis of the splenic artery. This is possible due to the tortuosity of the vessel.

SUBCLAVIAN ANEURYSMS

- May be dealt with by extra-thoracic resection, interposition vein graft, or aneuryssmorrhaphy.

CAROTID BODY TUMOUR

- Also known as chemodectoma, is an uncommon tumour arising from the chemoreceptor cells of the carotid body
- Presentation as a swelling in the neck with transmitted pulsation, in the region of the carotid bifurcation
- Diagnosis is by colour duplex and carotid angiography, with the latter displaying the 'blush in wine glass' appearance
- Metastasis is uncommon unless the lesion is very large
- Surgical excision is advocated in younger patients; however, in the frail and elderly a conservative approach is taken.

VASCULAR TRAUMA

- The majority of vascular trauma is the result of blunt injury, fractures or stabbing. A high index of suspicion is required and knowledge of classical associations important

- Vascular insufficiency may result from contusion of the arterial wall, intimal tear with local or propagated thrombosis, intimal tear with dissection and local or propagated thrombosis, puncture of arterial wall which may be complicated by haematoma and subsequent development of a false aneurysm. Rarely, simultaneous injury to an adjacent vein will result in an arterio-venous fistula forming
- Complete division of arterial wall, or soft tissue defect may include loss of a length of vessel.

Orthopaedic injuries associated with vascular trauma

- Supracondylar fracture of humerus – brachial artery
- Fracture of clavicle or first rib – subclavian artery
- Fracture of shaft of femur – superficial femoral artery
- Posterior dislocation of knee – popliteal artery.

Penetrating injury

- Knife wound
- Missile injury; low velocity or high velocity
- Iatrogenic injury, e.g. operative wound, arterial cannulation for blood sampling, angiography or angioplasty
- Blunt trauma, or crushing injury
- Traction injury, injury to subclavian artery following acute lateral flexion of cervical spine
- Acute deceleration injury may cause an aortic tear at junction of aortic arch and descending thoracic aorta
- Chemical injury may occur following accidental intra-arterial injection of anaesthetic or sclerosant agents. Injection of particulate matter may occur in intravenous drug abusers who crush tablets or aspirate benzodiazepines from capsules.

Principles of management (Fig. 5.4)

- Control haemorrhage with the application of direct pressure or pressure over the vessel proximal to the injury. Tourniquets are rarely required, but if necessary they should be applied carefully and relaxed every 5–10 minutes for a few seconds to prevent in situ thrombosis. Elevate the area if appropriate. Obtain intravenous access and resuscitate patient
- Classical signs of arterial occlusion are an indication for urgent exploration. Delay may result in ischaemic contracture or amputation. Delayed arterial occlusion is usually due to thrombosis, therefore regular reassessment of the distal circulation is required for at least 24 hours following any possible arterial injury
- Colour duplex may be useful in the acute situation, especially if traumatic arteriovenous fistula is suspected

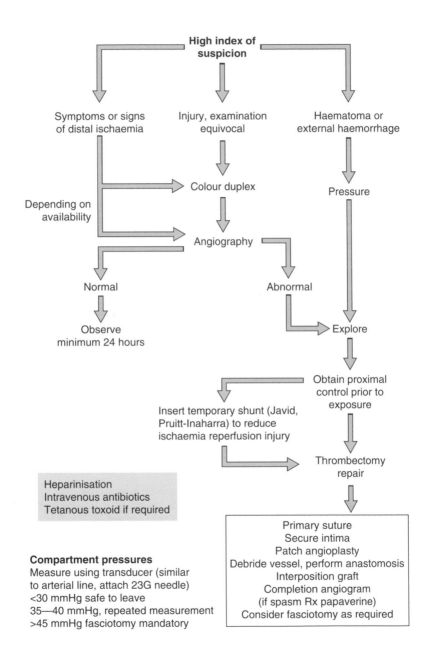

Fig. 5.4 Vascular trauma.

- Arterial spasm should not be diagnosed unless structural arterial damage has been excluded by surgical exploration or a normal arteriogram. Narrowing on angiography is due to contusion or thrombus until proven otherwise by exploration.

Fasciotomy

- If revascularisation is delayed significant tissue swelling may occur within fascial compartments leading to further ischaemia and ischaemic contractures or gangrene
- For an adequate fasciotomy all fascial layers should be incised via medial and lateral longitudinal incisions which are closed by delayed primary suture or skin grafting after 7–10 days when all oedema has subsided. In the leg, excision of a portion of the fibula decompresses all four compartments
- Subcutaneous fasciotomy via multiple small incisions provides inadequate compartmental decompression.

Venous injuries

- Major venous injuries are not frequent, simple ligation of large veins can lead to chronic venous insufficiency and surgical repair is favoured
- Thrombectomy may be required.

Fracture stabilisation

- Restoration of circulation takes precedence over fracture fixation
- A temporary inlay shunt may be used to restore flow until the fracture is stabilised and definitive repair carried out when stable
- Internal skeletal fixation is the ideal method of treating associated unstable fractures
- When wound contamination precludes its use skeletal traction or external skeletal fixation provide alternative methods.

Amputation

- The aim of amputation is removal of necrotic tissue, with subsequent tissue healing and return to mobility
- 5000 patients are referred to limb fitting centres having undergone an amputation for peripheral vascular disease
- Above-knee amputation, performed using a fish mouth incision, is associated with a 45% mortality within 2 years and only 20% of above-knee amputees achieve mobility
- Below-knee amputation has a 25% 2-year mortality and 40% of patients mobilise
- Below-knee amputation is classically performed creating a long posterior flap known as a Burgess flap, or using oblique incisions to create a skew flap; each technique has its supporters.

VENOUS DISEASE

VARICOSE VEINS

Varicose veins are **dilated tortuous superficial veins** affecting the lower limb. They are most commonly found in the distribution of the long saphenous vein, less frequently in the distribution of the short saphenous vein.

The aetiology is uncertain but an underlying weakness in the vein wall is likely. The commonest abnormality is incompetence at the sapheno-femoral junction.

Symptoms include aching on prolonged standing and itching over the gaiter area of the ankle.

Treatment with compression hose is sufficient for most patients. Surgery is performed to prevent the complications of varicose veins, namely varicose eczema, lipodermatosclerosis and venous ulceration. Thin-walled superficial varicosities can ulcerate or be punctured traumatically, resulting in brisk haemorrhage, this is successfully dealt with by pressure and elevation. Surgical treatment should be based on objective assessment of venous dysfunction. Many patients request surgery for cosmetic reasons.

Assessment

- Clinical – inspection and examination with the use of a tourniquet carrying out the Trendelenburg test to identify the level of reflux
- Reflux in the long saphenous vein can be demonstrated using the 'tapping test'. Tapping the proximal vein in the region of the sapheno-femoral junction will, in the presence of incompetent valves, cause a thrill detectable by a hand placed **distally** over the long saphenous vein
- Handheld Doppler insonation can detect reflux in the majority of sites with good sensitivity and specificity, except in the popliteal fossa. These two modalities are often sufficient in patients with primary varicose veins.
- Colour duplex – is an excellent tool in the assessment of patients with complex venous disease and can be used to map out any incompetent perforating veins
- Photoplethysmography is useful in identifying patients with venous pump dysfunction
- A history of previous deep venous thrombosis should be sought prior to any procedure that will remove portions of the saphenous veins
- Deep venous patency and function should be confirmed prior to surgery to prevent serious venous hypertension and its sequelae, because the venous return may depend on the superficial veins being present and patent.

Surgical treatment

Long saphenous territory

- Sapheno-femoral incompetence requires flush sapheno-femoral ligation, and many surgeons strip the long saphenous vein from groin *to* knee. Stripping the vein below the knee is associated with an increased risk of saphenous neuralgia
- Superficial varicosities can be successfully dealt with by multiple cosmetic stab phlebectomy.

Short saphenous territory

- These patients undergo flush sapheno-popliteal ligation in a prone position. Varicosities can be dealt with as for the long saphenous vein
- Incompetent perforating veins in the leg are treated by subfascial ligation. This can be carried out endoscopically
- Injection sclerotherapy is reserved for superficial varicosities in the leg, in the absence of sapheno-femoral or sapheno-popliteal incompetence. It is also useful for residual varicosities following surgery. The varicosity is marked, the limb is elevated and the vein partially emptied. The vein is cannulated and aspiration of blood confirms that the fine needle is within the vein lumen. The vein is then completely emptied and varicosity isolated by digital pressure. A small amount of sclerosant is injected and the vein walls opposed by a wedge of foam rubber, secured in place by a compression bandage. The compression must remain constant for 2 weeks and the patient encouraged to walk daily. Stockings alone are worn for a further 4 weeks.

Special cases

- Thread veins or spider veins: these may be successfully treated by micro-injection sclerotherapy, or laser coagulation.

VENOUS ULCERATION

- This is a significant problem affecting up to 100 000 patients at any one time in the UK, which places an exceptional burden on the NHS
- Adequate **compression therapy** will heal up to 74% of ulcers within 12 weeks. The current method of choice is the Charing Cross 4-layer bandage technique, this applies 40 mmHg pressure at the ankle, decreasing to 17 mmHg at the knee
- Colour duplex assessment of the venous system of the affected limbs is advisable
- Prior to commencement of therapy significant arterial insufficiency should be excluded by measuring the ankle brachial pressure index, an index of ≥ 0.8 in patients not suffering with diabetes mellitus is essential. Arterial insufficiency should be addressed, as healing is significantly impaired by ischaemia

- **Resistant ulcers** may require skin grafting or surgical intervention to treat venous reflux. In chronic ulcers, biopsy is advised to exclude malignant change. Significant arterial disease may have developed in chronic ulcers and mixed arterial and venous ulcers occur and are treated as described.

DEEP VENOUS THROMBOSIS AND PULMONARY EMBOLISM

Half the patients undergoing major abdominal, pelvic or hip surgery will develop a deep vein thrombosis (DVT) if no prophylactic measures are given. One-fifth of patients developing a DVT are likely to suffer a pulmonary embolism (PE).

Virchow's triad remains central to the pathogenesis of DVT:

- Alteration of venous blood flow: stasis, turbulence
- Endothelial damage, intraoperative trauma from manipulation and static compression
- Alteration of blood constituents: increased platelet adhesiveness and activation of procoagulants.

An aggregate of platelets with fibrin deposition produces a stable nidus of thrombus. If this is not cleared the thrombus is readily propagated.

The risk factors for DVT should be considered and presence of sufficient risk factors is an indication for prophylactic measures. The use of a scoring system to determine whether a patient is at low (< 5% risk), intermediate (5–40% risk) or high risk (> 40%) of venous thromboembolism may be helpful (Table 5.6).

Table 5.6 Scoring system to assess patients risk of venous thromboembolism

Patient factors	Score	Patient factors	Score
Age > 40	1	Duration of surgery < 60 min low risk	1
Age > 70	2	Duration of surgery > 150 min high risk	2
Pregnancy and puerperium	1	Postoperative immobility > 4 days	2
Obesity	1	Laparoscopic procedures	1
Oestrogen therapy and oral contraceptives	1	Sepsis	1
Thrombophilia	5	Varicose veins	1
Previous deep vein thrombosis or pulmonary embolism	5	Extensive burns and trauma, especially pelvic and femoral fractures	2
Surgical and pathological factors		Major surgery, especially abdominal and pelvic operations	1
Malignant disease	1	Myocardial infarction	1
Lower limb paralysis	1	Inflammatory bowel disease	1

Low risk score ≤ 2
Medium risk score 3–4
High risk score ≥ 5

Other factors to be considered:

- Increased euglobulin lysis time (ELT)
- Reduced antithrombin III concentration
- Congestive cardiac failure
- **High risk** should receive mechanical and chemical prophylaxis, that should be continued and be routinely screened for the presence of asymptomatic DVT.

Mechanical methods

- Static graduated compression of legs
- Electrical calf muscle stimulation
- Passive exercise of legs
- Intermittent external pneumatic compression of legs.

Chemical methods

1. Heparin: low-dose subcutaneous calcium or sodium heparin (5000 units 8- or 12-hourly) is given preoperatively and continued for 5–7 days. Low molecular weight heparin has been associated with a lower risk of haemorrhage in orthopaedic surgery than unfractionated heparin; however, this has not been shown in general surgery. There is no advantage using low molecular weight heparin in general surgical patients
2. Platelet inhibitory agents, e.g. aspirin, dipyridamole, sulphinpyrazone, Dextran 70, have all been used in the past but are not as effective as heparin combined with mechanical measures
3. Oral anticoagulant, e.g. warfarin, phenindione: these drugs need strict laboratory control and are incompatible with a number of other drugs. Significant haemorrhage may occur and the effects of these anticoagulants may be difficult to reverse.

No method of prophylaxis either chemical or mechanical is 100% effective: in very high-risk patients a mechanical method should therefore be combined with a chemical one.

Diagnosis of DVT
History and clinical examination are very unreliable as many patients with established venous thromboses are asymptomatic and have non-specific or equivocal physical signs. A high index of suspicion is necessary to make the diagnosis promptly.

Contrast venography
This provides the 'gold standard' against which other tests are compared. It accurately documents the extent of a thrombus and its nature. Ascending venography is used to show the calf and thigh veins; per-trochanteric injection may be used to demonstrate thrombi in the pelvic veins.

Table 5.7   Sensitivity and specificity of colour duplex in the diagnosis of acute DVT (%)

	Proximal DVT	Distal DVT
Sensitivity	100	87.5
Specificity	98.8	98.7

The use of contrast agents may be complicated by allergic reactions, thrombophlebitis and thrombosis.

Colour duplex
Colour duplex assessment of the venous system of the lower limb provides a sensitive and specific non-invasive alternative to contrast venography (Table 5.7).

D-dimer estimation
This is now becoming more widely available and provides a quick non-invasive method that can, within limits, exclude the need for duplex assessment in many cases.

Thermography
Infra-red camera detects areas of increased temperature. In the absence of inflammatory conditions these areas are related to the presence of an underlying thrombus.

Strain gauge and impedance plethysmography
Plethysmographic techniques measure the venous volume of the lower limb and venous emptying time. Suitable for detecting major proximal venous occlusion.

Radioactive (^{125}I-labelled) fibrinogen uptake
Useful tool for research investigations and as a routine screening test in high-risk patients. Only detects developing thrombi. Very sensitive method below the knee with an accuracy of 80–90%. Unreliable in the upper thigh. Cannot be used for pelvic vein thromboses. False-positive results occur in the presence of haematomata or recent surgical or traumatic wounds.

Traditional treatment of established DVT

- Bed rest
- Leg elevation – this must be HIGH ELEVATION! ≥ 50°
- Compression of affected leg
- Conventional bandaging
- Graded compression stockings
- Anticoagulants: anticoagulation is initiated with either i.v. heparin given by continuous infusion or by high-dose subcutaneous heparin for at least 5 days. Low molecular weight

heparins have the advantage of a once daily dose based on body weight and avoid the need for repeated APTT estimations. Warfarin is then given for 3–6 months in most cases
• Low molecular weight heparin and Warfarin are used in community based programme of DVT therapy
• Fibrinolysis: may be of use in patients with severe venous compromise
• Vein ligation and venous thrombectomy: indicated in the presence of severe ilio-femoral venous thrombosis with impending venous gangrene which does not respond to anticoagulants and where fibrinolytic agents are contraindicated. Ilio-femoral venous thrombectomy may be combined with ligation of the superficial femoral vein.

Diagnosis of PE
Only one-third of patients with clinical features compatible with a major PE have the diagnosis confirmed by angiography. Similarly, PE is often not diagnosed as it is clinically silent or its presentation atypical.

Electrocardiogram (ECG)
Massive pulmonary embolus is associated with signs of acute right ventricular strain. Typical ECG features include 'S1, Q3, T3' pattern with T-wave inversion in leads V1–V3.

Arterial blood gas analysis
May be non-specific but generally:

• Low arterial oxygen tension
• Low arterial carbon dioxide tension.

Chest radiography

• A number of abnormalities may be present but none is specific for PE
• Areas of decreased and increased pulmonary vascular markings
• Prominent hilar shadow, pulmonary atelectasis or consolidation, pleural effusion, elevated hemi-diaphragm.

Radio-isotope ventilation-perfusion lung scintigraphy
The regional distribution of inhaled radioactive gas (^{81} Kr) is compared with the distribution of radiolabelled particles (^{99}Tc-labelled macroaggregates of albumin) injected intravenously. Pulmonary emboli produce perfusion defects which are not associated with corresponding ventilation defects.

Pulmonary angiography (conventional or CT)
Definitive method of diagnosing pulmonary embolism. The extent and site of the obstruction to the pulmonary circulation is determined and the age of the embolus can be estimated.

Treatment of massive PE

Massive pulmonary embolism presents as collapse, syncope, acute right ventricular failure and cardiogenic shock. This is often fatal.

- IMMEDIATE RESUSCITATION
- External cardiac massage, with initial precordial 'blow'
- Endotracheal intubation
- Oxygen
- 8.4% sodium bicarbonate infusion to reverse metabolic acidosis
- Full anticoagulation (see above)
- Plasminogen activators
  - Streptokinase and urokinase can be used to accelerate the clearance of pulmonary emboli in the initial 24 hours
  - The efficacy of these thrombolysins is increased by their direct infusion into the pulmonary arteries via the catheter used for initial arteriography; however, this has not been shown to affect long-term survival.

Pulmonary embolectomy

- Open embolectomy (Trendelenburg's operation) ideally using cardiopulmonary bypass but if this is not available an attempt can be made using the normothermic venous in-flow occlusion technique
- Catheter embolectomy using a steerable cup-catheter inserted via the femoral or internal jugular vein and guided under fluoroscopic control.

Prevention of PE in patients with established DVT

- Anticoagulation as above
- Administration of plasminogen activators
- Defibrinating agents: ancrod (Arvin) is an enzyme derived from the venom of the Malayan pit viper. Given subcutaneously or intravenously it lowers serum fibrinogen levels by cleaving fibrinopeptide A from fibrinogen. Fibrinogen degradation products which are formed have significant anticoagulant activity
- Inferior vena caval ligation or plication
- Transvenous insertion of intracaval device
  - Used for patients with recurrent pulmonary emboli in whom anticoagulants are either contraindicated or ineffective
  - Can be inserted under local anaesthesia and is now used in preference to vena caval ligation or plication
  - Inserted via the internal jugular or femoral vein and usually placed just below the renal veins
  - Examples of the devices commonly used include the Mobin-Uddin umbrella filter, Kimray-Greenfield wire filter, Eichelter sieve and Pate clip
- Venous thrombectomy.

LYMPHATIC DISORDERS

Primary lymphoedema is a familial condition that may be congenital, when it is known as Milroy's disease, or may develop in adolescence, known as lymphoedema praecox. It may affect one or more limbs. Swelling is due to accumulation of protein-rich fluid in the limbs and accumulates during the day, and is worse following exercise. Basic treatment is supportive with compression hose and elevation. With advancing age the oedema may worsen and become woody hard and be present continuously. The patient must avoid any form of infection as this can aggravate the condition. Severe cases where the patient is becoming immobile can be treated by excision of all skin, subcutaneous tissue and deep fascia with skin grafting onto the bare muscle. This treatment is only used as a last resort.

SYMPATHECTOMY

Cervical sympathectomy is currently performed for hyperhidrosis of the hands or axillae or for peripheral vasoconstriction encountered with Raynaud's syndrome. Open cervical sympathectomy is an infrequently performed operation due to the use of thoracoscopic techniques. Thoracoscopic sympathectomy either diathermises or resects the second and third thoracic ganglia for conditions affecting the hands, and extends down to the third and fourth, and occasionally fifth thoracic ganglia for conditions affecting the axillae. Bilateral procedures may be carried out during the same anaesthetic.

Potential complications of thoracoscopic sympathectomy include pneumothorax, Horner's syndrome, compensatory sweating and recurrence.

Lumbar sympathectomy

This may be carried out as a radiological procedure using phenol, an extra-peritoneal laparoscopic approach, or by open techniques. For sympathectomy to be effective in the lower limbs there must be a reasonable blood flow to allow distribution of blood to the skin.

MINIMALLY INVASIVE VASCULAR SURGERY

Currently, minimally invasive techniques are becoming popular, such as subfacial endoscopic perforator surgery (SEPS), endoscopic saphenous vein harvesting, thoracoscopic sympathectomy and laparoscopic sympathectomy. Laparoscopic abdominal aortic aneurysm repairs have been carried out but are currently an experimental procedure. Other minimally invasive techniques could encompass also any endovascular procedure, such as endovascular aneurysm repair or angioplasty.

The use of an endovascular stent has become more commonplace. There are a variety of stents available, and they can be made of many different materials. The two main stent designs currently in use are those that require balloon dilatation and those that are made of a material that has a shape-memory and self-expands when exposed to body temperature (e.g. Memotherm stents that are made of nitinol). Stents have been inserted in many areas of the vascular tree, e.g. the coronary circulation, but currently for peripheral vascular disease their use is mainly in the aorto-iliac segments. Infra-inguinal use of stents has not currently been shown to be durable. Covered stents are also available and have the advantage that they may cover the opening of an arteriovenous fistula, seal a false aneurysm or cover roughened areas of atheroma that may lead to embolisation. They have also been used to secure and exclude dissections of the major vessels. Stents have been combined with thin-wall Dacron and PTFE grafts in the aorto-iliac segments.

Over 9000 endovascular aortic aneurysm repairs have been carried out. The current devices are either aorto-iliac where the graft passes from the aorta to the main iliac vessels, with exclusion of the other iliac artery to prevent aortic aneurysm sac expansion and rupture, and with an extra anatomical femoro–femoro cross-over graft to provide circulation to the contralateral lower limb. There are currently newer bifurcated devices with different deployment methods, and these are becoming more popular as they avoid an extra anatomical bypass. It is likely that, within 10 years, percutaneous stent grafting of abdominal aneurysms will become commonplace. Currently the problems associated with endovascular aneurysms appear to be due to incomplete exclusion of the aneurysm sac with potential expansion and rupture, these may be due to back bleeding from lumbar vessels or leakage at the proximal neck due to slippage or expansion of the neck of the aneurysm. Slippage and displacement can lead to rupture of the aneurysm or lower limb ischaemia due to kinking of the graft. At present many of these conditions can be managed by further endovascular procedures. The other limiting factor is the origin of the aneurysm with respect to the renal arteries. Some devices place uncovered stents over the renal vessel origins.

PRINCIPLES OF MANAGEMENT OF PROSTHETIC INFECTION

The use of prosthetic materials in vascular surgery is fraught with the danger of graft infection. Graft infection can lead to loss of limb or life. The principles of dealing with a graft infection are to remove the prosthetic material and revascularise the affected part using autogenous vein. Where long saphenous and arm vein is shown to be absent, harvesting of the brachial vein or superficial femoral vein has been used successfully to replace the infected graft. The superficial femoral vein is ideal as an aortic conduit as it has a large diameter and thick wall that is resistant to dilatation. Direct replacement with autogenous material can remove the necessity to create an extra anatomic bypass, e.g. axillo-bifemoral or axillo-popliteal grafts using prosthetic materials as these are also prone to the risk of graft infection.

MULTI-DISCIPLINARY APPROACH TO VASCULAR SURGERY

The practice of modern vascular surgery requires a multi-disciplinary approach and this is helped by regular surgical, radiological meetings. The management plan of each patient involves the radiologists and surgeon in clear dialogue as to the likely benefits of endovascular and operative interventions. For high-risk procedures, the surgeons will make themselves available for urgent reconstruction if this is required. The support services of physiotherapy and artificial limb fitting are also paramount if a patient is to be returned to the community with the best function.

FURTHER READING

Earnshaw J J, Murie J A 1999 The evidence for vascular surgery. tfm publishing
Rutherford R B (ed) 1999 Vascular surgery. 5th edn. WB Saunders, London
Davis A H, Baird J, Ulgatt M 1999 Essential vascular surgery, W B Saunders, London
Dotter C T, Judkins M P 1989 Transluminal treatment of arteriosclerotic obstruction. Description of a new technique and a primary report of its applications. 1964 [Classical article] Radiology 172: 904–920
Grüntzig A, Hopff H 1974 Percutaneous recanalisation after chronic arterial occlusion with a new dilator-catheter (modification of the Dotter technique). Dtsch Med Wochenschr 99(49): 2502–2510, 2511

6. Cardiac surgery

Paul Peters, Neil Moat

BASIC PRINCIPLES

PATIENT ASSESSMENT AND RISK STRATIFICATION

History and examination

Routine cardiac surgical patients are often referred with an accurate diagnosis and important investigations such as coronary angiography in place, but it is crucial to confirm both the history and examination findings. This not only re-establishes the diagnosis and severity of symptoms but also can reveal co-morbid conditions which may increase the risk of surgery, require further investigation or treatment or even preclude surgery. Particular attention should be paid to the assessment of those risk factors that may be modifiable in the period before surgery:

- Smoking
- Hyperlipidaemia
- Hypertension
- Obesity
- Control of diabetes mellitus
- Carotid disease.

Examination for the signs of commonly associated conditions or those that may complicate surgery will enable adequate operative planning:

- Respiratory disease
- History of transient ischaemic attack or stroke
- Peripheral arterial occlusive or aneurysmal disease
- Varicose veins (especially long saphenous) in patients with coronary artery disease.

Routine investigations

- Haematology: anaemia may exacerbate angina, may indicate occult bleeding in anticoagulated patients or haemolysis in valve disease
- Polycythaemia in patients with respiratory disease or cyanotic congenital heart disease
- Biochemistry: renal failure, dehydration or hypokalaemia following diuretics

- Electrocardiogram (ECG): rate or rhythm abnormalities, ventricular hypertrophy, ischaemia, recent or old infarction
- Chest X-ray: cardiomegaly, thoracic aortic or mediastinal abnormalities, respiratory disease or pulmonary oedema.

Symptom classification according to accepted definitions and identification of other factors such as diabetes, renal failure, hypertension, valvular disease with pulmonary hypertension, etc can be combined in scoring systems to allow calculation of approximate risk for the patient and the proposed operation.
Risk stratification allows:

1. Clear discussion of risks and expected benefits with the patient and relatives
2. Surgeon and institution to compare expected and actual outcomes with standardised figures.

Good communication (with colleagues and patients), preoperative recognition of special circumstances (re-do surgery, multiple cardiac pathology, comorbidity) and meticulous planning of procedures are crucial in achieving optimal surgical results.

SURGICAL ACCESS

Cardiac surgery is routinely performed via median sternotomy:

- Midline incision suprasternal notch to xiphisternum, division of tissues superficial to sternum
- Midline division of sternum with oscillating saw (re-do surgery or patients with high right heart pressures require special measures)
- Division or excision of thymic tissue/remnant
- Midline incision and elevation of pericardium.

Closure of sternotomy:

- Large drains to pericardium (and pleura/mediastinum if indicated)
- Six to eight steel wires or number 5 Ethibond sutures with apposition of deep and superficial bone tables
- Absorbable sutures to periosteum/fat and skin.

CARDIOPULMONARY BYPASS

Cardiopulmonary bypass (CPB) takes over the function of the heart and lungs allowing the heart to be arrested and isolated from the rest of the circulation, and surgery to be performed in a still, bloodless field (see Fig. 6.1).

- Full heparinisation (usually > 3 mg/kg or > 300 u/kg)
- Blood diverted from caval veins or right atrium to reservoir
- Pump and oxygenator CO_2/O_2 exchange
- Return at arterial pressure to distal ascending aorta or common femoral artery, flow rate according to body surface area nomogram

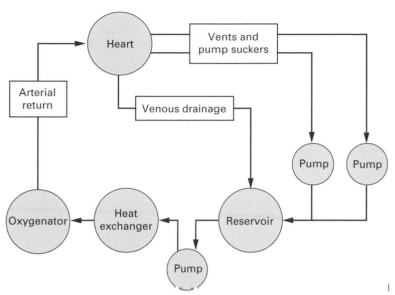

Fig. 6.1 Schematic cardiopulmonary bypass circuit.

- Temperature control by heat exchanger in circuit
- Isolation of heart possible by clamping ascending aorta proximal to arterial return cannula.

Meticulous deairing of the arterial circuit reduces but does not eliminate gaseous embolisation.
Complications of CPB are widespread, related to:

- Exposure of blood to non-physiological surfaces
- Abnormal forces on blood components in pumps, suckers and oxygenator
- Embolisation of gas, platelets and particles from bypass circuit.

Despite heparinisation, some clotting activation occurs, leucocytes are activated and platelets consumed and a systemic inflammatory response is initiated. Coagulopathy is common. Severe neurological injury occurs in up to 2% of patients (see below).

MYOCARDIAL PROTECTION

During aortic cross-clamping the heart is isolated, the coronaries are not perfused and therefore the heart is ischaemic. Many techniques for protecting the heart from the effects of ischaemia exist; none is perfect. An ideal strategy to protect the heart would ensure that myocardial oxygen demand/supply is balanced at all times. Reduction in oxygen demand may be achieved by reducing mechanical work or reducing metabolic activity either pharmacologically or by cooling. Electrical fibrillation effectively arrests the heart and reduces mechanical work but the heart is still metabolically active whilst ischaemic. This condition is tolerated well for 10–15 minutes before reperfusion is necessary. For procedures anticipated to last longer than this it is necessary to reduce the myocardial oxygen demand by other means to reduce the deleterious effects of ischaemia. Complete electrical arrest dramatically reduces myocardial oxygen demand and can be achieved by instilling a hyperkalaemic crystalloid or blood solution (cardioplegia) into the aortic root or directly into the coronary ostia if the aortic root is opened. Further protection is achieved by hypothermia, and therefore cold cardioplegia (4–10°C) can be used with topical cooling to reduce myocardial temperature. Moderate whole-body hypothermia (28–32°C) supplements myocardial protection and provides some cerebral protection also. Myocardial performance postoperatively is severely compromised by ventricular distension and a left ventricular vent can prevent this.

Myocardial recovery postoperatively can be improved by:

1. Adequate perioperative protection
2. Reduction in myocardial work
3. Maximising oxygen delivery.

CEREBRAL PROTECTION

Cerebral complications may be due to hypoperfusion or embolisation. Focal lesions are often transient with good prognosis, global cerebral ischaemia has a poor prognosis.

Risk factors

- Increasing age
- Re-do surgery
- Valve surgery
- Pre-existing cerebrovascular disease
- Ascending aortic calcification.

Risk may be minimised by:

- Preoperative recognition and treatment of carotid disease (simultaneous carotid endarterectomy and CABG is occasionally indicated)
- Hypothermia during bypass
- Meticulous deairing of the heart and aortic root.

If open access to the aortic arch or the origin of the head vessels is required, deep hypothermia (15–18°C core temperature) reduces cerebral metabolism to such an extent that complete circulatory arrest can be tolerated for 20–40 minutes (deep hypothermic circulatory arrest).

PERIOPERATIVE MONITORING AND SUPPORT

Minimum monitoring includes pulse oximetry/end-tidal CO_2, ECG, arterial pressure, right atrial pressure, urinary catheter.

Low-risk routine cases identified preoperatively who have uncomplicated surgery can be 'fast-tracked' with early extubation (< 2 hours) and transfer to a high-dependency unit. Complex cases, those with poor left ventricular performance or complications, may require ventilation, inotropic or even mechanical support best managed in an intensive care setting.

SURGERY FOR ACQUIRED HEART DISEASE

ISCHAEMIC HEART DISEASE

Ischaemic heart disease is a major cause of morbidity and mortality in the UK and even though there were around 25 000 operations for ischaemic heart disease in the NHS in 1995, requirement for coronary revascularisation still outstrips provision. The British Cardiac Society guidelines suggest that 1000 interventions (600 surgical and 400 percutaneous) per million population is a minimum target.

CORONARY ARTERY DISEASE (CAD) AND CORONARY ARTERY BYPASS GRAFTING (CABG)

Coronary artery disease
Atherosclerosis commonly occurs in the proximal coronary arteries (diffuse distal disease is less common but does occur in diabetes and hyperlipidaemia) and may present with slowly developing chronic stable angina on exertion, unstable angina, acute myocardial infarction (MI) or sudden death. Risk factors are those for atherosclerosis in general. Rate of progression of CAD is highly variable but may be altered by modification of risk factors (stopping smoking, treatment of hyperlipidaemia). Classification of symptoms is by functional limitation (Table 6.1). Atypical symptoms may be clarified by exercise ECG findings. Coronary angiographic findings (see Fig. 6.2) and knowledge of left ventricular (LV) function are critical in planning treatment.

Table 6.1 New York Heart Association functional classification of angina

Class	
I	No limitation of functional ability
II	Slight limitation: ordinary activity results in dyspnoea or angina
III	Marked limitation: less than ordinary activity results in fatigue, dyspnoea or angina
IV	Symptoms on minimal exertion or at rest

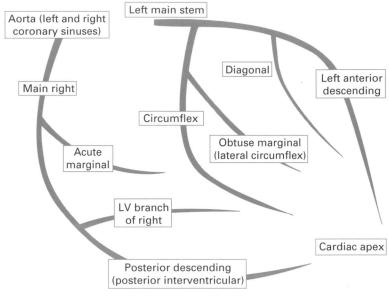

Fig. 6.2 Schematic normal coronary artery anatomy.

Coronary artery bypass grafting

CABG is indicated for symptomatic disease or for prognostic reasons (the existence of coronary stenoses carrying important prognostic implications):

- Class III–IV or unstable angina refractory to medical treatment (with coronary anatomy suitable for surgery)
- Class I–II angina with 3-vessel disease and impaired LV function
- Left main stem stenosis > 50%
- 2- or 3-vessel disease with severe proximal stenosis in the left anterior descending artery (LAD)
- Angioplasty and stenting are used in the treatment of 1- and 2-vessel CAD. Angioplasty alone has disappointing long-term results. Intracoronary stents improve the short-term results of percutaneous intervention but this has not yet been demonstrated beyond 2–3 years.

The aim of CABG is to bypass all major vessels with > 50% stenosis. Median sternotomy and cardiopulmonary bypass are routinely used, although as the LAD is relatively easily accessible on the front of the heart, various minimally invasive techniques are being explored to avoid the complications associated with CPB. None has yet been proven to be equal to standard techniques in long-term studies. Conduits routinely used are the left internal mammary artery (LIMA) as a pedicled graft to the LAD and segments of reversed long saphenous vein as aortocoronary grafts to other vessels. Free radial artery and gastroepiploic arteries are less commonly used.

Complications of CABG

- Bleeding requiring resternotomy 2%
- Stroke 1–2%
- Perioperative MI 3%
- Renal failure 2%
- Atrial fibrillation (usually temporary) 20–25%
- Overall hospital mortality 1–2% (elective CABG).

Risk factors include poor LV, unstable angina, older age, recent MI (especially within 1 week), increased bypass time and increased time of myocardial ischaemia.

CABG relieves symptoms, improves functional class and improves survival in patients with prognostically significant coronary stenosis.

- 60% of patients are free of angina at 10 years, but only 60% of vein grafts are patent at 10 years
- 5-year survival is 85%, 10-year survival 75%
- Mid- and long-term survival is further improved by the use of LIMA to LAD, which in survivors has a 90% 10-year patency

Postoperative low-dose aspirin and modification of risk factors (lipid lowering regimens, cessation of smoking, control of hypertension) improve graft survival.

SURGERY FOR STRUCTURAL COMPLICATIONS OF MYOCARDIAL INFARCTION

The usual causes of cardiovascular collapse following a completed MI are ventricular failure or arrhythmia. Occasionally structural failure of an infarcted muscular element can present as a severe complication within days of an acute MI which may be amenable to surgical intervention. These events have a high mortality without treatment but surgery is also high risk.

Post-infarction ventricular septal defect
Infarction of the interventricular septum can result in formation of a post-infarct ventricular septal defect (VSD). Mortality without treatment is high (> 90%). Surgical treatment is to patch the VSD. In early surgery (at presentation) myocardial tissues are friable and myocardial function is poor. Although in delayed surgery (e.g. at 6 weeks) fibrosis develops around the VSD and the remaining myocardium may have recovered, few patients survive this long. Early surgery is indicated following resuscitation and placement of intra-aortic balloon pump (see below – Management of the failing heart).

Acute mitral regurgitation

Rupture of an infarcted papillary muscle may result in severe mitral regurgitation often associated with a large anterior MI, leading to severe cardiogenic shock and pulmonary oedema. Surgical results are somewhat better than the prognosis without surgery of up to 75% 24-hour mortality.

Left ventricular aneurysm

The survivor of a large anterior MI may go on to develop a chronic left ventricular aneurysm, complicated by poor LV function and arrhythmias. Aneurysmectomy and CABG can improve both symptoms and survival. Operative mortality is up to 10% and late survival is only 65% at 5 years even with surgery.

VALVULAR HEART DISEASE

Rheumatic fever was a major cause of valvular heart disease but is now uncommon and, as the general population ages, degenerative valvular heart disease is increasing in importance. There were over 5000 operations in the NHS for valvular heart disease in 1995.

Echocardiography and cardiac catheterisation provide important information about valvular heart disease. Timing of surgery is critical. Careful follow-up allows surgery to be performed before irreversible ventricular dysfunction occurs.

PROSTHETIC HEART VALVES

Mechanical

- Usually bileaflet, occasionally tilting disc or ball and cage
- Lifelong anticoagulation INR 2.5–3.5 (aortic), 3–4.5 (mitral)
- Durability is excellent.

Biological

- Porcine xenograft, pericardial or human homograft (allograft)
- Require early anticoagulation only (3 months)
- All undergo structural degeneration
- Surviving patients require re-replacement for valve dysfunction at 10–15 years.

Choice of valve type for an individual patient is governed by several factors:

- If warfarinised for another reason (e.g. atrial fibrillation) then mechanical valve
- If anticipated survival of patient > 10–15 years then mechanical valve
- Contraindication to anticoagulation then biological valve
- In younger women the potentially teratogenic effect of warfarin in pregnancy must be weighed against the risks of re-do valve

replacement when choosing between mechanical and biological prosthesis.

AORTIC VALVE DISEASE AND AORTIC VALVE REPLACEMENT

Aortic stenosis
Aortic stenosis becomes severe when the normal valve area (2.5–3.5 cm^2) is reduced to < 1 cm^2 and is critical at < 0.75 cm^2. The LV hypertrophies (which can cause subendocardial ischaemia and angina even without CAD) and becomes stiff, increasing LV filling pressures leading to pulmonary oedema. Transvalvular gradients can be over 100 mmHg (there is virtually no gradient across a normal aortic valve) but in end-stage disease the gradient can be deceptively low as the LV fails. Surgery is indicated when symptoms occur (angina, syncope, heart failure) as this is associated with rapidly worsening prognosis and an increased risk of sudden death.

Aortic regurgitation
Aortic regurgitation (AR) from leaflet retraction or aortic root dilatation leads to volume overload of the LV with progressive LV dilatation and failure. Acute AR may be associated with type A dissection (see below) or endocarditis.

Aortic valve replacement
Aortic valve replacement is performed on CPB through the lower ascending aorta. The native valve is excised and the prosthetic valve sewn in place with non-absorbable sutures. Meticulous deairing of the left heart and aortic root is mandatory.

- Hospital mortality 3–5%
- Risks include older age, poor LV and poor functional status
- Complete heart block is a recognised complication
- 5-year survival 75%, 10-year 60%.

MITRAL VALVE DISEASE AND MITRAL VALVE REPAIR AND REPLACEMENT

Mitral stenosis
Mitral stenosis (MS) is usually rheumatic in origin, with thickening of leaflets and subvalvar apparatus and commissural fusion reducing the valve area from 4–6 cm^2 to less than 1 cm^2. Calcification often occurs. The left atrium enlarges, left atrial and pulmonary venous pressures rise producing pulmonary oedema. A rise in pulmonary vascular resistance can give rise to pulmonary artery hypertension and right heart failure. Dyspnoea, from pulmonary oedema, and cachexia are common. Surgery (usually valve replacement or repair but occasionally valvotomy or balloon valvuloplasty) is indicated for NYHA class III–IV symptoms.

Mitral regurgitation (MR)
Chronic MR may be due to:

- Leaflet prolapse due to degenerative disease (most commonly)
- Annular dilatation.

Acute mitral regurgitation (MR) may be due to:

- Endocarditis with destruction of leaflet tissue
- Ischaemia with papillary muscle or chordal rupture.

MR leads to dilatation of left atrium and LV and gradual LV failure. Surgery is indicated in acute MR, chronic MR with class III–IV symptoms or class I–II symptoms with deteriorating LV function. Repair rather than replacement is preferred although in rheumatic valves repair is rarely possible.

Mitral valve surgery
Mitral valve surgery is usually performed through the left atrium via median sternotomy on bypass. Right thoracotomy also gives good exposure of the mitral valve and a closed valvotomy may be performed through a left thoracotomy. Meticulous deairing of the left heart and aortic root is mandatory.

- Hospital mortality 3–6%
- Patients are usually in chronic atrial fibrillation.

ENDOCARDITIS

Active endocarditis should be treated with at least 4 weeks of appropriate antibiotics if the patient is well enough before valve replacement (if indicated) is contemplated. Implantation into an infected field may lead to prosthetic valve endocarditis (PVE), a catastrophic complication with a mortality of more than 50%. Similarly, antibiotic prophylaxis (see British National Formulary for current guidelines) covering all procedures in patients with prosthetic valves is critical in preventing PVE.

CARDIAC TUMOURS AND PERICARDIAL DISEASE

Cardiac tumours may be primary (benign or malignant) or secondary. Commonest are secondary deposits or local invasion by other thoracic malignancies (bronchogenic carcinoma, lymphoma). These may present with malignant pericardial effusion and tamponade (low cardiac output, raised jugular venous pressure, arterial paradox). The commonest primary cardiac tumour is atrial myxoma, benign (apart from its haemodynamic and potentially catastrophic embolic effects) and usually cured by open resection on bypass. Other cardiac primaries are rare.

Constrictive pericarditis may be tuberculous or idiopathic. Surgical treatment by pericardectomy is potentially hazardous due to obliteration of the normal plane between pericardium and epicardium.

THORACIC AORTIC ANEURYSMS AND DISSECTIONS

THORACIC AORTIC ANEURYSMS

Descending thoracic aortic and thoraco-abdominal aneurysms are usually atherosclerotic (but may be the result of a chronic dissection, or rarely infective, i.e. mycotic). A localised ascending aortic aneurysm may be atherosclerotic or associated with aortic stenosis (a form of post-stenotic dilatation); more generalised aortic root, ascending aortic and arch dilatation is associated with disorders such as Marfan's syndrome.

AORTIC DISSECTION

Hypertension and Marfan's syndrome are important risk factors for aortic dissection, in which an intimal tear allows blood to separate the inner and outer layers of media producing a false channel. Dissections involving the ascending aorta (De Bakey types I or II) are a surgical emergency as they can rupture into the pericardium or occlude the coronary arteries or innominate/carotid vessels. Those involving only the descending aorta (type III) are best treated medically unless the false channel occludes important branches producing limb or visceral ischaemia, or with time result in an aneurysm which continues to expand.

Replacement of the ascending thoracic aorta may be extended to replace the whole aortic root with a composite graft (aortic valve and Dacron tube) and reimplantation of the coronary ostia (Bentall procedure). If arch surgery is required, deep hypothermic circulatory arrest is employed.

MANAGEMENT OF THE FAILING HEART

REVERSIBLE HEART FAILURE

Support for heart failure thought to be reversible or recoverable (e.g. postoperative poor LV function) may be pharmacological:

- Catecholamines – dopamine, adrenaline
- Inodilators – dobutamine, milrinone

or mechanical:

- intra-aortic balloon pump (IABP): a sausage-shaped balloon is introduced into the descending thoracic aorta, usually via a femoral arterial route. The balloon is inflated (using helium) and deflated in time with the ECG; deflation occurs immediately before systole to reduce the pressure against which the left ventricle ejects (reducing left ventricular wall tension therefore

reducing myocardial work) and inflates in diastole increasing diastolic coronary perfusion (increasing myocardial oxygen delivery)
- ventricular assist device (VAD): various extra- or intra-corporeal pumping devices designed to reduce ventricular work by mechanically pumping blood from venous to arterial circulations. Modes used are LVAD (pulmonary veins/left atrium to aorta), RVAD (right atrium to pulmonary artery) or BIVAD (LVAD plus RVAD).

IRREVERSIBLE HEART FAILURE

The main surgical treatment of end-stage irreversible heart failure is cardiac transplantation.

- Improvements in immunosuppression particularly have improved prognosis of cardiac transplant recipients with > 85% 1-year and 60–70% 5-year survival
- Donor shortage limits the number of transplants performed. Xenotransplantation, long-term mechanical devices and skeletal muscle transformation are being explored as substitutes but at present have no clinical place
- Inotropes, IABP or VAD may support patients waiting for transplantation.

SURGERY FOR CONGENITAL HEART DISEASE

Congenital heart disease presents many complex problems for the cardiac surgeon, the full range of which cannot be covered here. Assessment and decision-making require a multidisciplinary approach. Many lesions require multiple-staged procedures progressing merely to palliation, whilst others are thought to be amenable to surgical cure. It is important to remember that in these patients decades of follow-up is required before the long-term sequelae of intervention become apparent. Many patients who had palliative treatment as infants or children are now presenting as young adults with complex cardiac lesions requiring further treatment. As an introduction some common lesions are discussed.

ATRIAL SEPTAL DEFECT (ASD)

- Communication between left and right atria, commonest is ostium secundum type
- Repair indicated if large left-to-right shunt
- Surgical treatment by patching the defect on CPB
- Some are amenable to closure by catheter-delivered device
- May present in adulthood with reversed shunt (Eisenmenger's syndrome).

PATENT DUCTUS ARTERIOSUS (PDA)

- Left-to-right shunt increases pulmonary blood flow, causing pulmonary oedema and LV volume overload
- Surgical ligation performed via thoracotomy.

TRANSPOSITION OF THE GREAT ARTERIES (TGA)

- Aorta arises from right ventricle and pulmonary artery from LV, survival depending on shunting through ASD or VSD (if present) or PDA
- Usual presentation is with closure of PDA at age 1–2 weeks
- Treatment by arterial switch procedure with good short-term results, although long-term prognosis is unknown as the operation was first performed regularly in the mid-1980s.

COARCTATION OF THE AORTA

- Severe stenosis of the thoracic aorta in the region of insertion of the ductus arteriosus. May present in infancy with failure to thrive or LV failure, or in later life with characteristic findings (upper limb hypertension, reduced or delayed femoral pulse, rib notching on CXR)
- Treatment in infancy by resection and end-to-end anastomosis or subclavian flap, in older patients by interposition graft via thoracotomy
- Non-critical coarctation may be treated by balloon dilatation.

TETRALOGY OF FALLOT

- The underlying abnormality leading to tetralogy (VSD, pulmonary stenosis, overriding aorta and right ventricular hypertrophy) is a malalignment of the septum of the right ventricular outflow tract with the rest of the ventricular septum
- The lesion is cyanotic due to reduced pulmonary blood flow and some patients are prone to severe cyanotic spells
- The condition may be palliated by a systemic-to-pulmonary shunt (see below) or corrected by patching of the VSD with relief of right ventricular outflow tract obstruction (which may render the pulmonary valve incompetent with unknown long-term consequences).

SYSTEMIC TO PULMONARY SHUNTS

- Palliation of some cyanotic conditions may be achieved by increasing pulmonary blood flow by the creation of a systemic artery-to-pulmonary artery shunt, the commonest of which is the modified Blalock–Taussig shunt. A 3.5–5 mm polytetrafluoroethylene tube graft is interposed between the subclavian artery and the ipsilateral pulmonary artery

- In neonates with cyanotic conditions, however, a PDA may be the only source of pulmonary blood flow and patency can be maintained by infusion of prostaglandin PGE keeping the baby alive until other treatment can be instituted.

THE FONTAN CIRCULATION

- In strict anatomical terms it is very rare to find a heart with only one ventricle but functionally univentricular hearts are more common. Such hearts can never have separate ventricles supporting the systemic and pulmonary circulations
- Staged procedures can allow the functional ventricle to support the systemic circulation whilst pulmonary flow is achieved by shunting blood to the pulmonary arteries directly from the right atrium or caval veins, a 'Fontan' circulation
- This can be well tolerated in the short- and medium-term but the long-term prognosis is poor.

FURTHER READING

Bojar R M 1994 Perioperative management in cardiac and thoracic surgery, 2nd edn. Blackwell, Boston

Kirklin J W, Barratt-Boyes B G 1993 Cardiac surgery, 2nd edn. Churchill Livingstone, New York

Information on risk stratification, outcomes and other educational information is available online at the web sites of the Society of Cardiothoracic Surgeons of Great Britain and Ireland (http://www.scts.org/) and the Cardiothoracic Surgery Network (http://www.ctsnet.org/).

7. Thoracic surgery

Paul Peters, Neil Moat

The range of thoracic disease presenting for surgical evaluation is extensive, ranging from management of critically ill trauma victims to tumour and reconstructive surgery. A methodical approach to patient assessment, investigation and planning of intervention is crucial in the process of performing appropriate surgery and achieving good results. The importance of chest physiotherapy in the pre- and postoperative management of thoracic surgical patients cannot be overstated.

PATIENT ASSESSMENT

1. Make the diagnosis
2. Determine whether or not the condition is amenable to surgical intervention
3. Decide whether or not that intervention can be performed with acceptable risk to the patient.

Diagnosis

History with special attention to timing and duration of symptoms, exercise tolerance, co-morbid conditions and features which may suggest increased risk (e.g. steroid use in chronic pulmonary conditions) or inoperability (e.g. metastatic disease in patients with a tumour).

Examination similarly for features of primary and co-morbid conditions, local tumour invasion (hoarseness, Horner's, superior vena caval obstruction) or metastasis (lymphadenopathy especially supraclavicular nodes, hepatomegaly, bony tenderness, neurology), nutritional status, paraneoplastic syndromes.

Non-invasive investigation

- Chest X-ray/computed tomography (CT) scan including all previous films which should be specifically sought if not immediately available
- Haematology and biochemistry (including liver and bone screen) and arterial blood gases.

Respiratory function tests

Many patients with thoracic disease amenable to surgery have chronic pulmonary disease with poor lung function and reduced respiratory reserve. The trauma of chest surgery with or without lung resection can have a profound impact on respiratory function. Ideally preoperative assessment would select out those patients in whom major surgery presents an unacceptable risk; unfortunately there is no absolute predictor of bad outcome.

- Arterial blood gases, simple spirometry and measurement of lung volumes can give an indication of likely risk. Simple exercise tolerance is also a useful guide (a patient who can climb two flights of stairs without stopping should tolerate most procedures, whereas inability to climb one flight carries a high risk)
- Respiratory function in a patient with preoperative collapse of a lobe or a lung may be improved by lung resection as ventilation may be unchanged whilst intrapulmonary shunting is reduced
- A preoperative FEV1 of > 2.0 L or > 60% of predicted values should be acceptable for all procedures
- An anticipated postoperative FEV1 of > 1300 ml or > 40% of predicted values should indicate acceptable risk. An anticipated postoperative FEV1 of < 800 ml carries a high risk (e.g. pneumonectomy with preoperative FEV1 of 1.5 L)
- Postoperative FEV1 can be calculated using quantitative radionuclide lung scanning:

  Postoperative FEV1 = preoperative FEV1 × (% contributed by remaining lung)

- Preoperative identification of risk factors that are modifiable before surgery can improve outcome
- Smoking cessation
- Preoperative physiotherapy with bronchodilators in reversible airways disease and antibiotics in acute or chronic chest infections
- Steroids should be weaned to the lowest dose compatible with disease control before surgery (with perioperative intravenous steroid cover)
- Nutritional status: both cachexia and obesity take time to correct but nutritional supplementation of the cachectic patient prior to surgery may improve outcome
- Identification of cardiac disease: a history of recent myocardial infarction, episode of heart failure, angina or arrhythmia increases operative risk (in lung resection a history of MI increases risk of cardiac complications from < 1% to around 6%). Treatment should be optimised and further assessment considered if there is evidence of ischaemic heart disease.

INTERCOSTAL DRAINAGE

Fluid or air in the pleural space may be drained percutaneously by needle aspiration but more complete and continuous drainage is secured by intercostal tube drainage. Size and site of drain may be dictated by circumstances but generally in adults a 28 French tube in the fifth intercostal space between anterior and posterior axillary lines is safe and effective both for air and fluid.

1. As with all procedures, inform the patient and get consent for the procedure, have assistance at hand (to replace the articles you drop while scrubbed) and position the patient so that you and the patient are comfortable and the site for insertion of the drain is accessible
2. Strict aseptic technique is critical. Local anaesthetic (10–15 ml of 1% lignocaine in an adult) even in a sedated patient or an emergency
3. Adequate skin incision, placement of purse-string and drain retention stitch, formation of intercostal track into pleura by blunt dissection
4. Drain placed along track into pleural space without force. A trochar may be used to direct position to apex or base, not to force the drain through the chest wall
5. Connect to underwater seal drain and continuous low pressure (–15 to –20 cm of water), high volume suction. Chest X-ray post placement and daily until removal
6. When full lung expansion is achieved and no air leak seen then suction is discontinued. With continued full expansion of the lung and no air leak or significant drainage for 24 hours the drain is removed (with patient performing Valsalva manoeuvre during actual removal)
7. The drain should not be clamped at any time.

CHEST TRAUMA

Follow basic principles: secure the airway, maintain ventilation and support the circulation. Maintain a high index of suspicion for immediately life-threatening conditions:

- Tension pneumothorax
- Flail chest
- Cardiac tamponade/aortic transection.

Chest X-ray, ECG and arterial blood gases can supplement diagnosis but occasionally early intervention is required on clinical grounds alone.

Understanding the mechanism of injury is important. Blunt and penetrating injuries may coexist (e.g. in blast injury or road traffic accidents), and blunt injury to the chest wall can cause penetrating injury to underlying lung from rib fracture. Iatrogenic injury is usually of the penetrating type (e.g. during placement of chest drains).

PENETRATING INJURY

Usually low-energy, e.g. knife or handgun wounds. Tissue damage occurs in the injury track only (as opposed to high-energy penetrating injuries where injury may be widespread due to internal shock wave energy transmission), but this track may involve chest wall, lung, mediastinum, thoracic inlet, diaphragm or intra-abdominal structures.

Suspicion of pneumothorax or haemothorax requires intercostal drainage. Uncontrolled air leak compromising ventilation, or continued substantial bleeding following initial drainage are rare but require surgical exploration.

Suspicion of cardiac injury may be raised by clinical evidence of cardiac tamponade (hypotension, raised jugular venous pressure, arterial paradox), ECG or chest X-ray findings. Subxiphoid ultrasound examination can confirm the diagnosis of tamponade and guide pericardiocentesis prior to surgical exploration. Embedded objects (knife, railing, etc.) should not be removed until a full assessment of deep tissue involvement is made, usually at surgery.

BLUNT TRAUMA

Blunt trauma (e.g. following a fall from a height or a road traffic accident) is often associated with multiple trauma and may result in chest wall flail segments, tracheobronchial, diaphragmatic or oesophageal rupture or thoracic aortic injury. Cardiac contusion may be associated with sternal fracture and can seriously impair cardiac function. Emergency thoracotomy is indicated if visceral rupture is suspected.

AORTIC TRANSECTION

Aortic transection, usually at the ligamentum arteriosum, characteristically occurs with severe deceleration injury, e.g. seat-belt wearers in a high-energy impact road traffic accident. X-ray finding of widened mediastinum requires CT scan or angiography, confirmation of the diagnosis requires surgery.

CHEST WALL DISEASE

PECTUS DEFORMITIES

Abnormal growth of costal cartilages causes the sternum to be depressed inward (excavatum) or to become prominent (carinatum). Underlying heart and lung tissues may be displaced in severe cases but function is almost always quite normal (however, carinatum deformity is common in Marfan's syndrome). Patients usually present in adolescence when body image becomes important. Surgical correction is for cosmesis only and should be delayed as long as possible (at least until late teens) as the deformity may recur with later growth. Correction requires surgical excision of costal cartilages 3–7 bilaterally. The sternum usually falls into an acceptable position; in excavatum deformities it may require splinting in place with a metal bar.

TUMOURS

Secondary tumours, especially to ribs, are much commoner than primary chest wall tumours which are rare but often have characteristic X-ray appearances. Diagnosis should be by excision biopsy with margins dictated by expected type according to radiology.

Benign (2–4 cm resection margin)

- Chondroma: painful mass, often anterior near costochondral junction. Lobulated, radiodense X-ray appearance
- Fibrous dysplasia: painless asymptomatic mass, often posterior rib in young adult. X-ray appearances of central fusiform mass with thinning of cortex and absence of calcification.

Malignant (excise whole rib plus > 4 cm margin above and below tumour)

- Chondrosarcoma: commonest malignant chest wall tumour (25% of all primary chest wall tumours, 80% occurring in rib, 20% sternum). Lobulated mass arising from medulla with cortical bone erosion and stippled calcification. Slow growing, chemo- and radio-resistant. Best treatment is with wide local excision with > 4 cm margins. Survival is good if surgical clearance is achieved
- Ewing's sarcoma, osteosarcoma and soft tissue sarcomas are rare. Treatment is wide local resection with adjuvant chemo- or radiotherapy.

Chest wall reconstruction should be planned in association with a plastic surgeon.

PLEURAL DISEASE

PNEUMOTHORAX

Spontaneous pneumothorax in:

- Young adults with tall, thin body habitus (often associated with apical bullae)
- Older patients with emphysema. Can cause severe respiratory compromise. May cause widespread surgical emphysema (which requires no treatment and resolves with drainage of underlying pneumothorax). These patients are at high risk of complications whatever treatment is employed especially if they are on steroids
- Ventilated patients with high airway pressures (e.g. adult or neonatal respiratory distress syndrome) can get multiple pneumothoraces.

Initial treatment is by intercostal drainage. Indications for surgery include:

- Failure of conservative management
- Two episodes of pneumothorax on the same side (as this is associated with a high incidence of further episodes).

Surgery may be open via limited thoracotomy or minimally invasive via thoracoscopy. Definitive treatment is parietal pleurectomy with tying or stapling of bullae where present. Two large (28 French gauge) intercostal drains are placed at surgery and are managed as above.

CHYLOTHORAX

Milky appearance, diagnosis confirmed by lab finding of chylomicrons, triglycerides and lymphocytes in fluid. May be congenital lymphatic abnormalities, trauma to thoracic duct (including operative trauma) or duct obstruction by tumour (typically lymphoma).

Conservative management is by intercostal drainage, nutritional support and medium-chain triglycerides in diet (reduces volume of chyle). Traumatic chylothorax may be treated by repair of the duct or by mass ligation of the duct at the aortic hiatus. Recurrent chylothorax may be palliated by pleurodesis. Chylothorax secondary to tumour involvement can be extremely resistant to treatment unless tumour control can be achieved.

MALIGNANT PLEURAL EFFUSION

Pleural secondary tumour deposits may cause persistent effusion with respiratory symptoms. Diagnosis is made by aspiration cytology or pleural biopsy (percutaneous or open). Palliation by pleurodesis (talc insufflation either open, thoracoscopic or via tube thoracostomy followed by intercostal drainage for at least 72 hours). If visceral tumour deposits have trapped the lung preventing full expansion, a pleuroperitoneal shunt may help provide palliation.

EMPYEMA

Pus in the pleural space secondary to pneumonia, lung abscess, chest or oesophageal trauma, surgery. Early empyema may resolve with adequate drainage and appropriate antibiotics. Once a visceral cortex has formed, trapping the collapsed lung, intervention is required. Operative decortication frees the lung to fill all potential pleural spaces. Longstanding empyema (or one in a debilitated patient) may not be amenable to decortication. Resection of a short segment of rib at the most dependent part with placement of a large-bore empyema drain into the cavity (draining into a stoma bag around the rib resection site) can, over a period of months, result in contraction of the cavity with eventual resolution of the empyema.

Rarely the cavity does not contract; thoracoplasty can collapse the chest wall onto the cavity or the empyema drain can effectively become permanent.

TUMOURS

Benign

- Fibroma
- Rare, may be associated with hypertrophic pulmonary osteoarthropathy.

Malignant

- Mesothelioma
- Increasing in incidence due to association with asbestos exposure and very long latency (20–40 years). A history of occupational asbestos exposure may entitle the patient to compensation
- Presents with chest wall pain or pleural effusion
- Open pleural biopsy often required as histology is notoriously difficult (differential being metastatic adenocarcinoma) and the consequences of the diagnosis profound
- Surgery (pleuropneumonectomy and resection of hemidiaphragm) is hardly ever curative
- Pleurodesis for effusion or radiotherapy for pain may palliate symptoms
- Mesothelioma is slow growing but inexorable (mean survival <1 year from diagnosis) and is uniformly fatal.

DISEASES OF THE TRACHEA, BRONCHUS AND LUNG

THE TRACHEA

TRACHEOSTOMY

- Indicated for management of prolonged ventilation, secretions (minitracheostomy may be adequate), emergency airway control or upper airway obstruction, e.g. in facial injury
- Vertical incision through second and third rings. Damage to first tracheal ring may result in subglottic stenosis, lower placement risks tracheoinnominate fistula
- Percutaneous tracheostomy under bronchoscopic control is used in some intensive care units.

Tracheal stenosis is often a postintubation phenomenon at the level of the sealing cuff (less common with low pressure cuffs) or at a stoma. Treatment is by bougienage or if recurrent and severe by resection of the stenotic segment.

Tracheal primary tumours are rare but invasion by bronchogenic, thyroid or oesophageal tumours is common.

TUMOURS OF THE BRONCHUS AND LUNG

The UK has more than 40 000 new cases of bronchogenic carcinoma per year. Smoking tobacco is a major risk factor for most lung cancers (others include asbestos, radiation, tuberculosis). A mass on a chest X-ray should be treated as carcinoma until proven otherwise. Complete surgical resection can result in cure (5-year survival) but less than 20% of patients are suitable for surgery at presentation on the basis of tumour type and clinical staging.

BRONCHOGENIC CARCINOMA

Pathology

- In smokers, multiple regions of dysplastic bronchial epithelium can be found ('field change')
- Squamous cell carcinoma: < 70% of tumours, may be radiosensitive
- Adenocarcinoma: < 15% of tumours. Less strongly related to tobacco use and less sensitive to radiotherapy
- Broncheoalveolar carcinoma: < 5% of tumours, relatively favourable prognosis
- Undifferentiated carcinoma: 15–30% of tumours. Large-cell type and small-cell type. Small-cell lung cancer is extremely aggressive and metastasises early. It is rarely amenable to surgery and in general terms is not a surgical lesion. Chemotherapy has a good early response rate but relapse is almost inevitable and 5-year survival is less than 3%
- The essential clinical differentiation to be made is between small-cell lung carcinoma (SCLC) and non-small cell lung carcinoma (NSCLC).

Diagnosis

Presentation may be with typical symptoms (cough, dyspnoea, chest pain, haemoptysis, anorexia and weight loss), symptoms due to metastasis (bone pain or pathological fracture, pleural effusion, neurological symptoms due to cerebral metastasis or nerve invasion, e.g. hoarse voice or Horner's syndrome) or endocrine abnormality (Cushing's, inappropriate antidiuretic hormone secretion).

Histology may be acquired from sputum cytology, fibre-optic bronchoscopy (washings, brushings, transbronchial biopsy), CT-guided biopsy, or frozen section histology during thoracotomy.

Pancoast syndrome comprises superior sulcus tumour, pain, Horner's syndrome.

Staging

- By TNM classification and stage grouping (Tables 7.1 and 7.2).
- Clinical staging requires knowledge of mediastinal lymph node status. Thoracic CT scan may reveal nodal enlargement but this does not correlate well with metastasis and therefore mediastinal node sampling at mediastinoscopy or anterior mediastinotomy can be an important staging procedure before thoracotomy
- Pathological staging achieved by mediastinal lymph node sampling at thoracotomy.

Table 7.1   TNM staging for lung carcinoma

Primary tumour	
T0	No evidence of primary tumour
Tis	Carcinoma in situ
T1	Tumour < 3 cm diameter, not extending to visceral pleura or beyond lobar bronchus
T2	Tumour > 3 cm diameter, involving main bronchus > 2 cm from carina, involving visceral pleura, or with lobar collapse
T3	Main bronchus < 2 cm from carina, collapse of entire lung, direct invasion of chest wall, diaphragm, mediastinal pleura or parietal pericardium
T4	Invasion of heart, great vessels, oesophagus, trachea or presence of a malignant pleural effusion
Regional nodes	
N0	No regional lymph node metastasis
N1	Involvement of ipsilateral hilar nodes
N2	Involvement of ipsilateral mediastinal nodes or subcarinal node
N3	Involvement of ipsilateral scalene or supraclavicular nodes or any contralateral nodes
Metastasis	
M0	No distant metastasis
M1	Distant metastasis

Table 7.2   Stage grouping of lung carcinoma

	TNM characteristics
Stage I	T 1 or 2, N0
Stage II	T 1 or 2, N1
Stage IIIA	T3 or N2
Stage IIIB	T4 or N3
Stage IV	All M1 disease

Treatment

Resectability and operability

- Stage I and II NSCLC lesions are resectable (but only stage I SCLC and this is controversial)
- Stage IIIB and IV lesions are unresectable
- Stage IIIA lesions may be resectable. Controversy surrounds the T3 tumour and the N2 (ipsilateral mediastinal) node group
- A patient is operable if the tumour is resectable and the risk of the procedure is deemed acceptable (see 'patient assessment' above).

Surgery
General anaesthetic, pre-intubation rigid bronchoscopy to assess proximal extent of tumour, double lumen endotracheal tube. Patient in full lateral position with posterolateral thoracotomy through fifth intercostal space. A suitable operative strategy has been described by Goldstraw (See Shields 1994):

1. Confirm the diagnosis (by frozen section histology if necessary)
2. Determine whether tumour can be removed by pneumonectomy (assess tumour clearance of bronchus, pulmonary artery and pulmonary veins at hilum)
3. Confirm staging by mediastinal lymph node dissection
4. Determine whether tumour can be removed by lesser resection, i.e. lobectomy or bilobectomy (assess tumour clearance of structures within hilum and in interlobar fissures). Perform the least resection to clear tumour.

After lobectomy two large (28 French) intercostal drains are managed routinely. Pneumonectomy may be closed without drainage or a single drain may be placed, clamped to reduce mediastinal shift and released for 5 minutes each hour to reveal bleeding or air leak and removed on postoperative day 1.
Complications following lung resection include:

- Cardiac complications or arrhythmias in < 30%, commonly atrial fibrillation
- Atelectasis and pneumonia in < 30%
- Bleeding
- Residual pleural air space
- Mortality 1–3%.

Following pneumonectomy, important complications include:

- Bronchopleural fistula in 1–3%
- Contralateral acute lung injury in 2–5% especially following increased intravenous fluid infusion
- Mortality 3–10%, risks include older age and right pneumonectomy.

Table 7.3   5-year survival following resection for lung carcinoma

Stage	5-year survival
I	50–60%
II	20–30%
III	5–15%

Long-term survival depends on stage and histology (see Table 7.3).

OTHER LUNG TUMOURS

Carcinoid

- 0.5–1% of lung tumours
- Slow-growing and slow to metastasise, may be without symptoms but typical symptoms include cough, haemoptysis and recurrent infections (carcinoid syndrome – flushing, wheezing; gastrointestinal symptoms – is rare)
- Histological diagnosis usually following resection
- Typical tumours are often cured by surgery (90% 5-year survival), atypical tumours more commonly have lymph node metastasis (up to 60% 5-year survival).

Hamartoma

- Benign; less than 1% of all lung tumours but more than 70% of benign lung tumours are hamartomas
- Only 4% of solitary pulmonary nodules are hamartomas
- A solitary pulmonary nodule should be regarded as potentially malignant until proven otherwise.

SURGERY FOR EMPHYSEMA

Much of the dyspnoea and respiratory compromise in emphysema is thought to be due to thoracic overdistension. Some patients may be improved by resecting severely bullous regions of lung, reducing distension and allowing respiratory muscles and relatively normal lung tissue to function more effectively. Results are variable, however, and lung reduction surgery for emphysema is still under evaluation.

SURGERY FOR PULMONARY METASTASIS

Surgical removal of pulmonary metastatic tumour deposits appears to prolong survival if:

- The tumour is slow-growing
- Control of the primary has been achieved
- There is no evidence of metastasis elsewhere.

Sarcoma and teratoma are occasionally suitable for pulmonary metastasectomy. Local resection rather than segmentectomy or lobectomy is appropriate as multiple metastases may be resected and repeated surgery has been described.

THE DIAPHRAGM

EVENTRATION

Usually an incidental finding in an asymptomatic patient, one hemidiaphragm is thinned out and raised with abdominal contents apparently in the thorax on chest X-ray. May mimic diaphragmatic hernia or rupture.

TRAUMA

Blunt trauma may cause diaphragmatic rupture, usually on the left, with herniation of abdominal viscera into the left chest with respiratory compromise and characteristic X-ray appearance (gas-filled loops in thorax). If laparotomy is planned for management of other injuries then repair can be attempted but thoracotomy is preferable. Phrenic nerve injury produces functional impairment even with successful repair. Penetrating trauma can lacerate the diaphragm with similar results and treatment, although function is less often impaired.

HERNIAS

Oesophageal hiatus hernia

- Dealt with fully in Chapter 12.

Bochdalek

- Congenital posterolateral defect usually on the left, often associated with ipsilateral hypoplastic lung.
- Presents with respiratory distress in the newborn infant requiring urgent resuscitation and surgical repair.

Morgagni

- Congenital anterior defect lateral to xiphisternum
- May be asymptomatic, with incidental finding of low anterior mediastinal mass on chest X-ray, or become symptomatic in adult life
- Repair transthoracically (especially if diagnosis uncertain) or transabdominally.

MEDIASTINAL MASSES

Chest CT is the investigation of choice, and the position of the mass (anterior, posterior, superior mediastinum) can suggest a likely differential diagnosis. Always consider aneurysm. Mediastinal lymph node enlargement is common:

- Consider infective causes, either acute (pneumonia) or chronic (tuberculosis, bronchiectasis)
- Secondary tumour deposits are common; mediastinal lymph node metastasis from bronchogenic carcinoma, oesophageal carcinoma, extrathoracic tumours
- Lymphoma; see below
- Sarcoidosis characteristically has bilateral hilar and paratracheal lymphadenopathy.

PRIMARY MEDIASTINAL TUMOURS

Thymoma

- Anterior mediastinum
- Symptoms may be due to mass effect (dyspnoea, cough, pain, venous obstruction) or may be asymptomatic
- May be associated with systemic disorders, most commonly myasthenia gravis (weakness and fatiguability of limb, ocular and bulbar muscles with antibodies to acetylcholine receptors)
- Although the relationship between thymoma and myasthenia is inconsistent (60% of patients with myasthenia have thymic hyperplasia, 10% have a thymoma and 60% of patients with thymoma have myasthenia), all patients with myasthenia should have a chest CT and 80% improve following thymectomy
- Diagnosis of thymoma is histological but needle or incision biopsy is not recommended as seeding of tumour cells may occur, so excision biopsy is required
- Diagnosis of malignancy is difficult and is based on invasion (which also determines staging) rather than cellular features
- Surgery is via median sternotomy with wide clearance of all thymic remnants and anterior mediastinal fat
- Surgical clearance carries a good prognosis but pleural dissemination of thymoma carries a poor prognosis
- Long follow-up is required (yearly CT scan, preferably on the same machine) as late recurrence may occur.

Germ cell tumours

- Usually anterior mediastinum (teratoma in men aged 20–35, seminoma in men aged 30–40), may be asymptomatic (benign) or with symptoms due to mass effect or local invasion (malignant)
- 2/3 teratoma, 1/3 seminoma, others are rare

- Occult testicular primary must be excluded
- Tumour markers (alpha fetoprotein, beta hCG) may be raised
- Diagnosis by biopsy (CT-guided fine-needle or by anterior mediastinotomy)
- Mature teratoma is usually well circumscribed and is cured by surgical excision
- Immature and malignant teratomas tend to metastasise early and have a poor prognosis
- Seminoma is rarely cured by surgery alone but in combination with chemo- and radiotherapy a high cure rate can be achieved.

Lymphoma

- Often anterior mediastinum
- 20% of mediastinal tumours in adults are lymphomas, usually associated with disease in extrathoracic sites, although occasionally restricted to mediastinal nodes
- Therapy is based on accurate histology acquired from adequate lymph node biopsy, with the specimen sent fresh to an expectant histologist
- Cure rates are high with multimodality therapy.

Thyroid

- Masses may extend retrosternally (therefore superior or anterior mediastinum) and occasionally require sternotomy to achieve clearance.

Neurogenic tumours

- Usually posterior mediastinum
- Uncommon but may be benign or malignant and may arise from peripheral nerves, sympathetic ganglia or mediastinal chemoreceptors
- A mass in the paravertebral gutter on chest CT may be of neural origin.

Oesophageal or bronchogenic duplication cysts or oesophageal tumours

- Either benign (leiomyoma) or malignant (carcinoma) may appear in the posterior mediastinum.

MINIMALLY INVASIVE THORACIC SURGERY

Postoperative pain following thoracotomy can occasionally be severe. Minimally invasive thoracic surgery aims to reduce the trauma of surgical intervention. The indication for performing a procedure with minimally invasive technique rather than open technique is that the procedure can be performed to the same technical standard and with reduced morbidity. It is not acceptable to perform a procedure with a minimally invasive technique where that involves technical compromise or an incomplete procedure. Procedures performed with video-assisted thoracoscopy include:

- Pleural biopsy, pleurodesis, pleurectomy
- Pericardial biopsy, pericardial window
- Lung biopsy, lobectomy (controversial in malignant disease)
- Lymph node biopsy
- Sympathectomy.

Contraindications to minimally invasive thoracic surgery include:

- Inability to tolerate singe lung anaesthesia
- Pleural adhesions.

As with all minimally invasive surgery, techniques should be learned under instruction in workshops before transfer to the patient.

FURTHER READING

Dojar R M 1994 Perioperative management in cardiac and thoracic surgery, 2nd edn. Blackwell, Boston

Shields T W (ed) 1994 General thoracic surgery, 4th edn. Williams & Wilkins, Baltimore

8. Urology

Johm Hines, Gillian L. Smith

URINARY TRACT INFECTION

Most acute urinary tract infections are caused by a single bacterial species. In chronic infections, two or more pathogens may be found. The most commonly isolated micro-organisms are aerobic Gram-negative rods (e.g. *Escherichia coli, Proteus* sp.) and Gram-positive cocci (e.g. staphylococci and enterococci). Urine culture and antibiotic sensitivity testing are central to the effective treatment of urinary infections. Risk factors are lower and upper tract obstruction, stones, foreign bodies, anatomical abnormalities and urothelial tumours. Urinary tract infection is more common in women because of the relatively short urethra and asymptomatic vaginal colonisation by bacteria.

PYELONEPHRITIS

- Usually an ascending infection
- Presents with fever, rigors, loin pain and tenderness, nausea and vomiting, lower urinary tract symptoms, malaise
- Pyelonephritis associated with upper tract obstruction may lead to septicaemic shock
- Investigations should include MSU, FBC, U&E, KUB film and ultrasound (or IVU)
- Treatment involves antibiotics to cover likely pathogens pending culture and sensitivity results. Intravenous administration is required for the first 24–48 hours
- Upper tract obstruction associated with pyelonephritis requires urgent drainage
- Predisposing factors such as stones or reflux should be treated following resolution of infection
- Chronic pyelonephritis may cause renal scarring.

CYSTITIS

- May be related to sexual activity in women
- Presents with frequency, urgency, dysuria, haematuria, fever, suprapubic pain and tenderness
- Imaging of the urinary tract and cystoscopy are required in all men with cystitis and women with recurrent cystitis
- Treatment involves oral antibiotics to cover likely pathogens pending culture and sensitivity results

- Predisposing factors such as stones or bladder outlet obstruction should be treated following resolution of infection
- Women with cystitis related to sexual activity should maintain a high fluid intake and void before and after intercourse.

PROSTATITIS

- Acute bacterial prostatitis is usually caused by aerobic Gram-negative rods or *Chlamydia trachomatis*. It presents with lower urinary tract symptoms and perineal pain. Antibiotic treatment should be continued for 4–6 weeks or longer
- Chronic bacterial prostatitis is difficult to cure. Associated recurrent urinary tract infections may require suppressive antibiotics
- Non-bacterial prostatitis is the most common prostatitis syndrome. Organisms are not found. Treatment is aimed at relieving symptoms using anti-inflammatory drugs and alphablockers
- Prostatodynia is clinically similar to non-bacterial prostatitis but there is no evidence of prostatic inflammation. Treatment is aimed at symptomatic relief. Some men benefit from psychological counselling.

HAEMATURIA

Blood in the urine (macroscopic or microscopic) *always* requires investigation. The same conditions cause both microscopic and frank haematuria and assessment therefore follows the same course.

The differential diagnosis is shown in Table 8.1.

Patients with disorders of coagulation, or on anticoagulant therapy who present with haematuria, may have significant urinary tract pathology. Their haematuria should not be ascribed to the bleeding diathesis without complete investigation.

Investigation

The following investigations are essential:

1. Urine microscopy and culture
2. Dipstick urinalysis for proteinuria

Table 8.1   Causes of haematuria

Neoplasms of the urinary tract
Calculi
Urinary tract infection
Prostatic disease
Renal parenchymal disease
Trauma
Bleeding diatheses
Loin pain–haematuria syndrome
Interstitial cystitis

---

3. Urine cytology
4. Imaging of the upper tracts. The choice lies between intravenous urography (IVU) and ultrasonography plus a plain KUB X-ray. An IVU is more sensitive for small upper tract transitional cell tumours
5. Diagnostic cystoscopy.

Measurement of serum creatinine and electrolytes is indicated in suspected renal disease. Serum levels of prostate-specific antigen (PSA) may be measured in male patients.

RENAL TUMOURS

Eighty to 90% are renal cell carcinomas; these arise from the proximal tubular epithelium. Five to 10% are transitional cell tumours; these arise from the urothelium of the renal pelvis. Less common tumours include angiomyolipomas, oncocytomas, lymphoma and metastases. Wilms' tumour (nephroblastoma) is the most common renal tumour of childhood.

RENAL CELL CARCINOMA

Epidemiology

- 11th most common cancer in men and 15th in women
- Incidence increases after 40 years of age
- Male:female ratio is 2:1
- More common in smokers
- May be hereditary as in the autosomal dominant Von Hippel–Lindau syndrome
- Associated with analgesic abuse.

Presentation

- Haematuria (60%) – the most common presenting symptom
- Loin pain
- Mass
- The classic triad of loin pain, a mass and haematuria is present in 10% of cases
- Systemic symptoms (hypertension, fever, raised ESR, anaemia, polycythaemia, hypercalcaemia, abnormal liver function tests) – so-called 'para-neoplastic' syndromes
- 30% of patients present with symptoms due to metastases.

Spread

- Local extension into perinephric fat, adrenal and adjacent organs
- Extension of tumour thrombus into the renal vein and inferior vena cava
- Lymph nodes (renal hilum and para-aortic)
- Haematogenous (lungs – 'cannonball secondaries', liver, bone).

Investigation

- CT or MRI scanning provides information about local tumour extension, nodal disease and renal vein or IVC involvement
- Chest X-ray is performed as the lungs are the most common site for distant metastases
- Serum creatinine must be determined prior to treatment
- Renal arteriography is reserved for patients in whom parenchymal-sparing surgery is being considered.

Staging
The tumour is staged by the TNM system.

T1	< 2.5 cm confined to kidney
T2	> 2.5 cm confined to kidney
T3a	Invasion of perinephric fat or adrenal
T3b	Extension to renal vein +/or IVC
T4	Extension beyond Gerota's fascia
Nx	Regional lymph nodes cannot be assessed
N0	No regional lymph node involvement
N1	Single lymph node < 2 cm
N2	Single node 2–5 cm or multiple nodes < 5 cm
N3	Node > 5 cm
M0	No distant metastases
M+	Distant metastases

Treatment

Localised disease

- Radical nephrectomy is the standard treatment
- Partial nephrectomy should be considered in solitary kidneys or bilateral tumours
- Embolisation may palliate local symptoms in patients with inoperable disease.

Metastases

- Chemotherapy and radiotherapy are ineffective
- Medroxyprogesterone acetate is used in metastatic disease with limited success
- Trials of immunotherapy with interferon and interleukin-2 are ongoing.

Prognosis

Stage	5-year survival (%)
Confined to renal parenchyma	60–70
Lymph node involvement	15–35
Metastases	5

TRANSITIONAL CELL CARCINOMA OF THE RENAL PELVIS AND URETER

Epidemiology

This tumour is uncommon. Risk factors are those for transitional cell carcinoma of the bladder.

Presentation

- Haematuria
- Hydronephrosis
- Routine upper tract imaging in patients with bladder tumours.

Treatment

Localised disease

- Nephroureterectomy removing a cuff of bladder around the ureteric orifice is the standard treatment
- Local resection can be considered for small, non-invasive ureteric tumours
- Lifelong urothelial surveillance is essential because of the risk of further transitional cell tumours.

Advanced disease

- Radiotherapy may be used in locally advanced disease
- Chemotherapy (M-VAC – see bladder cancer) may be used in metastatic disease.

BLADDER CANCER

Bladder cancer is the sixth most common tumour among men and the tenth most common among women. The male:female ratio is 3:1. In the UK, most cases are transitional cell carcinoma. Squamous cell carcinoma arises from areas of squamous metaplasia and is associated with *Schistosomiasis* and other chronic inflammatory conditions. Adenocarcinoma is rare. It arises from the urachal remnant or from an area of glandular metaplasia. Leiomyosarcomas occur occasionally. Rhabdomyosarcomas occur in childhood.

TRANSITIONAL CELL CARCINOMA OF THE BLADDER

Risk factors

- Previous transitional cell carcinoma
- Smoking
- Exposure to carcinogens, such as 2-naphthylamine, xenylamine and benzidine, in the dye, leather and rubber industries
- Cyclophosphamide
- Pelvic irradiation.

Presentation

- Painless haematuria is the most common presentation
- Irritative lower urinary tract symptoms
- Recurrent urinary tract infection
- Hydronephrosis due to obstruction of ureteric orifice (rare).

Investigation

The diagnosis is usually confirmed by flexible cystoscopy. Bladder tumours are occasionally diagnosed on IVUs performed for haematuria. In these cases, a rigid cystoscopy under general anaesthesia is more appropriate as a first-line investigation because it allows both confirmation of the diagnosis and resection of the tumour. All patients with new bladder tumours should have an IVU to exclude synchronous upper tract transitional cell carcinoma.

Staging

Bladder cancer is staged by the TNM system. The initial management of a new bladder cancer involves transurethral resection (TUR) and examination under anaesthesia (EUA). Staging (Table 8.2) of the tumour (T stage) is based on a combination of histology from the TUR specimen and findings on bimanual examination under anaesthesia after resection. A CT scan of the abdomen and pelvis and an isotope bone scan are also performed prior to radical treatment for invasive tumours.

Histological grade

G1 Well differentiated
G2 Moderately differentiated
G3 Poorly differentiated.

Table 8.2 Staging of bladder cancer

Stage		EUA
Tis	'Flat' carcinoma in situ	No mass
Ta	Non-invasive papillary tumour	No mass
T1	Invasion of lamina propria	No mass
T2	Invasion of superficial muscle	No mass
T3	Invasion of deep muscle +/– perivesical fat	Mobile mass
T4a	Invasion of adjacent organs	Mobile mass
T4b	Invasion of pelvic wall	Fixed mass
N0	No nodal involvement	
N1	Single involved pelvic lymph node < 2 cm	
N2	Single involved pelvic lymph node 2–5 cm or multiple involved pelvic lymph nodes < 5 cm	
N3	Involved lymph nodes > 5 cm	
M0	No distant metastases	
M+	Distant metastases	

Management

Management depends on the stage and grade of the tumour. In general, patients with superficial disease (Ta, T1) require a different approach to those with invasive disease (T2–T4). Note that, although T1 tumours are described as superficial rather than invasive, they are in fact invasive malignancies because the tumour has invaded the lamina propria.

Superficial tumours (Ta, T1)

Seventy percent of new bladder tumours are superficial. Initial management is by transurethral resection (TURBT). Following this treatment, 75% of patients are destined to develop recurrent disease, although only 10% progress to invasive tumours. For this reason patients must be kept under cystoscopic surveillance, although after 10 years some patients may be suitable for cytological surveillance.

Patients with recurrent superficial tumours can be treated with courses of intravesical chemotherapeutic agents such as mitomycin C and epirubicin. Single doses of these agents can also be administered after initial transurethral resection to prevent recurrence. Although these drugs reduce recurrence rates, they do not influence rates of progression to invasive disease or overall mortality. Recurrent tumours, especially poorly differentiated and carcinoma in situ, may also be treated by immunotherapy with intravesical BCG.

T1G3 tumours have a high risk of progression to invasive disease (40%) and therefore require more aggressive treatment. Management of these tumours is controversial. Therapeutic options include cystectomy, radiotherapy and transurethral resection with intravesical therapy.

Carcinoma in situ

Carcinoma in situ precedes invasive cancer and must be treated aggressively. Treatment with intravesical BCG or chemotherapy produces remission in most cases. Cystectomy should be considered if intravesical therapy fails.

Invasive tumours

Thirty percent of new bladder tumours are invasive.

Stage T2, T3, T4a   Radical cystectomy is the treatment of choice. This includes a hysterectomy and bilateral salpingo-oophorectomy in women (anterior exenteration) and involves cystoprostatectomy in men. After cystectomy, patients require urinary diversion (ileal conduit or continent diversion) or orthotopic reconstruction (e.g. Koch pouch to the urethra). Radiotherapy is an alternative. Salvage cystectomy may be required for relapse after radiotherapy.

Stage T4b   Palliative radiotherapy and/or chemotherapy.

Metastases Combination chemotherapy with methotrexate, vinblastine, doxorubicin and cisplatinum (M-VAC) produces complete remissions in 25% of cases but is highly toxic.

Prognosis

Stage	5-year survival (%)
T1 tumours	90–100
T2	55
T3	35
T4 tumours	10–20
Nodal involvement	6
Distant metastases	0

TRAUMA TO THE GENITOURINARY TRACT

RENAL TRAUMA

- 90% of cases result from blunt injury (road accidents, falls, sport) and 10% from penetrating trauma (stabbing, gunshots)
- There is a high rate of associated injuries, most commonly to the liver, spleen, pancreas and bowel
- Kidneys with pre-existing abnormalities such as hydronephrosis or tumour are at increased risk of injury from blunt trauma
- Pelvi-ureteric junction disruption and pedicle trauma are associated with deceleration injuries
- Most patients present with a history of injury followed by loin pain. Examination may reveal flank tenderness, ecchymosis or a mass
- Haematuria is absent in 10–30% of renal injuries. In particular, haematuria is often absent in pedicle injuries
- Most penetrating renal injuries and all gunshot wounds require exploration
- The management of blunt renal trauma is outlined in Figure 8.1
- Only 5% of blunt injuries require surgical exploration. The kidney should be explored through the midline allowing a complete examination of other organs as well as access to both renal vascular pedicles and kidneys. The vessels should be controlled before opening Gerota's fascia
- Nephrectomy is indicated for a severely traumatised kidney. Renal preservation may be appropriate in lacerations or when only part of the kidney is severely damaged
- Long-term complications of renal trauma include hypertension, arteriovenous fistula, PUJ scarring, pseudocysts, calculi, chronic pyelonephritis and loss of renal function.

URETERIC INJURIES

- Most ureteric injuries are iatrogenic, occurring in the course of urological, colorectal or gynaecological surgery

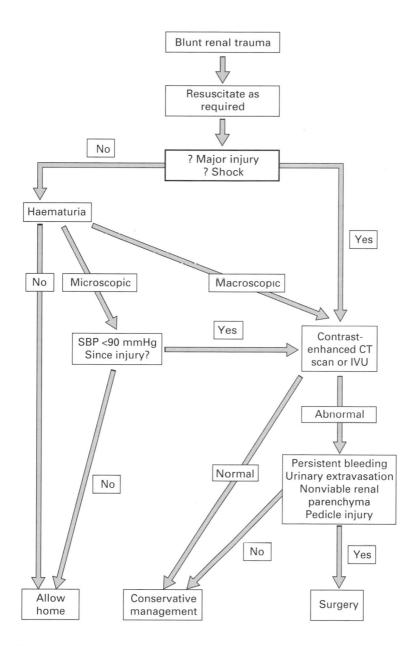

Fig. 8.1

- Injuries recognised intraoperatively can be repaired by end-to-end anastomosis, ureteric reimplantation, a Boari flap and psoas hitch or transureteroureterostomy, depending on the level and extent of the injury
- If the injury is recognised postoperatively, an IVU and cystoscopy are undertaken to determine the extent of the injury. Temporary stenting or nephrostomy drainage allow healing in some cases. Other patients require surgical intervention.

BLADDER INJURIES

Bladder injuries are comparatively rare and most commonly result from blunt trauma in road traffic accidents. Associated injuries are common.

Classification

1. Contusion
2. Intraperitoneal rupture. Intraperitoneal ruptures occur after indirect injury to a full bladder causing it to rupture at the dome, its weakest point
3. Extraperitoneal rupture. Extraperitoneal rupture is usually caused by a bony spike from the pelvis perforating the bladder wall.

Presentation

- Haematuria
- Patients may complain of inability to void and suprapubic pain
- There may be lower abdominal peritonitis
- There may be a suprapubic mass.

Investigation

- Plain X-rays to look for pelvic fracture
- IVU
- Cystogram (after excluding a urethral injury by ascending urethrography).

Management

- Intraperitoneal injuries require laparotomy, repair and drainage by suprapubic and urethral catheterisation
- Minor extraperitoneal injuries can be managed by catheter drainage, otherwise laparotomy is required
- Cystography to confirm healing should be undertaken prior to catheter removal.

URETHRAL INJURIES

Bulbar injuries

Straddle falls are the most common cause of bulbar urethral injury. Patients present with perineal bruising and blood at the meatus. If the patient voids, prophylactic antibiotics should be given and the patient followed up for the development of a stricture. Patients in retention require suprapubic catheterisation and antibiotic prophylaxis. A urethrogram should be performed after 5 days.

Membranous injuries

The membranous urethra is the most common site of urethral injury following blunt trauma. Approximately 10% of men with pelvic fractures have posterior urethral injuries. The usual injury is a partial tear. Occasionally, the puboprostatic ligaments are disrupted and the prostate is detached from the membranous urethra resulting in a complete tear with upward dislocation of the bladder and prostate.

The signs of membranous urethral injury are:

- Blood at the meatus
- Perineal bruising
- Inability to pass urine or a sensation of voiding without urine output
- High-riding prostate on digital rectal examination (DRE).

In suspected urethral injuries urethral catheterisation should not be attempted until a retrograde urethrogram (using water-soluble contrast) has been performed. If urethral injury is confirmed, bladder drainage is achieved by suprapubic catheterisation. Minor urethral lacerations usually heal spontaneously, but may result in stricture formation. Complete prostato-membranous disruption is usually managed by delayed open repair. The long-term complications of these injuries are impotence, urethral stricture and incontinence.

SCROTAL TRAUMA

Scrotal and testicular injuries usually result from blunt trauma. Blunt scrotal trauma may lead to scrotal wall haematoma, haematocele (bleeding within the tunica vaginalis) or testicular rupture due to disruption of the tunica albuginea. Most haematoceles are associated with testicular rupture, which can often be diagnosed by ultrasonography. If testicular rupture is diagnosed or suspected, early exploration and repair increase the chance of testicular salvage.

URINARY STONE DISEASE

Epidemiology

Urinary stones are common in the West, northern India and Pakistan, northern Australia and China. Stones have become more prevalent during the last century except for the periods around the two World Wars. This trend is associated with increasingly refined and calorific diets. The maximum incidence of stones is in the 3rd to 5th decades and they are three times more common in men. Urinary stones are associated with sedentary occupations, and 20% of doctors experience at least one attack of ureteric colic.

Conditions associated with urinary stones

Pregnancy   Renal colic is the most common non-obstetric cause of acute abdominal pain in the second and third trimesters.

Dysmorphia   Severe dysmorphic syndromes especially those associated with immobility are associated with urinary stones.

Obesity   Surgical bypass operations for obesity predispose to the formation of oxalate stones.

Renal malformations   Those associated with impaired drainage of the collecting system may be associated with stone formation.

Bladder outlet obstruction   Can be associated with bladder stones.

Foreign bodies   Stones may form on non-absorbable sutures and other foreign bodies such as catheters, stents, surgical clips and tumours.

Tuberculosis   Urinary tuberculosis is associated with stone formation.

Medullary sponge kidney (MSK)   Fifty percent of patients with MSK develop nephrolithiasis.

Renal tubular acidosis   A hydrogen ion excretion defect of the distal tubules that may be associated with calcium phosphate stones.

Primary hyperparathyroidism   Increased parathyroid hormone leads to increased calcium absorption from the gut and increased calcium mobilisation from bones resulting in hypercalciuria and calcium stone formation.

Stone formation

Urinary stones are polycrystalline aggregates of crystals (usually > 90%) and organic matrix (usually < 10%). The crystals are formed from calcium, phosphate, oxalate, urate and other ions. The matrix is composed mostly of protein, with small amounts of hexose and hexosamine. Stones form in supersaturated urine. The factors that affect supersaturation are pH, ionic strength, solute concentration and complexation of one ion to another. Increasing solute concentrations increase the likelihood of precipitation. In the stable zone of undersaturated urine no crystal nucleation occurs and crystals may dissolve. As solute concentrations increase, the point termed the solubility product is reached. Above this point, urine is in the metastable zone of supersaturation where stones can grow from previous crystals but no spontaneous nucleation occurs. As concentrations rise further the formation product is attained. Now urine is in the oversaturated zone where spontaneous crystal nucleation and rapid stone growth occur. Urine also contains natural stone inhibitors such as magnesium and citrate. Low concentrations of these may encourage stone formation.

Stone types

Calcium   Eighty-five percent of stones are calcareous. The calcium is combined with other ions such as oxalate and phosphate. They are radio-opaque.

Struvite   Composed of magnesium, ammonium and phosphate. Often seen as staghorn calculi. They are associated with urea-splitting organisms such as *Proteus* and resultant alkaline urine. They are radio-opaque.

Cystine   Associated with cystinuria, an autosomal recessive disease causing increased intestinal and renal tubular absorption of cystine, ornithine, arginine and lysine. They are radio-opaque.

Uric acid   Associated with gout and a low urinary pH. Radiolucent if purely uric acid.

Matrix   Associated with chronic urinary infections. They are radiolucent.

Clinical presentation

Pain   Upper tract stones cause renal or ureteric colic. Typical ureteric colic passes from the loin to the groin and may spread to the scrotum or labia. Less commonly, non-colicky pain is experienced. Stones causing upper tract obstruction tend to cause severe pain, nausea and vomiting. Large staghorn calculi are sometimes painless.

Haematuria   Usually microscopic but may be macroscopic.

Infection   Struvite stones are associated with *Proteus*, *Klebsiella*, *Pseudomonas* and *Staphylococcus* infections. Any type of stone may be associated with infection and stones are a cause of recurrent or intractable urinary infection. Infection associated with an obstructed upper tract (pyonephrosis) is a urological emergency.

Loin signs   Obstructed or infected kidneys may cause marked loin tenderness. If xanthogranulomatous pyelonephritis is present, a renal or perinephric abscess may develop which may point and discharge through the loin.

Renal impairment   Bilateral stones may be associated with impaired renal function. Unilateral upper tract obstruction may cause acute renal failure if the contralateral kidney is diseased.

Investigations

Urine Dipstick for pH and blood. MSU. Twenty-four-hour collections for calcium, oxalate, urate estimations in recurrent stone formers.

Blood Creatinine, urea and electrolytes if renal impairment is suspected. Serum estimation of calcium, urate, phosphate, which may be correlated with 24-hour urine collection results. Second-line blood tests may include parathyroid hormone estimation. Full blood count if urological sepsis is suspected.

Radiological Ninety percent or more of urinary stones are radio-opaque and can be seen on a plain KUB (kidneys-ureters-bladder) film. Ultrasonography will detect radiolucent stones. Intravenous (excretion) urography is the most important radiological investigation because it provides information about stones and urinary tract anatomy, and limited information about obstruction and renal function. Upper tract anatomy can be visualised further with retrograde ureteropyelography. CT scans can demonstrate calculi, although small stones may be missed between images. MRI images stones poorly. Radioisotope renography yields accurate information about obstruction and renal function.

Stone analysis Any retrieved stones should undergo constituent analysis.

Treatment

Ureteric stones Pain requires adequate analgesia (e.g. non-steroidal anti-inflammatory drugs which should be avoided if there is also renal impairment). Most ureteric stones up to 6 mm in diameter will pass spontaneously, although hold-up at the ureteric narrow points (the PUJ, pelvic brim and vesical intramural portion) may occur. Obstructing ureteric stones may require a ureteric stent. A stent can also be used to push the stone back to the renal pelvis to facilitate treatment. Obstruction can also be relieved by drainage of the renal pelvis with a percutaneous nephrostomy tube. Ureteric stones can be fragmented with in situ ureterscopic lithotripsy or retrieved by forceps or Dormier basket extraction. Extracorporeal shock wave lithotripsy (ESWL) can be used to treat those ureteric stones that are not obscured on imaging by bones. Associated infection must be thoroughly treated. Open ureterolithotomy is reserved for large or impacted stones that have not responded to other treatments.

Pelvicalyceal stones Staghorn calculi and large stones are best treated by percutaneous nephrolithotomy provided percutaneous access is possible. If not, open operation is required. Smaller stones may be amenable to dissolution with urinary alkalinisation. Non-functioning kidneys with associated stones are often best removed to prevent infection and to relieve symptoms.

Bladder stones These can usually be fragmented in the bladder endoscopically and evacuated. Large stones require open cystolithotomy. Consideration should be given to the treatment of attendant bladder outlet obstruction.

Asymptomatic stones Small asymptomatic renal stones may not require active treatment but should be kept under surveillance.

DISORDERS OF THE PROSTATE

BENIGN PROSTATIC HYPERPLASIA (BPH)

BPH is the most common benign tumour in men. It is typified by an increase in both stromal and glandular elements of the prostate leading to an increase in the size of the gland.

Epidemiology

- The risk of developing BPH increases with age. Seventy percent of men who reach 70 years of age develop histological BPH and nearly half of them experience lower urinary tract symptoms (LUTS)
- BPH is more prevalent in the West than the Far East. In the USA, BPH is more common in Blacks than Whites. South East Asians who migrate to the West acquire a higher rate of BPH than their counterparts remaining in the East
- A high dietary intake of soya and vegetables may reduce the risk of developing BPH
- BPH is associated with cardiovascular disease, hypertension and diabetes mellitus. BPH is less common in men with hepatic cirrhosis
- Transurethral prostatectomy (TURP) is the second most common operation performed on men aged over 65. Ten percent of males will eventually require prostatectomy if current treatment methods remain unchanged
- Because of the increasing longevity of the population as a whole, BPH is expected to become a bigger burden to health care services.

Pathogenesis

- The pathogenesis is uncertain but probably involves several factors. Ageing and the active metabolite of testosterone, dihydrotestosterone (DHT) are known to be involved
- Testosterone is converted to DHT by the enzyme 5α-reductase, which has increased activity in the prostates of men with BPH
- Oestrogens induce androgen receptors in prostatic cell nuclei and promote stromal cell hyperplasia
- Stromal–epithelial interactions influence the growth of prostatic cells. These are mediated by autocrine and paracrine growth factors or cytokines. Fibroblast growth factor, epidermal growth factor and insulin-like growth factor enhance prostatic cell division. Transforming growth factor-β reduces prostatic mitosis

Table 8.3   BOO symptoms

Obstructive	Irritative
Hesitancy	Urgency
Poor stream	Urge incontinence
Intermittent stream	Frequency
Incomplete emptying	Nocturia
Terminal dribbling	

- Decreased apoptosis (programmed cell death) may also occur in BPH.

Clinical BPH

- The LUTS associated with BPH present as the syndrome of bladder outlet obstruction (BOO). There is little correlation between symptoms and prostate size
- BOO symptoms fall into two groups, obstructive (voiding) and irritative (filling) (see Table 8.3)
- BOO symptoms can be objectively assessed by completion of a symptom index score. The best validated is the American Urological Association index which has seven questions (the AUA-7 index). The World Health Organization has added a further question about 'bothersomeness' to the AUA-7, to formulate the International Prostate Symptom Score (IPSS)
- LUTS are also affected by detrusor function, which declines with age
- Some men present with acute urinary retention
- Another group present with chronic retention, i.e. residual bladder volumes greater than 1 litre and LUTS. Men with chronic retention are prone to renal impairment
- The shape, size and surface contour of the prostate should be assessed by DRE. This may lead to a suspicion of prostate cancer (page 180)
- The presence of a palpable bladder should be noted
- A small proportion of men with BOO are prone to urinary infection
- Rarely BPH may lead to obstructive changes in the upper tracts and chronic renal failure.

Investigations

- Serum prostate specific antigen (PSA) (page 180), urea and creatinine
- Free urinary flow rates. Men with BOO typically have reduced maximum flow (Qmax)
- Assessment of post void residual volume by ultrasonography
- Upper tract imaging in men with a history of stones, renal impairment or haematuria

- Transrectal ultrasound (TRUS) can be used to measure prostate size and guide biopsies
- The presence of obstruction can only be determined accurately by performing pressure-flow studies (urodynamics or cystometrogram) and interpreting the results with the aid of pressure-flow nomograms such as the Abrams-Griffiths. Most men are managed without pressure-flow studies.

Treatment
Symptomatic BPH can be treated by surgery, other interventional methods or medically. Mild symptoms may not warrant treatment.

Surgical treatment (prostatectomy)

- Absolute indications are obstructive renal failure and recurrent acute retention of urine
- Relative indications are intractable symptoms, recurrent urinary infection, bladder stones and recurrent haematuria secondary to BPH
- Relative contraindications to surgery are poor anaesthetic risk, bleeding disorders, Parkinson's disease, dementia and sphincter weakness. Most men develop retrograde ejaculation after prostatectomy, which will reduce fertility, and this may also constitute a contraindication
- Open prostatectomy is usually reserved for glands over 100 g (< 5%). The prostate may be approached retropubically or transvesically
- TURP is usually performed on glands weighing less than 100 g
- Bladder neck incision is performed on small glands without a prominent median lobe
- Complications of TURP are haemorrhage (2–10%), incontinence (< 1%), sexual dysfunction (retrograde ejaculation in 60% and impotence in 5%) and urethral stricture. Transurethral syndrome comprises hypervolaemia, dilutional hyponatraemia and the neurological effects of intoxication with glycine (a neurotransmitter) which is used to irrigate the bladder during surgery
- The mortality rate from TURP is less than 1%
- TURP may be associated with late cardiovascular side-effects.

Interventional treatments
These are all recent developments and are still being assessed and perfected. It is not anticipated that all will become standard treatments.

- Transurethral microwave thermotherapy (TUMT)
- Vaporisation of the prostate using a Vaportrode™ powered by conventional diathermy generators
- Transurethral laser incision of the prostate (TULIP)

- Visual laser ablation of the prostate (VLAP)
- Interstitial laser coagulation of the prostate
- Transurethral needle ablation (TUNA) using radio-frequency energy
- Transrectal high intensity focused ultrasound (HIFU)
- Prostatic stents.

Medical treatments

- Selective α-blockers probably work by reducing tone mediated by sympathetic nerves in the bladder neck and prostate. However, there is some evidence that they may affect α-receptors in the CNS. They produce significant improvement in symptoms. Examples are indoramin, terazosin, alfuzosin and tamsulosin
- 5α-reductase inhibitors (e.g. finasteride) prevent the conversion of testosterone to DHT in the prostate. They are generally held to be less efficacious than α-blockers, but may help control prostatic bleeding.

PROSTATE SPECIFIC ANTIGEN (PSA)

- PSA is a glycoprotein with a molecular weight of 33 000
- It is a serine protease with the physiological role of lysing the ejaculate clot
- It is secreted predominantly by prostatic epithelial cells, both benign and malignant
- Insignificant amounts of PSA can be detected in other paraurethral glandular tissues in both men and women
- It can be measured in the serum by immunoassays. The most common method (Hybritech) has an upper limit of normal of 4 ng/ml
- It can be used as a tumour marker in prostate cancer and is especially useful when measured serially to assess treatment or disease progression
- Causes of a raised PSA are prostate cancer, BPH, prostatitis, UTI and instrumentation of the prostatic urethra or prostate.

PROSTATE CANCER

Prostate cancer is the most commonly diagnosed malignancy in men and is second only to lung cancer as a cause of male cancer death. The lifetime risk of microscopic prostate cancer is approximately 30%. Many of these tumours, however, never manifest clinically so that the lifetime risk of developing overt disease is 10% and of death from prostate cancer 3%. The incidence is increasing.

Epidemiology

- Prostate cancer is more common with increasing age and is rare before 50 years

- The disease is most common in the USA and Northern Europe and least common in the Far East
- In North America, Black men have a higher incidence than other racial groups
- The risk is increased in men with first-degree relatives who developed prostate cancer at a young age
- The disease is rare in men castrated before puberty, although the role of androgens in prostate carcinogenesis is incompletely understood
- There is a correlation between prostate cancer and red meat and fat consumption. Carrots and cereals may be protective.

Clinical presentation
In the UK, 60% of men have locally advanced disease and 50% metastases at presentation. There is currently insufficient evidence to support the introduction of population screening for prostate cancer using serum PSA levels.

Local disease

- Lower urinary tract symptoms
- Haematuria
- Suprapubic and perineal pain
- Erectile dysfunction
- Ureteric obstruction sometimes causing renal failure
- Haemospermia
- Rectal symptoms.

Metastases

1. Bone
   - Pain
   - Pathological fracture
   - Spinal cord compression
   - Anaemia due to marrow replacement
2. Lymph node
   - Lymphadenopathy
   - Lymphoedema
   - Ureteric obstruction
3. Other
   - Cachexia
   - Lethargy
   - Incidental finding in 10% of men undergoing TURP with presumed BPH.

Diagnosis

- DRE (digital rectal examination)
- Serum PSA: 33% of men with PSA > 4 ng/ml and 60% of men with PSA > 10 ng/ml have prostate cancer

- Prostate biopsy. This may be guided by transrectal ultrasound (TRUS).

Staging

- The local extent of the tumour may be assessed by DRE and TRUS
- Nodal status is assessed by CT scanning of the pelvis prior to radical treatment
- The presence of bony metastases is established by isotope bone scanning
- If the serum PSA is less than 20 ng/ml, nodal disease and distant metastases are rare. Imaging is therefore sometimes omitted.

Prostate cancer is staged according to the TNM classification.

T1 Tumour impalpable on rectal examination but present in tissue resected for presumed benign disease (T1a, T1b) or identified by needle biopsy (T1c)
T2 Tumour confined to prostate
T3 Extracapsular extension (including seminal vesicle involvement)
T4 Tumour is fixed or invades adjacent structures other than seminal vesicles
N1 Solitary pelvic lymph node < 2 cm in diameter
N2 Solitary pelvic lymph node > 2 cm in diameter or multiple nodes < 5 cm in diameter
N3 Pelvic lymph nodes > 5 cm in diameter
M0 No distant metastases
M+ Distant metastases.

Management

Localised disease (T1, T2)

- Radical prostatectomy
- Radiotherapy
- Watchful waiting.

There is at present a lack of adequate long-term follow-up data from randomised controlled trials comparing these options.

Locally advanced disease (T3, T4)

- Radiotherapy
- Androgen deprivation therapy (orchidectomy, LHRH agonists, e.g. goserelin, anti-androgen drugs, e.g. flutamide or maximal androgen blockade using a combination of LHRH agonists/orchidectomy and an anti-androgen). Intermittent deprivation may be useful in some men.
- TURP may be required for symptomatic BOO.

Table 8.4 10-year prostate-cancer-specific survival rates

	Radical prostatectomy (%)	Radiotherapy (%)	Watchful waiting (%)
Well-differentiated	94	90	93
Moderately differentiated	87	76	77
Poorly differentiated	67	53	45

Metastases

- Androgen deprivation therapy
- Radiotherapy for bony pain
- Palliative care.

Prognosis

Localised disease
The data in Table 8.4 are derived from a large population-based study analysed on an intention-to-treat basis and not from a randomised comparison of treatments. The data must therefore be interpreted with caution.

Metastatic disease
Five-year survival is 30%.

DISORDERS OF THE SCROTUM AND TESTIS

SCROTAL SWELLINGS

Scrotal swellings can be differentiated by following the algorithm in Figure 8.2.

Germ cell tumours of the testis

Testicular tumours are the most common malignancy in men aged 25–35 years. Cryptorchidism increases the risk by 8 times. Prompt diagnosis is important, as late presentation is associated with a worse prognosis.

Pathology

- Seminoma (42%)
- Non-seminomatous germ cell tumours (NSGCT) (58%)
- Mixed tumours (treated as NSGCT).

Clinical features

- Testicular swelling
- Testicular pain
- Back pain caused by retroperitoneal lymph node metastases

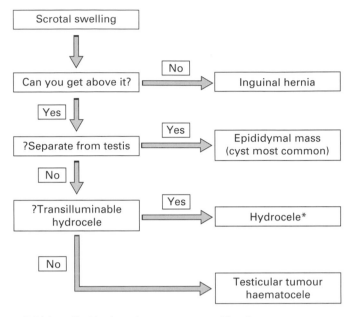

*Thick-walled hydroceles may not transilluminate.

Fig. 8.2 Differentiation of scrotal swellings.

- Gynaecomastia caused by tumour secretion of human chorionic gonadotrophin (rare)
- The diagnosis may be confirmed by ultrasonography.

Investigation

- Ultrasound
- Inguinal orchidectomy with pathological assessment of the testis
- CXR
- CT scan of the thorax, abdomen and pelvis
- Serum tumour markers (α-fetoprotein (AFP), β-human chorionic gonadotrophin (βhCG) and lactate dehydrogenase) before and after orchidectomy. βhCG or AFP or both are elevated in 70–80% of NSGCT at presentation. βhCG is elevated in 5–10% of seminomas.

Staging
The Royal Marsden Hospital Classification.

I   No evidence of metastases on CT scanning
IM Isolated elevation of markers post-orchidectomy
II   Infradiaphragmatic nodal involvement
III Supradiaphragmatic nodal involvement
IV Extralymphatic metastases (lungs, liver, bone, brain).

Treatment

Stage I Seminoma

- Inguinal orchidectomy and surveillance
- In some centres, prophylactic 'dog-leg' irradiation of the ipsilateral paraaortic and iliac lymph nodes is given.

Stage I NSGCT

- Inguinal orchidectomy and surveillance
- On surveillance, 70% of patients remain free from disease. Those who relapse receive chemotherapy.

Stage IM, II–IV

- Cisplatinum-based chemotherapy
- Surgical excision of residual masses
- Orchidectomy is not essential for diagnosis in patients with very high tumour marker levels and large volume metastases as it may delay chemotherapy.

Treatment should be undertaken in specialist cancer centres where overall cure rates are now in excess of 90%. Excellent survival rates have highlighted the importance of minimising the long-term side-effects of therapy which include renal impairment, pulmonary fibrosis, ototoxicity, peripheral neuropathy and infertility. Patients should be offered cryopreservation of sperm prior to treatment.

Hydrocele
A hydrocele is a collection of serous fluid within the tunica vaginalis. Most are idiopathic (primary). Trauma, inflammation or tumours of the testis may cause secondary hydroceles. Clinical diagnosis may be confirmed by ultrasonography. Symptomatic primary hydroceles may be treated by plication (Lord's operation), eversion (Jaboulay's procedure) or excision of the hydrocele sac. In secondary hydroceles, treatment is directed at the underlying cause.

Varicocele
A varicocele is a collection of dilated and tortuous pampiniform plexus veins and is present in 8% of young men. Left-sided varicoceles are more common, possibly because the left gonadal vein drains into the relatively high-pressure renal vein, whereas the right testicular vein drains directly into the IVC. There is an association between varicoceles and infertility. The diagnosis is essentially clinical but can be confirmed by ultrasonography. The indications for treatment are pain and infertility. Therapeutic options include embolisation under local anaesthesia or surgical ligation. Sudden onset of a left varicocele may indicate pathology in the left kidney.

TESTICULAR PAIN

Acute testicular pain is a common urological emergency usually caused by one of three conditions – torsion of the testis, torsion of the hydatid of Morgagni and infection.

Torsion of the testis

The testis twists on the spermatic cord leading to vascular occlusion. Infarction can ensue within several hours unless treated.

Presentation

* Most common in children and adolescents but may occur at any age
* Sudden severe testicular pain
* Diffuse central abdominal pain
* Vomiting
* Tender testis
* Scrotal erythema and oedema.

Management

* The diagnosis is clinical
* If torsion is diagnosed or suspected, urgent scrotal exploration is required
* If an untwisted testis is viable, fixation to the scrotal wall will prevent further torsion
* If a testis is not viable, an orchidectomy is performed
* The contralateral testis should also be fixed to the scrotal wall.

Torsion of the hydatid of Morgagni

This condition produces symptoms similar to testicular torsion. Distinction between the two is usually made at exploration at which the hydatid should be excised.

Infections of the testis and epididymis

Epididymitis

1. Acute epididymitis
   * Secondary to urinary tract infection. Infection spreads retrogradely from the urinary tract. Coliforms are the most common causative organisms. There may be associated bladder outlet obstruction
   * Sexually acquired. *Chlamydia trachomatis* is the usual cause. Gonococcal epididymitis may also occur
2. *Chronic epididymitis*
   * Bacterial
   * Tuberculosis.

Presentation

- Pain and swelling in the affected epididymis ± testis
- Signs of inflammation of the scrotal skin
- Fever
- Lower urinary tract symptoms.

Diagnosis

- Clinical
- May be confirmed by ultrasonography
- MSU may yield the causative organism
- Urethral swabs may detect *Chlamydial* or *Gonococcal* infection
- Three early morning urine specimens (EMUs) should be obtained if tuberculosis is suspected.

Treatment
Antibiotics active against likely pathogens should be administered. Ciprofloxacin is active against both coliforms and *Chlamydia*. Treatment should continue for 4–6 weeks.

Orchitis
Mumps and Coxsackie viruses may cause orchitis.

PENILE DISORDERS
SQUAMOUS CARCINOMA

- Rare in the West. Common in Africa and South America
- Peak incidence in the sixth decade
- Rare in those circumcised within a few days of birth. Later circumcision is not protective
- May be related to poor hygiene
- May be caused by sexually transmitted viruses
- Precancerous lesions include carcinoma in situ, erythroplasia of Queyrat, Bowen's disease
- Penile cancer usually presents within the preputial sac or on the glans in circumcised men
- Early superficial disease spreads to involve the corpora, urethra, prostate and surrounding structures
- Lymphadenopathy is common secondary to tumour or infection or both
- Distant metastases are rare
- Early distal disease may be treated by irradiation or partial amputation
- Advanced disease necessitates total penile amputation or radiotherapy. Chemotherapy should be considered
- Inguinal and iliac lymph node dissections are often required
- 5-year survivals: node negative – up to 90%, inguinal node involvement – 50%, iliac node involvement – 10%, distant metastases – 0%.

PEYRONIE'S DISEASE

- Presents as a painful erection with curvature of the erect penis (usually dorsally) and poor erection distal to the curve
- A tender fibrous plaque is often palpated on the dorsum of the penis
- It is associated with Dupuytren's contracture of the hand
- Spontaneous remission may occur
- Surgical correction (Nesbit's operation) leads to penile shortening and must not be attempted until progression of the deformity is complete. There are some reports that systemic vitamin E may be useful.

PRIAPISM

- The rare condition of painful prolonged erection
- Priapism is usually iatrogenic secondary to intracorporeal injections of papaverine or prostaglandin used to treat impotence. Patients receiving these injections are warned to seek urgent medical advice if their erection lasts longer than 4 hours
- Also associated with leukaemia, sickle cell disease, pelvic trauma and pelvic tumours
- Acutely, blood can be aspirated from the corpora which can also be irrigated with heparinised saline. Metaraminol or phenylephrine can be administered
- For priapism resistant to simple treatment, formation of a shunt between the glans and the corpora, or a saphenocorporeal shunt may be required.

HYPOSPADIAS

- Opening of the urethral meatus onto the ventral aspect of the penis
- Prevalence – 1 in 300 male births
- Associated with a hooded prepuce, chordee and feminisation syndromes
- Most require surgical correction. Surgery should be undertaken before the age of 2 years.

PHIMOSIS

- Contracted preputial opening preventing retraction of the prepuce over the glans
- Associated with balanitis, balanitis xerotica obliterans (BXO), diabetes mellitus, poor hygiene and penile cancer
- Treated by circumcision
- It is important to differentiate phimosis from congenital preputial adhesions and the long narrow prepuce of young boys, which usually resolve without treatment.

Table 8.5 Presentation of MED

Organic	Psychogenic
Slow onset	Sudden onset
Loss of early morning and nocturnal erections	Normal early morning and nocturnal erections
Normal libido	Reduced libido
Normal sexual development	Problems during sexual development
	Related to specific events

PARAPHIMOSIS

- A retracted prepuce that cannot be replaced over the glans
- Associated with phimosis and penile oedema
- Treatment involves preputial reduction by compression to reduce oedema followed by replacement of the prepuce ensuring that the constriction ring has been mobilised distally off the glans. Dorsal slit operations are rarely required. Interval circumcision may be necessary.

MALE ERECTILE DYSFUNCTION (MED)

- MED affects 5% of men in their forties and becomes more common with ageing
- The aetiology may be psychogenic, vasculogenic, neurological, endocrine, traumatic or drug-related (anti-hypertensives, antidepressants, etc.). Prostate cancer may present with MED
- The presentation is summarised in Table 8.5
- The presence of hypogonadism, groin pulses and prostate cancer should be noted on physical examination
- Investigation requires urine dipstick and serum glucose estimation. Hormonal profile and imaging of penile blood flow may be indicated
- Treatments for organic MED include intracavernosal therapy, vacuum devices, androgen replacement and surgery
- Treatments for psychogenic MED include psychosexual counselling, intracavernosal therapy and vacuum devices
- Sildenafil (Viagra) is a new oral therapy for MED.

FURTHER READING

Guidelines on management of men with lower urinary tract symptoms suggesting bladder outflow obstruction 1997 London: British Association of Urological Surgeons and the Royal College of Surgeons of England

Guidelines for the investigation and treatment of urological cancers in the United Kingdom 1996 London: British Association of Urological Surgeons

Chamberlain J, Melia J, Moss S, Brown J 1997 Report prepared for the Health Technology Assessment Panel of the NHS Executive on the diagnosis, management, treatment and costs of prostate cancer in England and Wales. *British Journal of Urology* 79(Suppl 3)

Tanagho E A and McAninch J W 1995 Smith's general urology, 14th edn. Lange: Connecticut

9. Organ transplantation

Chris Darby

Organ failure is a common occurrence and in some situations replacement of that organ can save life (heart, liver, lung) and in others preserve quality of life and prevent complications (renal, pancreas). However, any attempt to transfer tissue between individuals will fail without an understanding of the biological principles underpinning transplant surgery.

MAJOR HISTOCOMPATIBILITY ANTIGENS

All individuals inherit a unique tissue identity. In utero the body learns to identify self from a multitude of non-self antigens. In practice it is only necessary to consider matching donor and recipient for blood group and the major histocompatibility antigens (MHC) (see Table 9.1). Any individual expresses two copies of the antigens HLA A, B and DR. Therefore, any two individuals can be six antigen matched through to six antigen mismatched. Results of surgery will be influenced by the above, although for the different organs the importance and practicality of matching donor and recipient varies.

REJECTION

When a disparate graft is implanted the body will try to 'reject' it. This process has a recognition phase and an effector phase. Donor graft material is presented by recipient antigen processing cells as small fragments of protein (peptides) to recipient T-cells. These T-helper cells are activated and start a cascade of effector mechanisms to destroy the foreign material. For example, chemicals secreted by the T-helper cells (cytokines) recruit cytotoxic T-cells, induce B-cells to make antibodies and activate macrophages.

Table 9.1 Essential requirements for the donor organ

	Kidney	Liver	Heart–lung	Pancreas
Blood group matching required	+	+	+	+
HLA matching required	+	−+	−	−+
Maximum cold ischaemia time	48	20	6	12

HLA, human leucocyte antigen.

IMMUNOSUPPRESSIVE DRUGS

Immunosuppressive therapy is required to prevent rejection. A growing armamentarium of drugs is available. However, suppressing the immune system will be a balance between preventing rejection and the risk of potentially fatal sepsis and cancer formation. Additionally, all drugs have specific side-effects. Therefore, it is normal to use a lower dose of at least three drugs rather than a high dose of a single one.

- *Cyclosporine and Tacrolimus* are fungal derivatives that suppress T-cell production of cytokines. The principal specific complication of both is nephrotoxicity
- *Azathioprine* is an antiproliferative drug which interferes with the assembly of messenger RNA and DNA. Principal complications are bone marrow suppression and hepatotoxicity
- *Steroids* are anti-inflammatory drugs with a specific suppressive effect on T-cell and antigen-presenting cell function principally through a reduction in the production of interleukin I. Principal complications are growth retardation in children, bone disease, myopathy, cataracts, diabetes and peptic ulceration
- *Antibodies* are powerful intravenous preparations with specificity for the immunoreactive components of rejection. These can be polyclonal, raised against a wide range of human cell targets (e.g. anti-thymocyte globulin, ATG), or monoclonal against a specific target such as the T-cell receptor (e.g. OKT3). Principal complications are acute toxicity due to target cell lysis and marked immunosuppression with the risk of infections and late malignancy.

All drugs given to achieve immunosuppression will lead to a raised incidence of tumours, particularly in the skin and reticuloendothelial system (e.g. relative risk ratio to age-matched controls is 7.4 for non-Hodgkin's lymphoma). The incidence of non-lymphoid solid organ tumours is not raised markedly.

Infections with cytomegalovirus, Herpes virus, pneumocystis and Candida are increased.

General contraindications

Immunosuppression will reduce the ability to provide surveillance and eradication of malignant cells within the body. It is clear that metastatic disease can stay latent after previous apparently curative surgery. Therefore, it is common practice to decline transplantation in patients with a history of cancer within the last 5 years. Similarly, for patients with chronic viral infection, the risk of acceleration of disease should be considered carefully. Patients who are unlikely to withstand the operative and immunological insult inflicted by the intended procedure should not be offered transplantation.

DONATION

Organs are made available to recipients through cadaveric and living related sources.

CADAVERIC ORGANS

Patients who have died following intracranial haemorrhage or head injury, but are being ventilated on intensive care units, are the main source of donor organs. These patients have to undergo a rigorous, rigidly defined set of brain stem death tests carried out by two independent clinicians. Once the brain stem is dead there is no possibility of cortical function or respiration and the patient has died, although the heart will continue to beat for some days if ventilation is maintained. No patient satisfying brain stem death testing, where ventilation has been continued, has ever been reported to have regained cortical or brain stem function. At this time, consent for organ transplantation should be sought from the next of kin. After consent, tissue typing to ascertain the MHC status and blood group will be carried out. The deceased organ donor will be taken to theatre and the organs removed by a dedicated retrieval team.

LIVING RELATED AND UNRELATED ORGANS

Due to the chronic shortage of cadaveric organs, living organ donation is an attractive option. Furthermore, the quality and long-term function of living grafts is significantly better. Renal donation, through a loin incision, is well established and safe. More recently, partial hepatectomy and transplantation into paediatric recipients is practised. Living unrelated transplantation, usually from a spouse, is becoming increasingly common.

XENOGRAFTING

A theoretically attractive unlimited source of donor organs. Not practised currently. Has major ethical and immunological hurdles to cross.

ORGANISATION

A computer database of the blood group, MHC type and organ required, of all those awaiting transplantation, is kept centrally. When an organ is retrieved the donor is compared, with regard to the above, with the database and allocated appropriately. To maintain the integrity of the organ during this process and possible long distance transportation, the organ is flushed through with preservation fluid and packed on ice. Some organs can tolerate this period of preservation better than others (Table 9.1). Current practice dictates that there is insufficient time and choice of donor organ to allow for MHC matching of cadaveric liver and heart grafts other than for blood group.

SPECIFIC ORGAN TRANSPLANTS

RENAL TRANSPLANTATION

- Number currently waiting in the UK, 5370
- Number performed annually, circa 1800
- Quality of life is reduced on dialysis and renal replacement therapy costs between £12 000 and £18 000 per year
- Renal transplantation can be expected to restore health, ability to work and achieve renal replacement therapy at approximately £4000 per year.

Indications: renal
The more common indications are renal failure following:

- Glomerulonephritis
- Diabetes
- Pyelonephritis
- Atherosclerotic renal artery disease
- Polycystic kidneys
- Congenital obstructive uropathies.

Physical requirements

- Recipient age 2–70 years
- Recipient iliac vessels adequate for vascular anastomosis
- Bladder suitable for anastomosis. This may require bladder augmentation or construction of an ileal conduit
- A urinary tract free of sepsis.

Preparation

- Blood group match, MHC matching ideal is zero or one mismatch, acceptable down to three mismatch (out of six MHC loci)
- Correct renal function with preoperative dialysis if required
- Cross-match 2 units blood.

Donor

- Age 2–70 years
- No malignancy, sepsis or renal impairment
- Kidneys only:
  — Mobilise right and left large bowel mesentery
  — Mobilise small bowel mesentery to expose entire anterior aspect of aorta and inferior vena cava (IVC) to the level of the superior mesenteric artery
  — Catheter to aorta via the common iliac artery and catheter to IVC for drainage
  — Clamp or balloon occlusion to supra-coeliac aorta
  — Kidneys cold perfused and removed.

Surgery

- Prepare donor kidney under sterile conditions, at 4°C in theatre. Involves assessment for damage, cleaning off excess fat and preparing renal vein and artery for rapid anastomosis
- Muscle-cutting incision in either iliac fossa, extraperitoneal space expanded to expose, control and clamp external iliac artery and vein
- Anastomose renal vein end-to-side to external iliac vein
- Anastomose renal artery end-to-side to external iliac artery or end-to-end to internal iliac artery and release clamps
- Anastomose ureter to bladder.

Postoperative

- As for major surgery with continuous invasive monitoring
- Administer immunosuppressive regimen, for example cyclosporine, azathioprine and steroids.

Surgical complications

- Bleeding
- Ureteric leakage or stenosis
- Renal vein thrombosis
- Lymphocele around kidney.

Early immunological complications

- Rejection, maximal 5–14 days
- Diagnose clinically by weight gain, fall in urine output, increased temperature or a tender kidney. Also by rise in creatinine and percutaneous renal transplant biopsy
- Treat with high-dose steroids or antibody therapy
- Consider a change in baseline drugs
- Infection, often fungal or viral, in particular Candida and cytomegalovirus.

Results

- See Table 9.2 (p. 200)
- Renal transplantation has become a cost-effective, safe mode of treatment for end-stage renal failure
- Quality of life is improved considerably.

PANCREAS

- Number waiting currently in the UK, 60
- Number performed annually, circa 30.

The majority of pancreas transplants are performed as a combined procedure with renal transplantation. These patients have suffered renal failure secondary to diabetic nephropathy. As the diabetes itself is not life-threatening in the short term, the risks of adding this procedure to renal transplantation have to be carefully weighed against the expected benefits. Benefits may be: prevention of recurrent disease in the graft and secondary diabetic complications such as retinopathy and neuropathy. Theoretically, it would be more attractive to transplant the pancreas pre-emptively to prevent secondary complications. Confirmation of the efficacy of this stategy is awaited from American practice.

Indications: combined pancreas and renal

- Renal failure with brittle diabetes or progressive secondary complications despite tight sugar control.

Indications: pancreas only

- Previous successful renal transplantation plus diabetic complications
- Preventative in early diabetic renal failure and proteinuria
- Brittle diabetics with recurrent hypoglycaemic coma or insulin resistance.

Physical requirements

- As for renal transplantation plus:
- Recipient any age, usually between 25–40
- Both iliac vessels will need to be acceptable for anastomosis
- No active sepsis or peripheral leg ischaemia
- No significant cardiac disease
- Mobile patient.

Preparation

- Full cardiac and psychological assessment
- Blood group matching and HLA cross-matching as for the kidney. However, the reduced number of suitable donors widens the range of HLA discrepancy acceptable.

Donor

- As for renal transplantation plus:
- Age < 40
- No sepsis
- No trauma
- Non-diabetic
- Retrieval is usually with liver and kidneys
- For whole pancreas grafts:
  - After perfusion and liver retrieval, preserve origin of superior mesenteric artery (SMA) and stump of splenic vein and artery
  - Mobilise pancreas towards pancreatic head

— Dissect free a length of SMA into the small bowel mesentery below the pancreas
— Mobilise the second part of the duodenum and cross-staple just above and below the level of the pancreas
— Ligate common bile duct stump.

Surgery

Technique varies as it is possible to transplant either a segmental graft consisting of pancreas from the neck to the tail or the whole pancreas. Furthermore, the whole pancreas graft can be implanted with enteric drainage or bladder drainage of the exocrine secretions. Transplantation of the whole pancreas with bladder drainage will be described.

• First, bench surgery has to be performed upon the donor organ. The length of SMA below the pancreas is brought anteriorly and superiorly around the pancreatic body and anastomosed end-to-end to the short cut end of the splenic artery. A 3 cm segment of donor iliac vein is anastomosed end-to-end to the short cut end of the splenic vein to elongate it
• Make an intraperitoneal approach to iliac vessels through a right iliac fossa muscle cutting incision
• Position the pancreas with the duodenum inferiorly in the pelvis
• Anastomose the splenic vein to external iliac vein
• Anastomose the origin of the SMA to the external iliac artery
• Make an incision in the anti-mesenteric border of the duodenum and anastomose to the dome of the bladder.

Postoperative

• Correct fluid balance, temperature and preserve cardiac and renal function
• Correct bicarbonate loss
• Administer immunosuppressive regimen; for example: cyclosporine, azathioprine and antibody to avoid early steroid usage which may hinder sugar control.

Surgical complications

• Bleeding
• Splenic vein thrombosis
• Pancreatitis
• Peri-pancreatic collection or fistula
• Duodenum to bladder dehiscence.

Early immunological complications

• Rejection, maximal 4–14 days
• Diagnose clinically by increased abdominal pain and graft tenderness. Also by deterioration of measured urinary amylase,

which is an advantage of draining exocrine secretion to the bladder rather than enterically
- Blood sugar rise is a late sign
- Transplant biopsy can be performed percutaneously but is hazardous
- The renal transplant usually acts as an early marker of rejection and this is one of the major advantages of combined transplantation over pancreas alone
- Treat with high-dose steroids or antibody therapy
- Consider a change in baseline drugs
- Infection, often fungal or viral, in particular Candida, cytomegalovirus and pneumocystis.

Results
Results of pancreas transplantation are improving. It is still not clear if the procedure will be beneficial in the long term. Until this issue is resolved the usage of this procedure is likely to remain limited. (See Table 9.2, p. 200.)

LIVER TRANSPLANTATION
- Number waiting currently in the UK, 189
- Number performed annually, circa 640
- Many patients with acute or acute on chronic liver failure will die whilst waiting for a suitable donor.

Indications

- Some of the more common indications are:
  — chronic liver disease associated with hepatitis B and C
  — alcohol
  — drugs
  — autoimmune disease
- Cholestatic liver diseases such as drug-induced, primary biliary cirrhosis, sclerosing cholangitis and biliary atresia
- In-born errors of metabolism
- Some primary hepatic malignancies
- Hepatic venous occlusions such as the Budd–Chiari syndrome
- Acute liver failure, often viral or drug-induced.

Physical requirements

- Recipient any age
- Fit enough to tolerate major surgery
- Technical feasibility including need for native hepatectomy
- Patent recipient portal vein or superior mesenteric vein
- No irreversible brain injury
- No extra-hepatic malignancy

- Paediatric recipients can be transplanted with segmental grafts from what would have been oversized adult donors. This has helped with the shortage of paediatric donors
- Left segmental living related donation is now possible.

Preparation

- Blood group matching only
- Matching for organ size with recipient abdomen
- 20 units whole blood, fresh-frozen plasma and platelets.

Donor

- Age 2–65
- No malignancy, sepsis or liver impairment
- HIV and hepatitis virus-negative
- Retrieval is usually with kidneys:- laparotomy to identify hilar structures, cannula to portal vein, aorta and IVC. Cross-clamp supra-coeliac aorta, cold perfuse aorta and portal vein, vent venous blood from IVC. Complete dissection and remove liver preserving supra-diaphragmatic IVC and renal artery origins for cardiac and renal surgeons respectively.

Surgery

- Technique varies
- Recipient hepatectomy is often very difficult
- Portal vein and IVC blood shunted by veno–venous bypass to axillary vein during anhepatic phase
- Divide recipient common bile duct, hepatic artery and portal vein in hilum
- Clamp and divide supra-hepatic IVC and infra-hepatic IVC. Remove liver
- Place donor liver and anastomose supra-hepatic IVC, infra-hepatic IVC and portal vein. Remove clamps and shunt
- Reconstruct hepatic artery
- Join duct to duct to restore biliary continuity.

Postoperative

- Correct fluid balance, temperature, blood sugar and clotting. Preserve renal function
- Administer immunosuppressive regimen, for example:
  1. Tacrolimus plus steroids
  2. Steroids, azathioprine and antibody with subsequent tacrolimus, in those with renal impairment.

Surgical complications

- Bleeding
- Portal vein, hepatic vein or IVC thrombosis

- Hepatic artery thrombosis
- Biliary leakage or stenosis may be expected in up to 10% of cases.

Early immunological complications

- Rejection, maximal 4–14 days
- Diagnose clinically, increasing jaundice, fall in biliary output, temperature or tender liver. Also by rise in liver function tests, rise in prothrombin time and by percutaneous liver transplant biopsy
- Treat with high-dose steroids or antibody therapy
- Consider change in baseline drugs
- Infection, often fungal or viral, in particular Candida and cytomegalovirus.

Results

- See Table 9.2
- Liver transplantation is an effective treatment for end-stage liver disease and acute irreversible liver failure
- Transplantation for malignant disease has good early results but is severely limited by the high incidence of metastatic disease
- Results are improved by the liver's ability to regenerate. However, obliterative biliary disease can occur as a consequence of chronic rejection.

HEART

- Number waiting currently in the UK, 303
- Number performed annually, circa 300
- 30% die on waiting list.

Indications

- Cardiomyopathies that can be ischaemic, valvular, congenital, viral or idiopathic.

Physical requirements

- Recipient any age, usually below 65
- No irreversible renal, hepatic or lung disease, though combined transplant procedures can be performed.

Table 9.2   Approximate patient and graft survival at 1-year post-transplant

	Kidney	Liver	Pancreas	Heart	Lung
Patient survival at 1 year (%)	95	80	90	85	70
Graft survival at 1 year (%)	88	80	75	85	70

Preparation

- Blood group matching only
- Matching for organ size by weight match, plus 20% usually accepted.

Donor

- Age < 50
- No sepsis
- No history of ischaemic heart disease or cardiac trauma
- No usage of high-dose inotropic support
- Retrieval is usually with liver and kidneys: median sternotomy, pericardium opened and heart inspected closely
- Aorta cross-clamped and cold cardioplegia run into aortic root
- IVC cross-stapled and divided at diaphragm
- Pulmonary veins divided
- SVC cross-stapled and divided
- Pulmonary artery transected
- Aorta transected and heart removed
- Retrieve liver, then kidneys.

Surgery

- Technique varies. Prepare donor heart by fashioning right and left atrial cuffs. Trim aorta and pulmonary artery above valves
- Median sternotomy and establish bypass at 30°C
- Excise recipient heart by cutting through atrioventricular groove to establish right and left atrial cuffs. Divide aorta and pulmonary artery. Remove heart
- Anastomose left atrium then right atrium
- Anastomose pulmonary artery then aorta. Come off bypass.

Postoperative

- Correct fluid balance, temperature and preserve renal function
- Monitor and correct cardiac function with inotropes and anti-arrhythmic agents as required
- Administer immunosuppressive regimen, for example:
  1. Cyclosporine, azathioprine and steroids
  2. Steroids, azathioprine and antibody with subsequent cyclosporine, in those with renal impairment.

Surgical complications

- Bleeding
- Arrhythmia
- Coronary thrombosis.

Early immunological complications

- Rejection, maximal 4–14 days
- Diagnose clinically, failing cardiac function, temperature, arrhythmia or tachycardia. Also by deterioration of measured cardiac parameters and by transjugular endomyocardial transplant biopsy
- Treat with high-dose steroids or antibody therapy
- Consider change in baseline drugs
- Infection, often fungal or viral, in particular Candida and cytomegalovirus.

Results

- See Table 9.2
- Results are steadily improving and consequentially potential candidates far outnumber donors
- Chronic rejection often presents as obliterative coronary artery disease and is a major limiting feature.

LUNG (OR HEART–LUNG 30%)

- Number waiting currently, 353
- Number performed annually, circa 169.

Indications: combined heart–lung

- Cardiomyopathies that can be ischaemic, valvular, congenital, viral or idiopathic where there is irreversible cardiac and pulmonary disease.

Indications: lung only

- Pulmonary fibrosis and emphysema
- Pulmonary vascular disease (or combined with heart)
- Septic lung disease, e.g. cystic fibrosis (usually both lungs are transplanted).

Physical requirements

- Recipient any age, usually below 60
- No irreversible renal or hepatic impairment
- No active collagen vascular disease, which may recur in the graft
- Recoverable right ventricular cardiac function for lung transplantation
- Non-smoker
- No active lung infection.

Preparation

- Blood group matching only
- Matching for patient size to ensure the lung matches the estimated non-diseased chest capacity.

Donor

- Age < 50
- No sepsis or trauma
- Excellent lung function
- Normal chest radiograph
- No history of lung trauma
- Retrieval is usually with heart, liver and kidneys: median sternotomy, pericardium open and heart and lungs closely inspected. Heart and two separate lungs are to be retrieved
- Pulmonary artery and aortic root cannulated
- Aorta cross-clamped and cold cardioplegia run into aortic root
- SVC and IVC ligated and divided
- Atria are divided, providing a cuff both sides
- Pulmonary artery transected just above bifurcation
- Aorta transected and heart removed
- Lungs dissected free and trachea divided
- Retrieve liver, then kidneys.

Surgery

- Technique varies
- Posterolateral thoracotomy for single lung transplant
- For pulmonary vascular disease, sternotomy and bypass
- Excise recipient lung by dividing pulmonary artery, bronchus and pulmonary veins
- Bronchial anastomosis fashioned
- Side-biting clamp to left atrium, fashion atrial cuff and anastomose to donor left atrial cuff
- Pulmonary artery anastomosis performed
- Bilateral sequential lung transplants can be performed as above.

Postoperative

- Correct fluid balance, temperature and preserve cardiac and renal function
- Prevent lung contamination
- Administer immunosuppressive regimen, for example: cyclosporine, azathioprine and antibody to avoid early steroid usage which may hinder bronchial anastomotic healing.

Surgical complications

- Bleeding
- Bronchial dehiscence
- Pneumonitis
- Mediastinitis.

Early immunological complications

- Rejection, maximal 4–14 days
- Diagnose clinically, failing pulmonary function, temperature. Also by deterioration of measured oxygenation parameters, chest radiograph and by transbronchial transplant biopsy
- Problems may be caused by patchy rejection that may be missed on biopsy
- Treat with high-dose steroids or antibody therapy
- Consider change in baseline drugs
- Infection, often fungal or viral, in particular Candida, cytomegalovirus and pneumocystis.

Results

- See Table 9.2
- Results have improved with earlier assessment and transplantation.
- As with other organs recurrent disease and chronic rejection are continuing problems.

SMALL INTESTINE

- Number waiting currently in the UK, ?
- Number performed annually, circa 5
- There are a small number of patients undergoing small intestinal transplants and therefore this procedure should be considered experimental at present.

Indications

- Short gut syndrome following intestinal atresia, infarction by embolus or volvulus and multiple resections for Crohn's disease.

Physical requirements

- Established gut failure without recovery after total parenteral nutrition (TPN)
- Recipient any age, usually below 50
- No irreversible liver failure as many long-term TPN patients will develop liver impairment. If severe, combined liver and small bowel transplantation can be considered
- Loss of access or recurrent sepsis with home TPN.

Preparation

- Full liver and psychological assessment
- Blood group matching and HLA cross-matching as for the kidney. However, limitations of suitable donors widens the range of HLA discrepancy acceptable.

Donor

- Age < 40
- No sepsis
- Retrieval is usually with liver and kidneys
- The small intestine is retrieved including the ileocaecal valve
- The superior mesenteric artery and vein are preserved.

Surgery

- Technique varies
- A laparotomy is performed. The superior mesenteric artery is anastomosed to the side of donor aorta. The superior mesenteric vein is anastomosed to the superior or inferior mesenteric vein
- Both ends of the intestine are exteriorised as stomas.

Postoperative

- Correct fluid balance, temperature and preserve cardiac and renal function
- Correct bicarbonate loss
- Administer immunosuppressive regimen, for example: cyclosporine, azathioprine and antibody to avoid early steroid usage
- Irrigate stomas to wash through bowel.

Surgical complications

- Bleeding
- Mesenteric vein thrombosis
- Liver decompensation
- Intra-abdominal sepsis
- Stoma dehiscence.

Early immunological complications

- Rejection, maximal 4–14 days
- Diagnose clinically abdominal pain and stoma deterioration
- Trans-stomal biopsies can be performed by endoscopy
- Treat with high-dose steroids or antibody therapy
- Consider change in baseline drugs
- Graft-versus-host disease can occur due to the large lymphoid load carried by the graft in a heavily immunosuppressed host
- Infection, often fungal or viral, in particular cytomegalovirus.

Results

- Results are poor. In particular, there is a high mortality in most reported series circa 20%
- In survivors, early graft survival approaches 50%
- Results in combined liver and small bowel transplants that survive are probably best of all.

FURTHER READING

Ginns LC, Cosimi AB, Morris PJ 1998 Transplantation, Blackwell Science, Oxford

10. Breast

Julie Dunn

REFERRAL AND ASSESSMENT

GUIDELINES FOR GP REFERRAL TO BREAST CLINIC (Table 10.1)

- All patients with a discrete mass
- All patients with nipple retraction, distortion, eczema or change in breast contour
- All patients over 50 years with nipple discharge
- Unilateral clear or bloodstained nipple discharge and persistent bilateral, multiduct discharge in premenopausal women
- Persistent breast pain
- Asymmetrical nodularity which persists following menses
- Patients with family history of breast cancer in first-degree relatives.

ASSESSMENT OF BREAST DISEASE

HISTORY

Duration of symptoms, detected accidentally or by regular self-examination. Details of breast cancer risk factors may be obtained from patient by questionnaire completed before consultation, i.e. age at menarche, menopause, details of pregnancies and breast feeding, previous breast biopsies, age of onset of affected relatives and details of other cancers, e.g. ovarian, bowel, childhood tumours in patient and relatives.

Table 10.1 Referral pattern of patients with breast disease

Breast lump	36%
Breast pain	18%
Pain and nodularity	33%
Nipple symptoms	8%
Family history	3%

Fewer than 10% of patients referred to a Breast Clinic will have breast cancer.

Triple assessment

Will diagnose 99.8% of breast cancers in women with a discrete mass, comprises:

1. Clinical examination
2. Mammogram and ultrasound (US) scan for women over 35 years or US for women under 35 years
3. Fine-needle aspiration cytology (FNAC) or core biopsy of all palpable abnormalities.

Clinical examination

* Careful inspection precedes palpation
* Skin dimpling is not pathognomonic of breast cancer and may be due to fat necrosis, trauma, previous treatment or involution
* Callipers should be used to record the size of a discrete mass
* Palpation of axillary nodes is routine but known to be inaccurate.

Breast radiology

* Mammography involves oblique and craniocaudal views which are obtained with a radiation dose of under 1.5 mGY. Architectural distortion, densities and microcalcifications are detected. Additional compression or magnification views are taken to examine abnormalities in more detail. When the diagnosis of breast cancer is clinically obvious, mammography is still required to detect multifocal or contralateral disease
* Mammography is less useful in women under 35 years because the breasts are relatively dense; it is not routinely recommended
* US scan differentiates between solid lumps and cysts, is used in young women for assessment of breast lumps and nodularity and as an adjunct to mammography in older symptomatic women. It is used to provide serial measurements of tumours treated by tamoxifen or primary chemotherapy
* The role of magnetic resonance imaging (MRI) in breast assessment is now being explored. It avoids the risk associated with radiation but is too time-consuming for routine use at present. It may have a role in differentiation of recurrence from scarring in the breast following surgery and radiotherapy.

Fine-needle aspiration cytology

* A 21 or 23 gauge needle and syringe are used. Following aspiration of a cyst, the patient should be re-examined to exclude an underlying palpable mass and the cyst fluid discarded unless bloodstained. Bloodstained fluid is sent for cytology and FNAC taken from an underlying solid mass
* With a solid breast lump, several passes are made while applying suction, the material is smeared onto slides and air-dried or fixed

before staining and microscopic examination. A result may be obtained within minutes enabling clinicians to offer a rapid diagnosis service. If an inadequate smear is obtained, i.e. fewer than 5 clumps of epithelial cells, a further sample or core biopsy may be taken before the patient leaves clinic

- Core biopsy, under local anaesthesia using a 14 gauge spring-loaded device, has gained popularity recently because it differentiates invasive from in situ carcinoma and detects lobular carcinoma, which frequently produces inadequate cytology. Many women find core biopsy more comfortable than FNAC
- Preoperative diagnosis should be obtained in the majority of patients
- Frozen section biopsy of a suspected breast cancer before definitive surgery should be kept to a minimum. Frozen section examination of axillary lymph nodes allows selection of patients with nodal disease for full axillary dissection.

MANAGEMENT OF BREAST LUMP

- Following triple assessment the patient may be reassured and discharged, given the diagnosis of breast cancer, or a benign abnormality may be detected
- C1 cytology should be considered inadequate and further samples taken unless this is consistent with the clinical and mammographic findings of fatty or normal breast tissue
- C2 cytology from a discrete lump in a woman under 35 years – patient offered further examination in 3–6 months or removal if clinically and radiologically benign. Remove lump in women over 35 years
- C3 cytology may occur in women on oral contraceptive pill or hormone replacement therapy. Repeat biopsy or remove lump
- C4 cytology in woman with clinical and mammographic suspicious abnormality, repeat FNAC or core biopsy to obtain diagnosis of breast cancer prior to treatment. If not suspicious, excise mass to obtain definitive histology
- C5 cytology requires definitive treatment of cancer.

BENIGN BREAST DISORDERS

CONGENITAL ABNORMALITIES

- Supernumerary nipples occur in up to 5% of men and women usually just below the normal breast along the milk line
- Ectopic breast tissue usually occurs in the axilla, may be unilateral or bilateral and present during pregnancy. Absence of the breast (amastia) or nipple (athelia) is rare but hypoplasia of the breast is more common and is treated by augmentation of the smaller side. Some degree of asymmetry is normal but many patients require reassurance.

ABERRATIONS OF NORMAL DEVELOPMENT AND INVOLUTION (ANDI)

Prepubertal hypertrophy

Fibroadenoma

- The common fibroadenoma is typically a smooth, mobile, firm mass in young women but can occur at all ages
- Diagnosed by triple assessment (clinical examination, FNAC, US scan)
- 13% of all palpable breast lumps
- 30% decrease in size or disappear
- Advise excision in women over 35 years or over 4 cm in size through small incision along Langer's lines
- Offer choice of excision or reassessment to women under 35 years. The risk of cancer within a fibroadenoma is 1 in 1000 and is usually lobular carcinoma in situ.

Breast cyst

- 15% of breast lumps
- Often sudden onset and painful, usually in perimenopausal women
- Two types are recognised – type I cysts (high K^+/Na^+ ratio in breast cyst fluid) and type II cysts (low K^+/Na^+ ratio). Risk of relapse more common in type I or multiple cysts at presentation
- Diagnosis by FNA – fluid usually pale yellow to dark green sent for cytology only if bloodstained. Patient re-examined following aspiration – any palpable underlying mass requires FNAC and mammography
- Slight increased risk of breast cancer (two- to four-fold) in patients with multiple cysts.

Nipple discharge

- Differentiate between unilateral/bilateral, single/multiple ducts, clear/coloured/bloodstained
- Bloodstained, single duct discharge may be benign duct papilloma
- Bilateral, multiduct, coloured (cream to dark green) usually due to duct ectasia
- Milky discharge – physiological, mechanical stimulation, hyperprolactinaemia
- Clear/serous or bloodstained discharge treat with suspicion – smear cytology, mammography. Microdochectomy for single duct or major duct excision for multiple duct discharge.

Duct ectasia

- Dilatation and shortening of subareolar ducts, perimenopausal women

- Present with nipple discharge, slit-like nipple retraction or mass
- Cytology of nipple discharge may show foamy macrophages
- Leakage of duct secretions into periductal tissue causes inflammation, periductal fibrosis and nipple retraction
- Bacterial infection may be involved, including anaerobes
- Surgery to disconnect ducts if discharge troublesome or to evert nipple.

Periductal mastitis

- May occur without dilated ducts
- More common in cigarette smokers
- May develop into abscess or mammary fistula which requires antibiotics. Excision of fistula and tissue behind nipple/areola complex and recurrence is common.

Epithelial hyperplasia

- Increase in the number of cells lining the terminal duct lobular unit – mild, moderate or severe
- Only if atypia present (atypical hyperplasia) is condition associated with 4.5 times increased risk of breast cancer.

Gynaecomastia

- Occurs in puberty in 30–60% of boys and usually managed conservatively
- Drugs commonly responsible:
  — Digoxin
  — Spironolactone
  — Cimetidine
  — Phenothiazines
  — Steroids
  — Cannabis
  — Tricyclic antidepressants
  — Isoniazid
- Exclude testicular tumour by clinical examination and hormone assays if no cause found
- Other causes:
  — Cirrhosis
  — Hypogonadism
  — Hyperthyroidism
  — Renal disease
  — Klinefelter's syndrome
- FNAC to exclude carcinoma, reassurance, discontinue causative drug, treat medical condition
- Excision if persists or for cosmetic reasons (usually via circumareolar incision).

BREAST PAIN

- Breast pain with or without lumpiness is the commonest reason for referral to breast clinics
- 70% of women experience breast pain at some time in their lives
- 7% of breast cancer patients present with breast pain alone.

Cyclical breast pain

- Typically occurs in the outer part of the breast in the week preceding menses with relief of symptoms after the period
- Studies have not identified a hormonal cause
- Many patients with cyclical breast pain seem to benefit from evening primrose oil (gamolenic acid 6–8 capsules per day) – few side-effects (nausea) but require 3-month trial of treatment
- Second-line therapies – danazol 100 mg bd and bromocriptine 2.5 mg bd (gradually introduced), but side-effects
- Vitamin B_6, antibiotics and diuretics of no value
- Tamoxifen, goserelin (GnRH) beneficial but not licensed in the UK.

Non-cyclical breast pain

- Affects older women
- True breast pain must be differentiated from chest wall pain, referred pain (cervical/thoracic spondylosis), thoracic outlet syndrome, gallstones, cardiac/pulmonary disease
- Localised painful spot treated by local anaesthetic/steroid injection
- True non-cyclical breast pain – exclude carcinoma, reassure, bra advice, non-steroidal anti-inflammatory drug, stop HRT

BREAST INFECTION

Breast abscess

- Early antibiotics for breast infection
- No response to antibiotics – FNA for MC+S and cytology to exclude breast cancer (inflammatory breast cancer presents with enlarged, inflamed breast but less pain than abscess)
- Treat with repeated aspiration and antibiotics unless skin necrotic. If skin necrotic, requires incision and drainage (peripheral incision in neonates and children)
- *Staphylococcus aureus* commonest organism in lactating and non-lactating infections but *Streptococcus* and anaerobes (*Bacteroides*) also involved.

Periareolar infection

- See periductal mastitis.

Tuberculosis

- Rare, breast or axillary sinus
- Requires combination of surgery and antituberculous drugs.

BREAST CANCER

Epidemiology

- 20 000 new patients per year in UK, prevalence 2%
- Affects 1 in 11 women in UK, modal age 58 years
- Commonest cause of death among women between 40 and 50 years
- Incidence rising but mortality rate now falling since late 1980s.

Risk factors

- Increasing age
- Geography – developed country and higher socio-economic group
- Menarche before 11 years, menopause after 54 years
- First child over 30 years
- Family history – first-degree relatives, early onset, bilateral disease
- Atypical hyperplasia
- Contralateral breast cancer
- Exposure to radiation
- Exogenous hormones
- Lifestyle – high intake of saturated fat, alcohol, body weight.

BREAST SCREENING

- Mammography is best screening tool available but only detects 95% of breast cancers
- National Breast Screening Programme, introduced in England and Wales in 1988 following Forrest report, aims to achieve 25% reduction in mortality by 2000
- Women aged 50–64 years invited on 3-yearly cycle. Women over 65 years no longer receive invitation but may request screening
- Two views now taken at first visit with single oblique view on subsequent rounds (two views detect 24% more cancers, with 15% lower recall rate)
- Recall rates for assessment should be below 7% on first screen and 3% on subsequent screens. Assessment includes further mammographic views, clinical examination and ultrasound scans. FNAC or core biopsies are taken from palpable lesions. Ultrasound-guided or stereotactic biopsies are required for impalpable lesions but if the diagnosis is not

established a wire localisation biopsy is performed. A hooked wire is placed close to the abnormality by a skilled radiologist and the area around the wire tip is excised by a surgeon through a small cosmetic incision. Diagnostic benign biopsies should weigh less than 20 g and an X-ray of the biopsy is taken before closing to ensure accurate removal of the lesion

- The cancer detection rate at the first screen (prevalence round) should be at least 50 per 10 000 women screened and at the second (incidence round) should be 35 per 10 000. Fifty percent of tumours should be less than 15 mm and 10–20% ductal carcinoma in situ (DCIS). There should be a higher incidence of special type cancers with good prognosis, e.g. tubular, medullary, mucoid, papillary
- The risk from the radiation delivered during mammography is estimated as one extra cancer per year after 10 years for every 2 million women screened
- Cancer detection rates among women 40–49 years is 2.9/1000 compared with 12/1000 in women over 65 years
- Screening women with a strong family history of breast cancer has a detection rate of 8/1000 but is not provided nationally at present
- Interval cancers occur in the first, second or third year following screening and consist of true interval cancers (not present on the previous films), false-negatives (present on the previous films), or occult cancers (not present on the current films). The incidence of interval cancers is 5–7.5/10 000 in first year, 9.3–10.5 in the second and 13.5–18 in the third year. A 2-year screening interval may be better than 3 years.

Management of breast cancer

- Multidisciplinary specialist treatment in Cancer Centres and Cancer Units is recommended following the 1994 Calman report on reorganisation of cancer services in the UK. The team includes radiologists, pathologists, surgeons, oncologists, psychologists with an interest in breast disease and breast care nurses. The patient and partner are involved in the decision-making and are fully informed of the treatment options and complications.
- The TNM classification which is incorporated into the UICC stage is a clinical assessment and hence inaccurate, but prognosis is related to the stage at presentation (Tables 10.2 and 10.3). A full blood count, liver function tests and chest X-ray are performed on all patients. Routine bone scan and liver ultrasound are not recommended as the majority of patients presenting with early disease do not have detectable metastases. Scans are usually restricted to patients with metastatic symptoms or advanced disease at presentation.

Table 10.2   TNM classification of breast cancer

T_{is}	Carcinoma in situ
T_1	< 2 cm
T_2	> 2 cm–< 5 cm
T_3	> 5 cm
T_{4a}	Involvement of chest wall
T_{4b}	Involvement of skin (ulceration, direct infiltration, peau d'orange, satellite nodules)
T_{4c}	T_{4a} and T_{4b}
T_{4d}	Inflammatory cancer
N_0	No regional node metastases
N_1	Palpable ipsilateral axillary nodes
N_2	Fixed ipsilateral axillary nodes
N_3	Ipsilateral internal mammary node involvement
M_0	No evidence of metastasis
M_1	Distant metastasis (includes ipsilateral supraclavicular nodes)

Table 10.3   UICC classification of tumours, 1987

UICC stage	TNM classification
I	T_1, N_0, M_0
II	T_1, N_1, M_0; T_2, N_{0-1}, M_0
III	Any T, N_{2-3}, M_0; T_3, any N, M_0; T_4, any N, M_0
IV	Any T, any N, M_1

Pathology

- Breast cancers develop in the terminal duct lobular unit
- Cancers are classified as in situ (cancer cells within the basement membrane) or invasive (basement membrane breached).

Invasive carcinoma

- Cancers are named on the basis of their morphology and growth pattern rather than structure of origin, i.e. ductal carcinoma does not necessarily arise from the duct
- The majority of invasive carcinomas are ductal of no special type (NOS) which are given a histological grade 1, 2 or 3. This is a score derived from the degree of nuclear pleomorphism, presence of tubule formation and number of mitoses. Grade 3 tumours are associated with a poor prognosis
- Vascular and lymphatic invasion are other markers of more aggressive disease
- Lobular carcinoma is more frequently diffuse or multifocal or bilateral.

Carcinoma in situ

- DCIS
- 4% of symptomatic cancer, 20% of screen-detected cancers
- Usually impalpable, detected as heterogenous, branching microcalcification on mammogram
- Classified into solid, cribriform, papillary, comedo ± necrosis and low or high grade
- Widespread DCIS requires mastectomy and reconstruction but patients with small foci of DCIS should be entered into national trials and the optimum treatment is not known. Axillary surgery is not required
- LCIS (lobular carcinoma in situ)
- Usually incidental finding following breast biopsy, not visible on mammogram
- Associated with increased risk of breast cancer on either side of 1% per year
- Increased surveillance or bilateral mastectomy.

Treatment of early breast cancer

Surgery

- Wide local excision combined with radiotherapy or mastectomy offer similar long-term survival. The majority of patients are offered the choice between wide local excision or mastectomy
- A wide local excision should achieve tumour clearance with 1 cm margins and good cosmesis. The margins should be marked with sutures and re-excision performed for incomplete excision or close margins
- Mastectomy is still recommended for large tumours (relative to the size of the breast), tumours involving the nipple, multifocal or diffuse disease and extensive DCIS. All breast tissue is removed but no chest wall muscles are taken, i.e. radical mastectomy is not performed. Reconstructive surgery is offered to all women requiring mastectomy and this may be an immediate or delayed procedure
- Node status is the most important prognostic marker
- All patients with invasive cancer require axillary surgery to stage the disease and to remove diseased lymph nodes to reduce the risk of axillary recurrence
- An axillary sample currently involves removal of lower axillary tissue (at least four lymph nodes). If the nodes are involved further axillary treatment is indicated, i.e. axillary clearance or axillary radiotherapy
- An axillary clearance removes axillary contents below the level of the axillary vein (level 1 below the pectoralis minor, level 2 behind and level 3 above). Only level 3 clearance is a full clearance – the head of pectoralis minor may be divided to improve access.

Complications of axillary clearance

• Wound infection
• Seroma (30%)
• Impaired shoulder mobility
• Intercostobrachial nerve numbness or paraesthesiae
• Lymphoedema.

Ideally axillary clearance would be restricted to those patients likely to benefit from the procedure, i.e. those with involved nodes. Frozen section examination of nodes during surgery or sampling of the sentinel node identified by injection of the tumour with dye or radioisotope may become more commonplace in the future.

Retrospective studies suggest survival benefit for premenopausal women operated on in the luteal phase of the menstrual cycle (second half). Prospective studies are now in progress.

Radiotherapy

• Following wide local excision, a 5-week course of radiotherapy to the breast with a boost to the tumour bed is commenced 6 weeks following surgery (40–50 Gy)
• After mastectomy radiotherapy is recommended for patients with a high risk of local recurrence – large tumour > 4 cm, grade 3, skin or chest wall involvement, lymphatic and vascular invasion
• Axillary radiotherapy is indicated following an axillary sample which produces metastatic nodes. Axillary radiotherapy following level III axillary clearance is contraindicated because of the unacceptably high rate of lymphoedema
• Skin inflammation is a common short-term complication. Other complications have become rare with improved delivery techniques – brachial plexus neuropathy, pulmonary fibrosis, excess cardiac deaths following left-sided treatment, second malignancies.

Systemic treatment
This may be given as adjuvant therapy following surgery and/or radiotherapy or as a primary treatment (neoadjuvant).

Tamoxifen

• Binds to oestrogen receptors and has partial oestrogen agonist activity
• Effect greatest in women with oestrogen receptor (ER)-positive tumours but up to 15% of ER-negative patients respond
• Beneficial in premenopausal and postmenopausal women regardless of node status but not statistically significant in premenopausal women with ER-negative tumours

- Dose of 20 mg daily for 5 years at present
- 40% reduction in contralateral breast cancer
- Side-effects include hot flushes, weight gain, gastrointestinal symptoms, visual disturbance (retinal and corneal deposits) and increased risk of endometrial carcinoma.

Chemotherapy

- Combinations of drugs are used, e.g. cyclophosphamide, methotrexate and 5-fluorouracil (CMF) in a 21- to 28-day cycle over 6 months
- Four cycles of anthracycline-based regimens, e.g. doxorubicin (Adriamycin) or epirubicin and cyclophosphamide may be more effective but have more side-effects. Chemotherapy produces the most significant benefits in node-positive premenopausal women. This may be related to ovarian ablation induced by the chemotherapy (in 50% of women)
- Side-effects must be weighed against potential long-term survival improvements. Nausea and vomiting, alopecia, fatigue, increased susceptibility to infection and mouth ulcers are common
- Chemotherapy in postmenopausal women is not routine in the UK but is more common in the USA and may be offered on an individual basis following discussion of the risks and benefits
- High-dose chemotherapy with bone marrow harvest and autologous transplantation is offered to women with more than ten involved axillary nodes in the USA and is available in the UK within clinical trials in specialist units. The treatment has a mortality of 5% and considerable morbidity but survival benefits have been reported.

Neoadjuvant chemotherapy

- Patients with large tumours and inflammatory cancer are offered primary chemotherapy rather than surgery
- The tumour may decrease in size and become amenable to conservative surgery or completely regress when biopsy is usually taken to confirm response
- Response rates of 70% are seen with 5-year survival up to 50%.

Ovarian ablation

- Achieved by surgery, radiotherapy or luteinising hormone releasing hormone (LHRH) agonist
- Benefits in premenopausal women similar to chemotherapy (25% reduction in mortality)
- Results of combination of ovarian ablation and chemotherapy awaited.

Management of advanced disease

- Advanced disease is no longer curable by local treatments
- 50% of breast cancer patients will develop local/regional recurrence and/or metastatic disease.

Local recurrence

- Majority of patients present with symptoms of recurrence between follow-up appointments – value of follow-up clinics now questioned
- Diagnosis confirmed by FNAC and/or radiology – gadolinium-enhanced MRI may help to differentiate between post-surgical or radiotherapy scarring and recurrent disease
- Staging investigations to detect simultaneous distant metastases
- Local re-excision/mastectomy for localised breast or axillary recurrence
- Tissue transfer, rotation flap or skin graft for symptomatic disease over larger area, e.g. chest wall
- Radiotherapy if maximum dose not exceeded previously
- Second-line hormone therapy
- Regional chemotherapy via internal mammary, lateral thoracic or subclavian arteries. Less effective following radiotherapy.

Metastatic disease

- Bone and soft tissue metastases have better outcome than liver, lung or brain secondaries
- Second-line hormone therapy including rechallenge with tamoxifen:
  — Medroxyprogesterone acetate or megestrol 160 mg
  — Oral aromatase inhibitor, e.g. anastrazole 1 mg
  — LHRH agonist
- Oophorectomy in premenopausal women
- Chemotherapy
- Taxoids
- Derived from Yew tree, stabilises microtubule assembly and inhibits cell division; used for anthracycline-resistant disease.

Bone

- 80% of patients with secondary disease
- Radiotherapy to painful bone metastases
- Prophylactic orthopaedic surgery to impending pathological fractures including spinal surgery for cord compression
- Bisphosphonates for hypercalcaemia, healing lytic metastases.

Brain

- 50% single metastases, some resectable – MRI investigation of choice
- Radiotherapy, steroids and anticonvulsants.

Palliative care

- Control of pain, nausea, breathlessness, constipation and psychological support.

FAMILIAL BREAST CANCER

- 5–10% of breast cancer dominantly inherited with variable penetrance
- Usually early onset, bilateral, increased incidence of other tumours in relative, e.g. bowel, ovarian, childhood malignancies
- Family history clinics now common within Breast Clinics to offer risk assessment, increased surveillance including earlier mammographic screening, counselling and genetic testing. Benefits and risks of cumulative radiation unknown
- BRCA 1 (chromosome 17q21)
- 30–40% breast cancer families, 90% breast/ovarian families
- Large gene (100 kb DNA) with wide spectrum of mutations makes screening difficult
- Mutation carriers have 85% lifetime risk of breast cancer
- BRCA 2 gene on chromosome 13q24
- p53 gene on chromosome 17p associated with Li–Fraumeni syndrome
- High-risk individuals offered tamoxifen prevention trial or prophylactic bilateral mastectomy with reconstruction.

FURTHER READING

Dixon J M (ed) 1995 ABC of breast diseases. BMJ Publishing Group, London
Early Breast Cancer Triallists' Collaborative Group 1992 Systemic treatment of early breast cancer by hormonal, cytotoxic or immune therapy. Lancet 339: 1–15, 71–85
Harris J R, Lippman M E, Morrow M, Hellman S 1996 Disease of the breast. Lippincott-Raven, Philadelphia

11. Endocrine surgery

Michelle E. Lucarotti

HYPERPARATHYROIDISM

Hyperparathyroidism is the most prevalent cause of hypercalcaemia and is the second commonest cause of hypercalcaemia in hospitalised patients after malignancy. It has a prevalence 1:1000 of the population and is the commonest in the fifth and sixth decade of life, and particularly postmenopausal females.

Presentation
Often an incidental finding, or discovered as part of the investigation of:

- Urinary tract calculi
- Bone and joint pain
- Gastrointestinal symptoms – constipation, anorexia, peptic ulceration
- Pancreatitis
- Polydypsia, polyuria
- Hypertension
- Depression, lethargy, confusion, dementia.

Diagnosis
The diagnosis is dependent upon the findings of:

- Persistent hypercalcaemia and the presence of an inappropriate serum level of parathormone
- Radiological features – osteitis fibrosa cystica
- A positive steroid suppression test. Steroids will suppress calcium in all cases of hypercalcaemia except primary hyperparathyroidism.

Relevant anatomy

- The normal parathyroid glands are 3–6 mm in length, orange/tan in colour
- Superior parathyroids arise from the fourth branchial pouch approximately, where the middle thyroid vein crosses the recurrent laryngeal nerve near the inferior thyroid artery after the latter has started to branch
- The inferior parathyroids arise from the third branchial pouch with the thymus and normally descend to approximately the lower pole of the thyroid gland

- Inferior glands may be found in the anterior mediastinum or adjacent to or within the thymus
- Although the normal number of parathyroid glands is four, supernumary glands occur in 2% of patients and may be found in the region of the neck or thorax.

CLASSIFICATION OF HYPERPARATHYROIDISM

1. Primary
   a. Single adenoma 85%
   b. Multiple adenomata 5%
   c. Diffuse hyperplasia of all parathyroid glands 10%
   d. Parathyroid carcinoma < 1%
2. Secondary
   a. The response of parathyroid glands to hypocalcaemia from some cause, often chronic renal disease
   b. All glands are enlarged
3. Tertiary
   a. Chronic stimulation of all the parathyroid glands by hypocalcaemia eventually renders them autonomous, resulting in hypercalcaemia.

Operative strategy

1. Preoperative localisation of parathyroid glands is valuable when planning surgery, several techniques are available:
   - Technetium Tc99n sestamibi scanning
   - Ultrasound (US)
   - Magnetic resonance imaging (MRI)
   - Computed tomography (CT) with contrast
   - Selective venous catheterisation (reserved for re-exploration).
2. Parathyroid exploration should be bloodless and systematic. Scrupulous haemostasis is required to prevent 'staining' of tissues which may impair recognition of parathyroid tissue. All four glands should be identified.
3. Identification may be aided apart from recognition of parathyroid tissue by:
   - Preoperative intravenous infusion of methylene blue 5 mg/kg body weight in 500 ml 5% dextrose infused over 1 hour immediately prior to surgery
   - Biopsy of a normal gland and frozen section histological examination of the abnormal gland.
4. In 15% of cases the glands may occupy ectopic sites, these include: adjacent to great vessels, adjacent to or within the carotid sheath, within the thyroid gland, behind the larynx, pharynx or oesophagus, or within the anterior or posterior mediastinum.
5. A single adenoma is excised with a biopsy of normal gland for histological comparison.

6. In hyperplasia either a three-and-a-half gland removal is performed or a four gland removal with a half gland auto-transplantation into the forearm to avoid further neck exploration. A complication of the latter technique is temporary or permanent hypocalcaemia.
7. Serum calcium 4–6 hours postoperatively is mandatory as occasionally temporary hypocalcaemia may occur before the 'normal' glands increase their output of parathormone.

FURTHER READING

Akerstrom M D, Rudberg C, Grimelius M D et al 1992 Causes of failed primary exploration and technical aspects of re-operation in primary hyperparathyroidism. World Journal of Surgery 16: 562–569

Kaplan E L, Yashiro T, Salti G 1992 Primary hyperparathyroidism in the 1990s. Choice of surgical procedures for this disease. Annals of Surgery 215(4): 300–317

Kohri K, Ishikawa Y, Kodama M 1992 Comparison of imaging methods of localisation of parathyroid tumours. American Journal of Surgery 164(2): 140–145

Nicholson M L, Veitch P S, Feehelly J 1996 Parathyroidectomy in chronic renal failure: comparison of three operative techniques. Journal of the Royal College of Edinburgh 41(6): 382–387

Petti G H, Kirk G A 1996 Parathyroid imaging. Otolaryngology 29: 681–691

Reid R K 1996 Hyperparathyroidism. Otolaryngology 29: 663–679

Rice D H 1996 Surgery of the parathyroid glands. Otolaryngology 4: 693–699

THYROID GLAND

THYROID NODULES

The appearance of a thyroid nodule is the commonest presentation of thyroid cancer. True solitary thyroid nodules are malignant in 10% of cases. Dominant nodules in multinodular goitres require evaluation for malignancy. Multiple nodules have a 3% incidence of malignancy. History of irradiation increases malignancy by 30–50%. The risk of malignancy in a solitary nodule is 20–35% in males, and 40% in children and adolescents. Thyroid cancer may present with cervical node metastases, the so-called 'lateral aberrant thyroid'.

Careful evaluation of the thyroid nodule requires:

- History of hoarseness
- Pain
- Shortness of breath
- Exposure to radiation
- A positive family history increases suspicion (consider MEN syndromes).

In addition to clinical examination, diagnosis is helped with a combination of fine-needle aspiration cytology and US which will differentiate between solitary or multiple nodules. This is supplemented with CT and MRI if any question of nodal involvement. Laryngoscopy is useful to document vocal cord function and possible involvement of the recurrent laryngeal nerve.

THYROID TUMOURS

Benign tumours

Papillary adenoma
Papillary adenomas are exceptionally rare. Even when there is no evidence of capsular invasion or vascular invasion present it is best to regard papillary tumours as well differentiated papillary carcinomas.

Follicular adenoma
This may be differentiated from a carcinoma by the absence of capsular or vascular invasion. It is suspected when very cellular and many mitoses even when invasion cannot be seen.

The Hurthle cell adenoma contains large acidophylic granular cells showing minimal signs of follicular formation. It contains very little colloid. They are not currently thought to be premalignant.

Teratoma
A rare tumour exclusive to young infants, it is invariably benign. Presence of calcification is diagnostic.

Malignant tumours

Papillary carcinoma
Papillary carcinoma accounts for 60–80% of all thyroid carcinomas. Most specimens are mixed papillary and follicular. They have a good prognosis with a survival rate > 90% over 20 years. Metastases are more common if primary tumour is > 1 cm in size. Tumours commonly multifocal and bilateral. Fifty percent spread to lymph nodes at presentation but has less effect on mortality than primary tumour site. Local invasion is more common if tumour is > 3 cm and spread is into strap muscles, trachea, larynx, oesophagus or recurrent laryngeal nerves. These more aggressive tumours have a 15-year survival of 15%.

Treatment is controversial but in experienced hands a total thyroidectomy has the advantage of removing all possible involved thyroid tissue as the disease is often bilateral and multifocal. Some authors argue that a unilateral approach is indicated as it carries considerably less potential morbidity and in most cases the prognosis is very favourable with suppressive doses of thyroxine.

Patients with impalpable cervical lymph nodes require no further treatment.

Prophylactic cervical lymph node dissection and external beam radiotherapy are of no proven value.

Recurrent disease is generally treated by local excision which may be repeated as required.

Suppressive doses of thyroxine are given to all patients regardless of when total thyroidectomy has been performed as papillary tumours are TSH-dependent and thyroxine reduces the incidence of recurrence. Involvement of cervical lymph nodes does not affect overall prognosis.

Follicular carcinoma

Follicular carcinoma accounts for 10–18% of thyroid carcinomas. It is usually single, solid and encapsulated. Most are more than 3 cm in diameter at presentation. Lymph node metastases have occurred in 5% at presentation. Prognosis is related to the extent of vascular invasion.

Tends to occur in an older age group. Peak incidence is in fifth and sixth decades. Commonly metastasises to the bone and lung.

Treatment is controversial. Total thyroidectomy is advocated by many authors because of the poorer prognosis and the ability post total thyroidectomy to trace recurrence and metastases with radioactive iodine. Therapeutic treatment with radio-iodine is also more effective after removal of all normal thyroid tissue. Some authors advocate a unilateral lobectomy for small tumours with little vascular or capsular invasion as these tumours are usually unifocal.

All patients should receive suppressive doses of thyroxine. Prognosis depends on the histological grade of the tumour and its degree of vascular invasion. Patients with marked vascular invasion have a 60% 5-year survival rate compared to over 90% in those with only slight invasion.

Hurthle cell tumours

These are a variant of follicular tumours and are sometimes classified as a separate entity. They behave unpredictably. They may be entirely benign or may invade into the thyroid, lymphatics and regional lymph nodes. They account for 3–7% of epithelial tumours of the thyroid.

Total unilateral lobectomy is recommended for 'benign' Hurthle cell adenomas and total thyroidectomy for the clearly malignant ones. Most Hurthle cell tumours do not concentrate iodine and therefore radioactive iodine is of little help in treating metastases.

Medullary carcinoma (MTC)

Medullary carcinoma accounts for 5–10% of all thyroid neoplasms. Arises in sporadic form in over 80% (and as part of an MEN syndrome in 20%). It is a tumour of the para-follicular or C cells of the thyroid, which secrete calcitonin, which has a major role as a biochemical marker for MTC. May occur in both MEN II A and more rarely in MEN II B.

MEN II A is an autosomal dominant syndrome consisting of MTC, phaeochromocytoma and parathyroid neoplasia. The RET proto-oncogene responsible for MEN II A has been localised to a centromeric chromosome 10 locus.

Screening for MEN syndrome RET mutations can be detected by molecular biology techniques, specifically those based on polymerase chain reaction (PCR) methodology. Once identified, children can be screened with annual pentagastrin stimulation tests (provocation test for calcitonin).

Metastases from MTC have been identified as early as 6 years. A total thyroidectomy is advocated for children older than 5 years who have confirmed genetic mutation.

Treatment of MTC Total thyroidectomy and dissection of the lymph nodes of the anterior compartment of the neck.

Prognosis It has a 50% 5-year survival rate.

Anaplastic carcinoma
Anaplastic carcinoma accounts for 5–14% of primary thyroid neoplasms. It is characterised by rapid growth of a mass in the neck. Peak incidence in the seventh decade, and 30% arise in a longstanding goitre. Anaplastic carcinoma is resistant to most forms of treatment. Tracheostomy for palliation of symptoms is sometimes useful.

Lymphoma
Quite uncommon – less than 2% of thyroid malignancies. It is commonest in the sixth decade. Female to male ratio is 4:1. Majority are non-Hodgkin's B-cell type. Treatment is chemotherapy and radiotherapy achieving a 5-year survival in 70%.

FURTHER READING

Austin J R, El-Naggar A K, Goepfert H 1996 Thyroid cancers II: medullary, anaplastic, lymphoma, sarcoma and squamous cell. Otolaryngology Clinics of North America 29(4): 611–627

Cady B 1984 Surgery of thyroid cancer. British Journal of Surgery 71: 976–979

Dunn J M, Farndon J R 1993 Medullary thyroid carcinoma. British Journal of Surgery 80: 6–9

Goldman N D, Coniglio J U, Falk S A 1996 Thyroid cancers I: papillary, follicular and Hurthle cell. Otolaryngology Clinics of North America 29(4): 593–609

Halliday A, Lynn J 1996 Thyroid. In: Surgical Oncology, Allen-Mersh T G (ed). Chapman and Hall, London, pp. 101–109

Har E L G, Hadar T, Segal K et al 1986 Hurthle cell carcinoma of the thyroid gland. Cancer 57: 1613–1617

Shvero J, Gal R, Avidor I et al 1988 Anaplastic thyroid carcinoma. Cancer 62: 319–325

Silverman J F, West R L, Larkin W et al 1986 The role of fine needle aspiration biopsy in the rapid diagnosis and management of thyroid neoplasm. Cancer 57: 1164–1170

Singer P A 1996 Evaluation and management of the solitary thyroid nodule. Otolaryngology Clinics of North America 29(4): 577–591

Multinodular goitre
Surgery reserved for symptoms, cosmetic reasons, suspicion of malignancy or thyrotoxicosis. Sub-total thyroidectomy is the

treatment of choice. No evidence that postoperative thyroxine suppresses recurrent growth of the gland which may result in a hazardous re-exploration many years after the primary operation. Patients may become hypothyroid many years postoperatively and, if not given prophylactic thyroxine replacements, thyroid function requires regular surveillance.

Thyrotoxicosis

Aetiology

- Autoimmune Graves' disease
- Toxic multinodular goitre
- Toxic nodules.

Clinical features

- Typically it affects young females
- Smooth goitre with a bruit
- Secondary thyrotoxicosis tends to occur in the older patient
- Other symptoms:
  — Weight loss
  — Heat intolerance
  — Tremor
  — Anxiety
  — Diarrhoea
  — Menstrual irregularities.

Signs

- Exophthalmos
- Lid lag
- Lid retraction
- Tachycardia or atrial fibrillation
- Ophthalmoplegia
- Pretibial myxoedema
- Proximal myopathy.

Treatment

- Initially, medical therapy is used: carbimazole – an initial dose of 15 mg tds reduced to 10 mg tds; propranolol for symptomatic control
- Spontaneous remission may occur in 50% of patients after withdrawal of carbimazole following a year of treatment.

Indications for surgery, which usually requires sub-total thyroidectomy

- If patient relapses after carbimazole withdrawn
- Poor response to antithyroid drugs
- Poor compliance

- Large goitre
- Severe thyrotoxicosis in the young patient
- Thyrotoxicosis during pregnancy
- Patient preference.

Complications of thyroidectomy

- Recurrent laryngeal nerve palsy 1%
- External laryngeal nerve palsy 1–5%
- Hypoparathyroidism 1–2%
- Recurrent hyperthyroidism 1–5%
- Hypothyroidism 20%.

Radio-iodine

- Reserved for patients over the age of 40 years
- Predominantly used in the elderly and for recurrent thyrotoxicosis following sub-total thyroidectomy
- Hypothyroidism occurs in 20% at 1 year and in 50% at 10 years so thyroxine replacement is required with T4.

Treatment of ophthalmic complications
Methyl cellulose eye drops, 5% guanethidine eye drops and in severe cases, lateral tarsorrhaphy.

For severe progressive ophthalmic complications

- Immunosuppression with high-dose corticosteroids – prednisolone 60 mg/day, azathioprine may be added or used as an alternative
- Total thyroidectomy, pituitary ablation and orbital irradiation is used in 'malignant' exophthalmos.

FURTHER READING

Gardiner K R, Russell C F 1995 Thyroidectomy for large multinodular goitre. Journal of the Royal College of Edinburgh 110(6): 867–870

Krainings J L, Marechaud R, Gineste D et al 1993 Analysis and prevention of recurrent goitre. Surgical Gynecology and Obstetrics 176(4): 319–322

Nies C, Silta H, Zielhie A 1994 Parathyroid function following ligation of the inferior thyroid artery during bilateral subtotal thyroidectomy. British Journal of Surgery 81(12): 1757–1759

Rojdmark J, Jarhult J 1995 High long-term recurrence rate after subtotal thyroidectomy for nodular goitre. European Journal of Surgery 161(10): 725–727

CARCINOID TUMOURS

They are rare with an incidence 1.5 in 1 000 000. Arise from entero-chromaffin cells, which are part of the amine precursor uptake and decarboxylation (APUD) system. The entero-chromaffin cells synthesise, store and secrete amines, notably serotonin.

Primary sites include:

- Vermiform appendix 45%
- Small gut (mainly ileum) 30%
- Large gut (mainly rectum) 20%
- Lung and bronchus 10%
- Other sites include ovary, biliary tree and stomach 10%.

Tumours more than 2 cm are clinically malignant. Most carcinoids of the appendix and rectum are benign and incidental findings. Colonic and non-appendiceal small gut tumours usually behave in a malignant fashion with hepatic metastases. Even malignant carcinoids with metastases may progress very slowly.

Presentation

Most often it is an incidental finding. An abdominal mass with or without small bowel obstruction. Gastrointestinal haemorrhage. Carcinoid syndrome.

Diagnosis

Twenty four-hour urinary 5-hydroxyindole acetic acid (5-HIAA). Urinary profile for 5-hydroxy-tryptophan may be helpful for carcinoid tumours of gut origin which lack the decarboxylase necessary to synthesise serotonin (gastric carcinoids in particular).

Monoclonal antibody isotope scanning may identify a primary lesion if the syndrome is present.

Carcinoid syndrome

- Facial flushing attacks precipitated by exercise, emotion or alcohol
- Episodic watery diarrhoea
- Hepatomegaly
- Bronchoconstriction
- Telangiectasia of the face
- Right-sided heart failure due to pulmonary stenosis and tricuspid regurgitation.

Treatment

1. Somatostatin analogue will abolish 80% of carcinoid syndrome symptoms.
2. Cytotoxic treatment consists of 5-fluorouracil and streptozotocin but it is relatively ineffective.
3. Hepatic artery embolisation provides sustained symptomatic relief but no survival advantage.

Management

Surgery
Depends upon site:

Appendix   Appendicectomy is all that is required unless the tumour is more than 2 cm or involves the base of the appendix or the meso-appendix when a right hemicolectomy is indicated.
Small gut   Segmental resection.
Rectum   If the tumour is less than 2 cm a local excision is indicated but if the tumour is more than 2 cm a more extensive resection is indicated.

FURTHER READING

Allison D J, Modlin J M, Jenkins W J 1977 Treatment of carcinoid liver metastases by hepatic artery embolisation. Lancet ii: 1323–1325
Coupe M, Levi S, Ellis M et al 1989 Therapy for symptoms in the carcinoid syndrome. Quarterly Journal of Medicine 271: 1021–1036
Makridis C, Oberg K, Juhlin C 1990 Surgical treatment of mid-gut carcinoid tumours. World Journal of Surgery 14: 377–385
Moertel C G 1983 Treatment of the carcinoid tumour and the malignant carcinoid syndrome. Journal of Clinical Oncology 1: 727–740

PANCREATIC TUMOURS OF ENDOCRINE ORIGIN

These are rare, with an incidence < 1 in 100 000. They are associated with clinical syndromes due to excess of specific hormones. Most prevalent is insulinoma (two-thirds of patients).
Zollinger–Ellison (Z–E) syndrome (hypergastrinaemia) is diagnosed with increasing frequency and it is the most common hormone excess in MEN I.
Vipoma and glucagonoma syndromes are rare manifestations of adult cell neoplasms and even less common is the somatostatinoma.
Rarity and variable presentation cause considerable delay in diagnosis.

INSULINOMA

They are usually solitary benign tumours unless with MEN I when they are multiple in 76% of patients.

Differential diagnosis

- Post-prandial or reactive hypoglycaemia
- Drug-induced fasting
- Hypoglycaemia (including exogenous insulin administration)
- Hormonal enzyme deficiencies
- Malnutrition
- Acquired liver disease.

Whipple's triad

1. Signs and symptoms of hypoglycaemia occurring during periods of fasting or exercise

2. At the time of symptoms the blood sugar level is 50 mg/dl
3. The symptoms are reversed by intravenous administration of glucose.

Diagnosis
Depends upon fasting insulin levels compared with glucose level. Normal: < 0.3 insulin to glucose ratio. In insulinoma: the ratio is > 1.

Lesion localisation is helped with a combination of angiography, selective venous catheterisation of portal, superior mesenteric and splenic veins for collection of blood specimens and insulin level gradients, and intra-operative ultrasound.

CT and MRI will only identify the tumour in 20–30% of cases but will identify liver metastases.

Operative strategy

- Frequent blood glucose estimations during operation
- Watch for hyperglycaemia for 2–3 weeks postoperatively
- Enucleation of single surface tumours
- Frozen ooction to exclude malignancy
- Distal pancreatectomy, or Whipple's for malignant lesions only
- Sub-total pancreatectomy is used for MEN I-associated tumours with enucleation of pancreatic head tumours
- Malignant insulinoma therapy is supplemented with cytotoxic treatment with Streptozotocin (a beta-cell toxin), caution is required as it is nephrotoxic.

Postoperative complications

- Pancreatic fistulae
- Pancreatic pseudocyst formation
- Pancreatitis.

GASTRINOMA

Zollinger–Ellison syndrome (described in 1955) consists of severe gastric hypersecretion and peptic ulcer disease associated with non-beta-cell tumour of the pancreas.

Secretin test
This is suitable to diagnose a gastrinoma patient with a gastrin level in an indeterminate range. When secretin is injected into a patient with a gastrinoma, a large increase in serum gastrin occurs. Little or no gastrin elevation occurs in patients without gastrinoma.

Localisation

- 80–90% of all gastrinomas occur in an area centred around the head of the pancreas and duodenum. The majority occur in the

pancreas but may occur in the duodenum but rarely in the gastric, antrum or splenic hilum
- Duodenal gastrinoma accounts for 30–40%. They may be only 1–2 mm and are often only found at duodenotomy
- 60% of gastrinomas are malignant and size and histological appearance do not reflect biological behaviour
- Arteriography has a sensitivity of 60%
- Hypertonic duodenogram and upper GI series are also useful
- Trans-hepatic portal venous sampling
- It is no longer necessary to offer total gastrectomy with H_2 receptor blockers or H_+-K_+-ATP-ase inhibitors can be used instead
- Treatment of metastatic disease is with streptozotocin.

GLUCAGONOMA

- Presents with diabetes and skin rash
- Diagnosed by demonstrating elevated serum glucagon
- Localised by CT and angiography
- Typically the rash is necrotising and migratory
- The lesion may be malignant
- There is an increased susceptibility to venous thromboembolism
- Palliation is by somatostatin and streptozotocin.

VIPOMA

- Vipoma is a neuro-endocrine tumour, which secretes vasoactive intestinal polypeptide (VIP)
- 90% lie within the pancreas
- 10% are found in neural tissue of autonomic nervous system
- 80% are simple, primary pancreatic neoplasms
- 50% of pancreatic tumours are malignant
- Presentation is usually with the triad of:
  1. Watery diarrhoea
  2. Hypokalaemia
  3. Achlorhydria
- Diagnosis requires demonstration of raised levels of serum VIP
- Localisation is by CT and selective angiography
- Treatment requires correction of dehydration and electrolyte imbalance and 85% are cured with a sub-total pancreatectomy
- In advanced disease, 50% respond to streptozotocin.

FURTHER READING

Bloom M A, Polak J M 1980 Glucagonomas, VIPomas and somatostatinomas. Clinical Endocrinology and Metabolism 9: 285–297
Bottger T C, Webster W, Beyer J et al 1990 Value of tumour localisation in patients with insulinoma. World Journal of Surgery 14: 107–114

Carter D C 1987 Pancreatic endocrine tumours. British Medical Journal 2954: 593–594

Edis A J, McIlrath D C, van Heerden J A et al 1976 Insulinoma. Current diagnosis and surgical management. Current Problems in Surgery 13: 1–45

Friesen S R 1982 Tumours of the endocrine pancreas. New England Journal of Medicine 306: 580–590

Grama D, Eriksson B, Martensson H et al 1992 Clinical characteristics, treatment and survival in patients with pancreatic tumours causing hormonal syndromes. World Journal of Surgery 16: 632–639

Grant C C, van Heerden J A, Charboneau J W et al 1988 Insulinoma: the value of intraoperative ultrasonography. Archives of Surgery 123: 843–848

Metz D C, Pisegna J R, Fishbevin V A et al 1993 Control of gastric acid hyper secretion in the management of patients with Zollinger–Ellison syndrome. World Journal of Surgery 17: 468–480

Stavri G T, Pritchard G A, Williams J, Stamatakis J D 1992 Somatostatinoma of the pancreas with hypercalcaemia. A case report. European Journal of Surgical Oncology 18: 298–300

MULTIPLE ENDOCRINE NEOPLASIA (MEN)

MEN I

The 3 Ps:

1. Pituitary
2. Parathyroid
3. Pancreatic islet cell tumours.

Infrequent associations include adreno-cortical, thyroid adenomas, carcinoid tumours, ovarian tumours and multiple lipomas. It is inherited in an **autosomal dominant** fashion.

Parathyroids are involved in 85% of patients; 40% have multiple adenomas compared with 2–4% in sporadic cases.

Presenting symptoms are usually due to pituitary (acromegaly) or pancreatic (insulinoma – hypoglycaemia, gastrinoma – duodenal ulcer) tumours because hypercalcaemia is asymptomatic.

MEN II

This is subdivided into MEN II A and MEN II B.

Men II a

This is a combination of medullary carcinoma of the thyroid (MTC) and phaeochromocytoma with infrequent association of parathyroid adenoma. MEN II A is inherited in an autosomal dominant fashion.

Men II b

MTC, phaeochromocytoma, marfanoid habitus and multiple mucosal neuromas affecting lips, eye lids, tongue and oropharynx with ganglioneuromas of gastrointestinal tract.

FURTHER READING

Grama D, Skogseid B, Wilander E 1992 Pancreatic tumours in multiple endocrine neoplasia type I: clinical presentation and surgical treatment. World Journal of Surgery 16: 611–619

Malmaeus J, Benson L, Johansson A et al 1986 Parathyroid surgery in the multiple endocrine neoplasia type I syndrome: choice of surgical procedure. World Journal of Surgery 10: 668–672

Matthew C G P, Chin K S, Easton D F et al 1987 A linked genetic marker for multiple endocrine neoplasia type 2a on chromosome 10. Nature 328: 527–528

Mignon M, Rusziewski P, Podevin P et al 1993 Current approach to the management of gastrinoma and insulinoma in adults with multiple endocrine neoplasia type I. World Journal of Surgery 17: 489–497

ADRENAL SURGERY

PHAEOCHROMOCYTOMA

This is rare with an incidence of 3 per million population.
It may be remembered as the 10% tumour!

* 10% are familial associated with MEN II
* 10% are malignant
* 10% are bilateral (25% in children)
* 10% outside adrenals (25% in children). Extra-adrenal locations include the organ of Zuckerkandl, para-aortic and para-vertebral regions and urinary bladder.

Clinical features are due to increased levels of circulating catecholamines secreted by the tumour.
    Phaeochromocytomas **only** account for 0.1% of all cases of hypertension.

Clinical features

* The principal feature is hypertension, in 50% this is persistent and 50% paroxysmal. The hypertension is frequently associated with headaches, palpitations, nausea, vomiting, abdominal pain and acute anxiety states
* Symptoms may be precipitated by exertion, emotion and various drugs including anaesthetic agents
* There is impaired glucose tolerance and hyperglycaemia.

Diagnosis
Vanillylmandelic acid (VMA) level greater than 35 mmol per 24 hours.

* Total plasma cathecholamine level greater than 1 microgram per litre
* Urinary adrenaline excretion greater than 20 micrograms per 24 hours
* Urinary noradrenaline excretion greater than 70 micrograms per 24 hours.

Localisation is achieved with a combination of CT, MRI, scintigraphy using 131 I-meta-iodo-benzyl-guanidine (MIBG), vena caval catheterisation and selective venous sampling with measurement of plasma catecholamine level.

Preoperative management

- All patients should have a serum glucose performed
- All patients should be checked for MTC by measurement of calcitonin
- Oral alpha-blocking agent should be instigated if there is biochemical evidence of phaeochromocytoma prior to localisation. The drug of choice is phenoxybenzamine with a gradual increase in dosage over 7–14 days starting with 10 mg 12-hourly
- If significant tachycardia occurs with alpha-blockade then a beta-blocker should be used such as propranolol
- Beta-blockers should not be given to a patient who has not first received alpha-blocking agents because of the risk of worsening hypertension.

Surgical management

- A lateral approach through the 11th rib bed may be used unless the tumour is very large or bilateral in which case an anterior transperitoneal approach is used
- Intraoperative hypertensive crises are treated with nitroprusside
- Avoidance of direct manipulation of the gland before venous ligation
- Hypotension usually occurring after the tumour has been devascularised is treated with volume expansion.

FURTHER READING

Bouloux P M G, Farees H M 1995 Investigation of phaeochromocytoma. Clinical Endocrinology 43: 657–664

Dow C J, Palmer M K, O'Sullivan J P et al 1982 Malignant phaeochromocytoma: report of a case and a critical review. British Journal of Surgery 69: 338–340

Hall A S, Ball S G 1993 Phaeochromocytoma. Netherlands Journal of Medicine 43: 829–838

Karet F E, Brown M J 1994 Phaeochromocytoma: diagnosis and management. Postgraduate Medical Journal 70: 326–328

Zarrilli L, Marzano A, Porcelli A et al 1991 The surgical management of malignant phaeochromocytoma. Journal of Nuclear Biology and Medicine 35: 266–268

ADRENO-CORTICAL TUMOURS

Adrenal adenoma is more common than carcinoma in a ratio of 3:1. Carcinomas are rare, occurring at a rate of 1 in 1 000 000 per year.

CONN'S SYNDROME

- 72% are due to a benign cortical adenoma secreting aldosterone
- 27% are due to bilateral cortical hyperplasia
- 1% are due to multiple or bilateral adenomas
- Carcinoma is exceptionally rare.

Diagnosis
Usually achieved with CT, IVU and tomography, and MRI.

ADRENAL CARCINOMA

Presentation

- Usually enlarged, non-functioning neoplasm
- Peak incidence in fourth decade
- Cushing's syndrome in 50%
- Virilisation is present in 30% and feminisation in 12%
- 40% have metastases at presentation
- Usually greater than 5 cm at presentation.

Treatment

- Adrenalectomy: via an anterior or thoraco-abdominal approach
- Chemotherapy with O-P'DDD (mitotane), a cytotoxic agent ablating adrenal tissue.

CUSHING'S SYNDROME

Aetiology

- Pituitary 90%
- ACTH-dependent 85%
    — ectopic
    — alcoholism, depression, etc.
- ACTH-independent 15%
    — adenoma 75%
    — carcinoma 25%.

Pathology

- 80% due to a basophilic micro-adenoma of the pituitary (Cushing's disease)
- Prolonged stimulation may occasionally cause the adrenal glands to become autonomously overactive and suppress the original pituitary adenoma – so-called bilateral adrenal macronodular hyperplasia
- 50% of Cushing's syndrome is due to adrenal causes
- Ratio of adrenal carcinoma to an adenoma is 1:3
- Adrenal carcinoma carries a poor prognosis, with 40% having metastases at presentation.

Diagnosis

- Elevated plasma cortisol with loss of normal diurnal variation
- 24-hour urinary cortisol excretion
- Insulin tolerance test. Patients with Cushing's disease fail to increase their circulating cortisol levels in response to hypoglycaemia
- Dexamethasone suppression test (failure to depress morning cortisol in response to dexamethasone confirms the diagnosis of Cushing's syndrome).

Differentiation of Cushing's syndrome and disease

Radio-immunoassay plasma ACTH

- If ACTH very low or undetectable, patient has an autonomous adrenal tumour
- ACTH is high in Cushing's disease and fairly high in ectopic ACTH syndrome.

Metyrapone test

- Large increase in plasma ACTH and urinary corticosteroids confirms Cushing's disease.

High-dose dexamethasone suppression test

- A 50% suppression of plasma and urinary corticosteroids occurs in Cushing's disease but not other causes of Cushing's syndrome.

Localisation of adrenal abnormality

- Ultrasound
- CT
- Selective venous catheterisation. Adrenal venous blood is sampled and plasma cortisol measured
- Arteriography
- Scintigraphy: 131 I-iodo-cholesterol is taken up by benign tumours.

Surgical management

- Transphenoidal pituitary microsurgery is the treatment of choice in Cushing's disease with a success rate of 85%. This has replaced bilateral adrenalectomy which is reserved for failed microsurgical hypophysectomy
- The adrenal is approached anteriorly through a gable or transverse incision or posteriorly through the 11th or 12th rib bed for bilateral disease. The lateral approach is usually appropriate for tumours greater than 5 cm in diameter
- It is usually possible to stay extra-pleural and extra-peritoneal. The thoraco-abdominal approach is only rarely needed for very large tumours.

Complications of adrenalectomy

Morbidity (up to 40%)

- Intra-operative injury to adjacent or contiguous structures
- Postoperative infection
- Thrombo-embolism increases to 11% in Cushing's syndrome
- Adrenal insufficiency.

Mortality (2–4%) due to:

- Pulmonary emboli
- Sepsis
- Myocardial infarction.

Postoperative management

All patients who have adrenal insufficiency require corticosteroids often for as long as 12 months.

FURTHER READING

Atkinson A B 1991 The treatment of Cushing's syndrome. Clinical Endocrinology (Oxford) 34: 507–513

Grondal S, Cedermaru B, Eriksson B 1990 Adrenocortical carcinoma. A retrospective study of a rare tumour with a poor prognosis. European Journal of Surgical Oncology 16: 500–506

Henley D J, van Heerden J A, Grant C S et al 1983 Adrenal cortical carcinoma: a continuing challenge. Surgery 94: 926–931

Lucarotti M, Farndon J R 1993 Cushing's syndrome. Current Practice in Surgery 5: 172–177

Schwartz R W, Sloan D A, Kenady D E 1991 Diagnosis and treatment of primary adrenal tumours. Current Opinion in Oncology 3(1): 121–127

Seddon J M, Baranetsky N, van Boxel P J 1985 Adrenal incidentalomas. Urology 25: 1–7

Venkatesh S, Hickey R C, Sellin R V et al 1989 Adrenal cortical carcinoma. Cancer 64: 765–769

12. Upper gastriontestinal surgery

Mark Vipond

OESOPHAGEAL CANCER

Incidence and geography

Approximately six-fold increase in the last 25 years in Western developed countries. Incidence now $\approx 12/10^5$ (UK). This change is probably related to an increased incidence of Barrett's oesophagus so that in the West the incidence of adenocarcinoma now equals squamous cell carcinoma and lower third tumours predominate. Areas of high incidence of squamous cell carcinoma include Iran, Transkei and China and are probably secondary to dietary factors. Smoking and alcohol are also risk factors and reflect the male:female incidence of 5:1 Oesophageal carcinoma is also associated with a previous history of Plummer–Vinson syndrome (post-cricoid carcinoma), corrosive injury and achalasia.

Pathology

Squamous cell carcinoma	(50%)	Upper and middle third
Adenocarcinoma	(50%)	Lower third
		Arise in Barrett's in two-thirds.

Spread

- Direct extension to mediastinal pleura, pericardium, aorta
- Lymphatic
  — submucosal (therefore longitudinal resection needs to be extensive)
  — nodal
- Blood-borne to lung, liver (rarely bone or brain).

Clinical features

- Dysphagia: often present several months before presentation and tumours are frequently advanced at presentation. Circumferential involvement is required to produce liquid dysphagia
- Weight loss
- Anorexia
- Odynophagia
- Bleeding
- Reflux symptoms
- Hoarse voice. RLN palsy
- Aspiration.

Diagnosis and investigation

1. Barium swallow: typically shows shouldered stricture with irregular mucosa
2. OGD and biopsy/brush cytology: essential for histological diagnosis. Identifies level and length of tumour.

Staging

1. Chest X-ray: lung metastases
2. CT thorax and abdomen: to detect metastatic disease. Poor for local invasion or lymph node staging
3. Endoluminal ultrasound: over 90% accuracy for depth of tumour invasion and detection of local lymph node involvement
4. Bronchoscopy: detects tracheo-bronchial involvement in middle and upper third tumours
5. Laparoscopy/mediastinoscopy: mediastinoscopy rarely used and of limited value. Laparoscopy indicated if doubt about peritoneal involvement or liver metastases and may be combined with laparoscopic ultrasound
6. TNM staging (see Table 12.1)

Treatment

The only hope for cure is major resectional surgery. Selection is vital to avoid patients being inappropriately subjected to radical treatment. This requires accurate staging and assessment of cardiorespiratory status and co-morbid disease. Sixty percent of patients will have advanced disease or be unfit for major surgery and require palliation alone.

Palliation

The aims of palliative treatment are to:

1. Restore swallowing
2. Relieve pain
3. Improve or maintain quality of life: this should be done with low morbidity and mortality. The options available are tailored to the individual patient:
   - Dilatation
   - Oesophageal intubation – rigid or metal self-expanding stents
   - Laser or Argon plasma coagulation
   - Alcohol injection
   - Radiotherapy – for squamous cell carcinoma
   - Palliative care team.

Surgical resection

The aims are radical resection of tumour with associated lymph nodes. Because of submucosal lymphatic spread 10 cm clearance of tumour is required proximally. Three approaches are in common use.

- Ivor-Lewis oesophagectomy: abdominal and right thoracic approach with intra-thoracic anastomosis
- Trans-hiatal oesophagectomy: abdominal and left neck incision. Distal oesophagus dissected under direct vision through hiatus. Remainder of intra-thoracic oesophagus dissected bluntly and blindly. Gastric tube brought through oesophageal bed for anastomosis in the neck.

(These two approaches are suitable for distal third tumours.)

- McKeown three-phase oesophagectomy: abdominal, right thoracic and left neck incision. Essential for middle and upper third tumours to enable wide resection of tumour and associated lymphatics.

Adjuvant therapy
There is no proven role for either postoperative chemotherapy or radiotherapy. Trials of neo-adjuvant chemo-radiotherapy are occurring and there is some evidence that it may downstage disease.

Prognosis (Table 12.1)
Overall 5-year survival is < 5% with the median survival for non-resected patients 6 months. Five year survival for any stage post-resection is 15%.

Table 12.1 Prognosis by stage for oesophageal carcinoma

	Stage	Proportion at presentation (%)	5-year survival (%)	Median survival (months)
I	$T_1N_0M_0$	9	60	> 60
II	$T_{2-3}N_0M_0 T_{1-2}N_1M_0$	24	30	30
III	$T_{3-4}N_1M_0$	42	15	14
IV	$T_{any}N_2M_{0-1}$	25	2	6

MOTILITY DISORDERS

Swallowing is initiated by a voluntary coordinated movement of the lips, tongue, palate and cricopharynx. The bolus of food is moved from the mouth to the pharynx, from which the sequence is involuntary, with relaxation of the cricopharyngeal sphincter. A ring of muscular contraction passes down the oesophagus at 30–50 mm/second. The lower oesophageal sphincter (LOS) relaxes as soon as swallowing is initiated and returns to a 'closed' state as the peristaltic wave passes through. Patients with motility disorders present with one or more of:

- Dysphagia
- Odynophagia
- Chest pain – often very similar to cardiac chest pain

- Heartburn
- Regurgitation.

Investigation

History and examination are essential to exclude secondary motility disorders (scleroderma, neuropathies and myopathies) and structural problems (tumour, stricture and gastro-oesophageal reflux disease).

1. Endoscopy: usually normal in motility disorder but food residue may be present (e.g. achalasia). Important to exclude tumour or stricture
2. Barium swallow: bolus swallow using barium-coated marshmallow may detect abnormal peristalsis and contractions.

If these investigations are normal it is reasonable to treat with a proton pump inhibitor (PPI) for 2–3 months. If symptoms persist further investigation is required.

3. 24-hour ambulatory pH and manometry: 24-hour manometry is the most reliable method to detect oesophageal motility disorders.

HYPERMOTILITY DISORDERS

Diffuse oesophageal spasm

- Uncommon disorder presenting with chest pain and dysphagia (may mimic myocardial infarction (MI))
- Frequent spastic responses to swallowing with high amplitude and long oesophageal contractions. There is some normal peristalsis and LOS relaxes normally
- Aetiology unknown
- Drugs to reduce smooth muscle contraction (nitrates, nifedipine or verapamil) are used with variable success
- Balloon dilatation or long longitudinal myotomy may be performed.

Nutcracker oesophagus

- Most commonly seen in non-cardiac chest pain
- Manometry shows normal peristalsis but mean amplitude > 180 mmHg (normal 30–120 mmHg) and there may be long duration contractions
- Treatment is with smooth muscle relaxants or balloon dilatation
- Myotomy is seldom required.

HYPOMOTILITY DISORDERS

Scleroderma

- Connective tissue disorder that may affect the smooth muscle of the oesophagus (CREST syndrome)

- Presents with dysphagia and complications of reflux (Barrett's oesophagus or stricture)
- Barium studies show reduced peristalsis and endoscopy shows oesophagitis or stricture
- Manometry reveals decreased oesophageal contraction amplitude and aperistalsis in the affected region with diminished LOS pressure
- pH studies may also be abnormal showing acid reflux secondary to poor oesophageal clearance
- Acid reflux is treated with PPI
- Prokinetics (e.g. cisapride) may help in early stages
- Dilatation for strictures.

SPHINCTER PROBLEMS

Achalasia

- Aetiology is unknown but similar to Chagas' disease caused by the protozoan *Trypanosoma cruzi*. There is complete aperistalsis with or without failure of the LOS to relax
- Incidence is 1.10^5 affecting all ages, with equal sex distribution
- As the disease advances there is dilatation of the oesophagus
- Presents with dysphagia and may cause aspiration
- Histologically there is loss of ganglion cells in the myenteric (Auerbach's) plexus
- Endoscopy shows a dilated oesophagus. This is confirmed by barium swallow with a typical smooth tapered (parrot's beak) narrowing above the gastro-oesophageal junction
- Manometry shows complete aperistalsis of oesophageal body with failure of LOS relaxation
- Smooth muscle relaxants have been used with minimal success
- Endoscopic balloon dilatation is the treatment of choice. If this fails after two procedures, surgery is indicated
- Heller's cardiomyotomy is performed dividing muscle fibres for at least 5 cm on the oesophagus
- 15% of patients will develop reflux post-surgery and the procedure may be combined with an anti-reflux operation
- Local injection of *Botulinum* toxin has recently been shown to be a useful treatment and may be helpful in patients unfit for surgery
- There is an increased risk of carcinoma in both treated and untreated achalasia (< 5%).

Pseudo-achalasia

Similar findings on manometry to primary achalasia but is secondary to a structural oesophageal problem such as carcinoma of gastro-oesophageal junction. Thus endoscopy is necessary in all patients diagnosed as achalasia.

Hypertensive lower oesophageal sphincter

- Presents with chest pain and dysphagia
- Manometry shows normal peristalsis but LOS pressure is > 45 mmHg (normal 10–25 mmHg)
- Treatment is by balloon dilatation or operative cardiomyotomy.

DIVERTICULA

Mucosal pouches from the oesophageal lumen. Majority are pulsion and secondary to motility disorders with increased intraluminal pressure acting against a chronic obstruction.

Pharyngeal pouch (Zenker's diverticulum)

- Dysfunction of cricopharyngeus muscle
- Pouch forms between the lower cricopharyngeal and upper thyropharyngeal fibres (Killian's dehiscence)
- Treatment is surgical with excision of the pouch and cricopharyngeal myotomy. Endoscopic treatment is possible with the jaws of a linear stapler placed in the oesophageal lumen and the pouch. This produces an anastomosis of the diverticulum to the back of the oesophagus.

Epiphrenic diverticulum

- Occurs in the distal oesophagus and is secondary to a motility disorder
- No treatment is required
- The main danger is perforation during endoscopy.

WEBS

Plummer–Vinson (Patterson–Kelly) syndrome

- Thin web immediately above the cricopharyngeal sphincter that can be seen anteriorly indenting the barium column on contrast swallow
- Clinical features include glossitis, dysphagia and iron-deficiency anaemia
- The web is stretched or ruptured by endoscopy
- Condition has malignant potential.

Kramer–Schatzki ring

- Web at upper border of gastro-oesophageal junction often above hiatus hernia
- May cause dysphagia and responds to dilatation.

OESOPHAGEAL RUPTURE

SPONTANEOUS (BOERHAAVE'S SYNDROME)

Forcible vomiting, usually with a full stomach, leads to distal oesophageal rupture. This causes mediastinal, and sometimes pleural, contamination. Patients present with chest pain, dysphagia and shortness of breath. There may be surgical emphysema. Diagnosis is confirmed by water-soluble contrast swallow.

Initial management is to stop oral intake, give broad-spectrum antibiotics and insert a chest drain if there is an associated pneumothorax. At operation the tear is identified and repaired if feasible. Adequate drainage to the contaminated area is provided by mediastinal and pleural drains. To isolate the oesophagus an oesophagostomy and gastrostomy may be added. The patient is fed enterally by jejunostomy and serial contrast swallows performed until the area of tear has sealed.

IATROGENIC

Flexible endoscopy	0.02%
Rigid oesophagoscopy	0.1%
Therapeutic dilatation	0.9%
Balloon dilatation	2–5%
Oesophageal intubation	8–11%

Diagnosis confirmed by water-soluble contrast swallow. Principles of treatment are similar with nil by mouth and broad-spectrum antibiotics. Definitive management depends on underlying disease and the patient's general fitness. For carcinoma, immediate resection is preferable; if the patient is unfit then a stent may be placed. For benign disease and a small tear, conservative treatment is reasonable; if there is no progress then operative repair as for spontaneous rupture is indicated.

GASTRO-OESOPHAGEAL REFLUX DISEASE (GORD)

Prevalence is at least 5% of the population. The majority do not seek treatment or are helped by simple measures and self-medicate. A significant minority require continuous drug therapy.

Symptoms

- Heartburn
- Epigastric and retrosternal pain
- Regurgitation
- Respiratory symptoms from spillover of refluxate.

Pathophysiology
Several mechanisms exist to prevent reflux. GORD occurs with failure of one or more components:

- Normal oesophageal motility
- LOS intrinsic pressure
- Positive pressure on intra-abdominal oesophagus
- Mucosal rosette; pinchcock effect of crus; angle of His
- Normal gastric emptying.

Investigation

Endoscopy

- ≈ 50% have oesophagitis but there is no correlation between severity of symptoms and degree of oesophagitis
- Biopsy to identify Barrett's.

Barium swallow

- Not generally helpful and no longer routine
- May see reflux with video studies and demonstrate severe oesophagitis.

24-hour ambulatory pH and stationary manometry

- Manometry with ten wet swallows to determine oesophageal motility, the level and resting pressure of LOS
- Small pH electrode with digital recorder placed 5 cm above manometrically-determined LOS
- 24-hour recording with patient marking meals and symptom episodes
- Acid reflux event is fall of oesophageal pH to < 4
- Positive recording shows correlation of symptoms with objective measure of pH < 4
- The total time oesophageal pH < 4 should be < 4%.

Management

1. Stop smoking and reduce alcohol
2. Lose weight
3. Raise head of bed
4. Avoid precipitating foods
5. Simple antacids.

If oesophagitis is present, a 4-week course of PPI is given and then reduced to the simple measures above. If symptoms relapse, long-term PPI is required.

Anti-reflux surgery
Indications are:

- Breakthrough symptoms despite long-term PPI
- Volume reflux causing respiratory symptoms
- Complications of GORD such as Barrett's or stricture.

A wide range of operations have been described. The most frequently performed with longest objective follow-up is Nissen fundoplication, now performed laparoscopically. This procedure involves:

1. Posterior crural repair
2. Division of short gastric vessels
3. Mobilisation of intra-abdominal oesophagus
4. 360° wrap of fundus around distal oesophagus over large (54–60 F) bougie
5. Wrap 2 cm long and loose.

- 85% of patients have symptomatic and objective relief of reflux
- 10–15% are troubled by gas bloat or dysphagia but the majority resolve by 3 months.

HIATUS HERNIA

Protrusion of viscus through oesophageal hiatus, usually abdominal oesophagus and upper stomach. Distinction by endoscopy and barium swallow/meal.

Type I Sliding (axial)	(80%)	Abdominal oesophagus and upper stomach move up and down together
Type II Para-oesophageal (rolling)	(10%)	Abdominal oesophagus below hiatus but gastric fundus herniates alongside
Type III Combined	(10%)	

SLIDING HIATUS HERNIA

Frequently asymptomatic but may be associated with GORD. Usually no treatment is required but otherwise for GORD and then general measures apply.

PARA-OESOPHAGEAL HIATUS HERNIA

Patients are often elderly and infirm. Symptoms are usually post-prandial and include lower chest and upper abdominal discomfort, respiratory embarrassment, dysphagia (20%) and bloating. They are associated with anaemia, and acute strangulation may occur. The patient often adapts to the symptoms by eating small frequent meals.

Surgery is indicated for incapacitating symptoms, acute strangulation or perforation. The hernia is reduced, a crural repair performed and the stomach fixed intra-abdominally.

BARRETT'S OESOPHAGUS

Acquired condition believed to result from chronic gastro-oesophageal reflux. Contents of refluxate (acid and bile salts) injure the oesophageal squamous mucosa and induce columnar metaplasia.

Definition
Circumferential columnar-lined oesophagus for more than 3 cm in the tubular oesophagus.

Prevalence

- Affects 10% of patients with symptomatic reflux undergoing endoscopy
- Incidence has increased in the last 25 years and this parallels the increased use of endoscopy
- Median age at diagnosis is 60 years and male:female ratio is 3:1
- From post-mortem studies it is estimated that 19/20 cases go unrecognised.

Diagnosis

- Endoscopic appearance is of salmon-pink velvety appearance of distal oesophagus. However, the endoscopic appearance can be subtle and is unreliable
- Diagnosis is histological and thus relies on biopsy. This shows intestinalisation of the oesophageal mucosa with columnar epithelial lining and gland formation
- Changes are classified as non-dysplastic or dysplastic with the latter subdivided into low-grade or high-grade.

Complications

1. Ulcer
2. Stricture
3. Adenocarcinoma: the natural history and time scale of malignant transformation is difficult to determine but overall risk is increased $\approx$ 40-fold with an incidence of $\approx$ 1:150 patient-years.

Surveillance
With the increased incidence of carcinoma in Barrett's oesophagus there would appear to be a strong case for surveillance. However, there are several reasons against such a policy:

- Adenocarcinoma does not develop in the majority of patients with Barrett's
- Overall survival of patients with Barrett's is no different from that of the general population
- Evidence is lacking that there is a natural progression from CLO to low-grade, high-grade dysplasia and then carcinoma. Indeed, it is possible that regression may occur before the final step.

Surveillance should be restricted to patients who would be candidates for surgical resection. A current recommendation would be quadrantic biopsies at 2-cm intervals:

No dysplasia   every 2 years
Low-grade dysplasia   every 6 months
High-grade dysplasia   every 3 months.

Treatment
The mainstay of treatment is PPI, which provide excellent symptomatic remission. Oesophagectomy is the treatment of choice once invasive carcinoma is found. Some surgeons advocate oesophagectomy for high-grade dysplasia as ≈ 40% of these patients will have underlying invasive carcinoma – such a decision has to be weighed carefully against the morbidity and mortality of the operation.

OESOPHAGEAL STRICTURE

- Peptic (secondary to GORD)
- Barrett's
- Corrosive.

For peptic and Barrett's stricture, multiple biopsy is required to exclude carcinoma. Most respond to dilatation and long-term PPI. Repeat dilatation may be required and, for intractable stricture, endoscopic intubation or surgical resection.

CORROSIVE STRICTURE

Caustic injury to the upper gastrointestinal (GI) tract is produced by strong alkaline (lye) or acidic agents. The patient presents with a combination of chest and epigastric pain, dysphagia, fever, shock, haematemesis. There may be laryngeal and pulmonary symptoms secondary to acute laryngeal and tracheal oedema.

The airway is cleared and protected. Intravenous fluids, analgesia and broad-spectrum antibiotics are given. A water-soluble contrast study is performed to exclude perforation. If intact, careful endoscopy determines the degree of burn and ulceration.

Once the patient is stable some advocate stent placement to prevent stricture. Perforation requires oesophagectomy. Late stricture occurs in 30% and responds to repeated dilatation. Overall mortality is 5–10%.

NON-VARICEAL UPPER GI HAEMORRHAGE

Common upper GI emergency. Incidence of acute bleeding ≈ 100/10^5 adults per year. One-third of upper GI bleeds in patients over 60 years are associated with non-steroidal anti-inflammatory drugs (NSAIDs). Overall mortality is 10%.

Aetiology

Duodenal ulcer	30%
Gastric ulcer	15%
Erosions	10%
Oesophagitis	5%
Mallory–Weiss tear	5%
Varices	5%
Malignancy	5%
Other: Dieulefoy lesion Telangiectasia AV malformation Aorto-duodenal fistula	5%
No diagnosis	20%

Presentation

Upper GI haemorrhage manifests in three ways with symptoms and signs of hypovolaemia of varying degrees:

- Haematemesis
- Melaena
- Fresh per rectal bleeding.

Management

1. Clear and maintain airway
2. Intravenous infusion and correction of hypovolaemia
3. Monitor fluid replacement by CVP and urinary catheter
4. Transfuse and correct clotting as required.

Once stable, a full history and examination is obtained with particular emphasis on nature of blood loss, drug history, previous peptic ulceration, signs of chronic liver disease.

Endoscopy is required to identify the cause of bleeding. This should be performed urgently if there are signs of continued bleeding and may require general anaesthesia with cuffed endotracheal tube. If the patient is stable, endoscopy is performed within 24 hours. Endoscopy identifies the cause of bleeding, stigmata of rebleed and allows therapeutic intervention (Fig. 12.1).

Treatment

Majority of cases of upper GI haemorrhage will resolve spontaneously with supportive measures alone. Oral or intravenous H_2 receptor antagonists (H_2RA) or PPI have no effect on acute bleeding.

Oesophagitis and hiatus hernia
Major bleeding is rare. Endoscopic injection therapy is required only for an ulcer that has eroded a vessel. Once acute bleeding has stopped, long-term PPI is required.

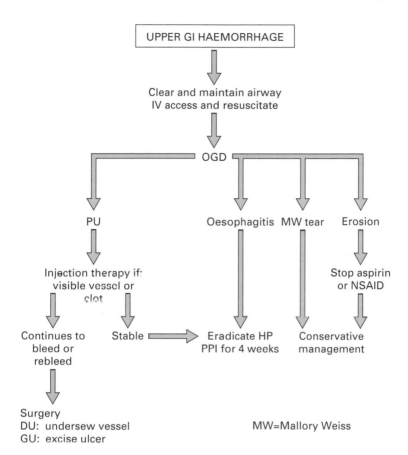

Fig. 12.1 Algorithm for the management of upper GI bleeding.

Mallory–Weiss tear
Classic history of vomiting or retching preceding haematemesis.
Usually located on gastric side of oesophagogastric junction. Stops
spontaneously in > 90% and rebleeding is rare. If surgery is
required the tear is underrun via a gastrotomy.

Peptic ulcer
Rates of hospitalisation, surgery and mortality (8%) have not
changed in 25 years. Aspirin, NSAIDs and warfarin are independent
risk factors, particularly in the elderly. Endoscopy allows
visualisation and assessment of the ulcer which is classified as:

• Flat ulcer
• Adherent clot

- Visible vessel
- Active bleeding.

The risk of rebleeding is increased with:

- Age > 60 years
- Haemoglobin < 10 g/dl
- Hypovolaemic shock
- Adherent clot or visible vessel.

Endoscopic haemostatic therapy is required for patients at increased risk of rebleeding or ulcers with a visible vessel or active bleeding. This can be provided by laser photocoagulation, bipolar diathermy or heater probe – all are equally effective but are complex and may be associated with perforation. Injection therapy with 1:10 000 adrenaline is simpler and just as effective. It has been shown to reduce rebleeding and surgery rates in randomised trials though has no effect on overall mortality. There is no additional benefit with the use of a sclerosant such as ethanolamine. If the patient rebleeds after injection therapy it can be repeated but 50% of these patients will continue to bleed. There is no benefit from second-look endoscopy in a stable patient.

The indications for surgery are:

- Continued uncontrolled bleeding
- Failed endoscopic therapy.

DU: Gastroduodenotomy, underrun vessel and pyloroplasty
GU: Ulcer excision and gastric closure
　　Partial gastrectomy (for large antral ulcer).

There is no place for definitive ulcer surgery in the acute bleed. Most patients who subsequently relapse with peptic ulcer can be controlled with PPI.

Erosions
Acute gastric erosions are associated with NSAIDs, aspirin, stress (burns, pancreatitis, major surgery) and alcohol. Prophylaxis with sucralfate should be give to prevent stress-induced erosions. Bleeding is rarely massive and usually stops with supportive measures. If there is massive uncontrolled haemorrhage then total or near-total gastrectomy is required which carries a high mortality.

GASTRIC CANCER

Incidence and geography
Declining incidence over the last century, particularly in the West, now ≈ $16/10^5$ (UK). Male:female incidence is 2:1. Areas of high incidence remain in Japan, Eastern Europe and Andes. Environmental factors are important, particularly a diet rich in nitrosamines such as cured meat and fish. Offspring of Japanese

migrants to the USA have the risk of the host country. Other associations are lower socio-economic class (III and IV), blood group A, pernicious anaemia ($\times$ 3), atrophic gastritis, hypogammaglobulinaemia ($\times$ 50), post-gastrectomy ($\times$ 2). Increased prevalence of *Helicobacter pylori* (HP) in areas with high incidence and this is thought to be a co-factor through the development of atrophic gastritis.

The site of gastric cancer is moving proximally (Table 12.2).

Table 12.2 Chronological change in anatomical site of gastric carcinoma

	Proximal third	Middle third	Distal third
1955	20%	30%	50%
1985	40%	15%	45%

Pathology
Tumours are adenocarcinoma and can be classified on macroscopic appearance (Borrman classification):

I   Fungating
II Excavated
III Ulcerative and raised
IV Linitis plastica.

The Lauren classification relies on histological appearance and reflects different clinical features of the two types (Table 12.3).

Early gastric cancer
Malignant tumour limited to mucosa or submucosa. More commonly found in distal third of stomach and has excellent 5-year survival of 95%.

Spread

- Direct extension to pancreas, liver, retroperitoneum
- Lymphatic

Table 12.3 Comparison of intestinal and diffuse type gastric carcinoma

Features	Intestinal	Diffuse
Prevalence	53%	33%
M:F ratio	2:1	1:1
Mean age (years)	55	48
5-year survival	20%	< 10%
Macro	Fungating	Ulcerative, infiltrative
Micro	Well-differentiated, glandular	Poorly-differentiated, ring cells
Aetiology	Diet, environmental, HP	Unknown

- Blood-borne to liver, lungs
- Transcoelomic – peritoneal and omental seedlings.

Clinical features

- Dyspepsia
- Weight loss
- Anorexia
- Gastric outlet obstruction
- Anaemia or bleeding.

Dyspepsia is a very common symptom and any patient over 45 years with new-onset dyspepsia should be referred for endoscopy. In Japan, mass screening is performed by double-contrast barium meal and endoscopy in patients over 40 years. This has led to 50% of identified cancers being early gastric cancer. This approach is not economic in the UK which has a much lower overall incidence of gastric cancer.

Investigation

1. Barium meal: shows polypoid, ulcerating or infiltrative lesion
2. OGD and biopsy/brush cytology: essential for histological diagnosis. Low threshold for biopsy of any lesion to detect early cancer.

Staging

1. Chest X-ray: lung metastases
2. Liver ultrasound: liver metastases
3. CT scan thorax and abdomen: instead of CXR and US to detect lung or liver metastases. Poor for local, lymphatic or transcoelomic spread
4. Endoluminal ultrasound: best modality for T and N stage; slightly less accurate than in oesophagus but still 80%
5. Laparoscopy: identifies local invasion and peritoneal/omental seeding. Allows biopsy of suspicious liver lesions.

Treatment

The only hope for cure is surgical resection. As with oesophageal cancer, selection is vital to avoid patients being inappropriately subjected to radical treatment. Forty percent of patients will have advanced disease or be unfit for major surgery and require palliation alone.

Palliation

Aims are to lessen symptoms with minimum morbidity and improve quality of life. Palliative care and nutrition team provide control of pain, nausea and vomiting. Surgery is indicated for gastric outlet obstruction or bleeding. Resection provides the best palliation at the expense of increased risk of morbidity and mortality. For unresectable distal tumours gastrojejunostomy provides symptomatic relief. Recanalisation by endoscopic intubation is rarely feasible and gives poor function.

Surgical resection
There is a large difference between Japanese and Western results for curative resection. To some extent this is due to the initial disease stage and a 'stage-migration' effect from better pathological reporting. The principal difference in the Japanese approach is the extent of lymph node dissection. Draining gastric nodes are divided into three tiers (N1, N2, N3) in relation to the primary tumour. Resection is described by the extent of lymph node dissection (D1, D2, D3) and in Japan is generally at least D2. Pancreatectomy and splenectomy may be performed but are associated with an increased morbidity and mortality.

Distal third tumours require an 80% partial gastrectomy and proximal or middle third tumours a total gastrectomy with appropriate node dissection. Operative mortality should be < 5%.

Adjuvant therapy
There is no proven benefit from postoperative chemotherapy or radiotherapy. Neo-adjuvant chemotherapy, given either systemically or intraperitoneally, is the subject of controlled trials.

Prognosis (Table 12.4)
Overall 5-year survival is 10% with the median survival of non-resected patients 6 months. Five-year survival for any stage after 'curative' resection is 50% (compared with 75% in Japan).

Table 12.4   Prognosis of gastric carcinoma

Stage		Proportion at presentation (%)	5-year survival (%)
IA	$T_1N_0M_0$	1	95
IB	$T_1N_1M_0T_2N_0M_0$	4	90
II	$T_1N_2M_0T_2N_1M_0T_3N_0M_0$	7	70
IIIA	$T_2N_2M_0T_3N_1M_0T_4N_0M_0$	10	50
IIIB	$T_3N_2M_0T_4N_1M_0T_4N_2M_0$	15	20
IV	$T_{any}N_{any}M_1$	60	2–5

PEPTIC ULCER DISEASE

Dramatic change in surgical practice in last 20 years. Elective operations have almost disappeared but incidence of complications of ulcers has not changed. Majority of peptic ulcer (PU) are treated in the community since the introduction of H_2RA, PPI and HP eradication therapy.

Aetiology

- Diet: no strong evidence for role of diet
- Acid/pepsin:
  — DU: associated with increased HCl secretion which may be related to larger parietal cell mass
  — GU: no association
- Smoking: more prone to develop PU and more likely to die from complications
- NSAID
- *H. pylori*: colonises gastric epithelium and mucus. Prevalence of HP mirrors that of PU. Causative role in > 95% of non-NSAID DU, but only 10% of HP-positive patients will develop an ulcer
- Blood group O
- Associated diseases: chronic liver disease, hyperparathyroidism, chronic renal failure.

Clinical features

Classical picture of epigastric pain which wakens patient at night and is relieved by food or antacids is rare. Generally vague recurrent upper abdominal pain and dyspepsia. Appropriate to treat young patients empirically. Any patient with recurrent dyspepsia and patients over 45 years require endoscopy (Fig. 12.2).

Investigation

1. OGD
   - Confirms ulcer and excludes other disease
   - GU requires multiple biopsy to exclude malignancy and repeat endoscopy and biopsy to confirm healing
2. HP
   - Antral biopsy and histology
   - Antral biopsy and culture
   - Carbon-isotope urea breath test
   - ELISA serology.

Treatment

1. Test for and eradicate HP. One-week course of PPI + amoxycillin + metronidazole is successful in 90%. All patients with DU require eradication therapy. Re-infection is < 0.5% in developed countries, ulcer recurrence is very rare, minor haematemesis is unlikely to rebleed
2. Stop NSAID: if not possible, most ulcers will heal with H_2RA or PPI
3. H_2RA ⎫ both effective;
4. PPI   ⎭ PPI better for GU
5. Dietary habits and smoking.

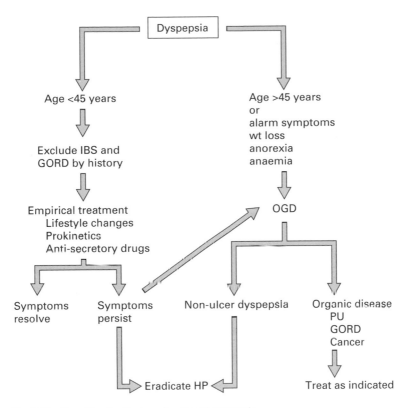

Fig. 12.2   Algorithm for the investigation of dyspepsia.

Refractory ulcer
Defined by lack of evidence of healing at 8 weeks for DU; 12 weeks
for GU. Repeat OGD and biopsy to exclude cancer. Confirm
eradication of HP and, if still present, repeat treatment with a
different combination. Ensure no NSAIDs and stop smoking.

Resistant ulcer
This includes refractory ulcer and those that relapse. Exclude
Zollinger–Ellison syndrome. Treatment lies between long term PPI
or surgery.

Zollinger–Ellison syndrome
Presents with epigastric pain and resistant ulceration together with
diarrhoea, weight loss (40%), oesophagitis (33%). Due to excess
gastrin production from gastrinoma. Two-thirds are multifocal,
two-thirds malignant and one-third have metastases at
presentation.

Either part of MEN 1 (30%) – generally multifocal within pancreas, or sporadic (65%) – often extra-pancreatic.

Diagnosis   Elevated fasting serum gastrin – false-positives may occur in achlorhydric states.

Treatment   The aims of treatment are to control acid production secondary to high gastrin and, if feasible, remove the primary tumour.

1. Excess hormone production
   * High-dose PPI
   * Parietal cell vagotomy may be added
2. Gastrinoma
   * Resection if tumour is localised, otherwise general measures with high-dose PPI are required.

Surgery for peptic ulcer

Indications

1. Resistant ulcer
   DU: Best operation is not known. Balance between low ulcer recurrence and operative morbidity. Highly selective vagotomy gives poor results in patients with ulcers refractory to PPI and HP eradication. Choice lies between selective vagotomy and antrectomy with Bilroth I or Roux-en-Y reconstruction or 80% gastrectomy and Roux-en-Y
   GU: For prepyloric ulcers or those associated with DU disease, operation is as for DU. Lesser curve ulcer requires excision and HSV or Bilroth I partial gastrectomy.
2. Perforation
   Conservative therapy with NG aspiration and antibiotics may be successful. However, the outcome is less good in those over 70 years and thus surgery is the preferred option.
   DU: Omental patch and peritoneal lavage which may be performed laparoscopically. Followed by HP eradication. Definitive ulcer surgery has no role in acute perforation
   GU: Excision of ulcer and closure.
3. Severe haemorrhage
   Discussed in section on upper GI bleeding.
4. Pyloric stenosis
   Endoscopic balloon therapy is an attractive, minimally invasive option; however, there is a 50% recurrence at 2 years. Surgical option is pyloroplasty or gastrojejunostomy if the duodenum is very scarred. Antrectomy is a more aggressive option.

GASTRITIS

ACUTE

Acute inflammation of the stomach can occur with chemicals (salicylate, NSAIDs, acid, alkali), thermal injury, radiation, uraemia, stress, Gram-negative shock. Characterised by oedema and leucocyte infiltrate which may lead to ischaemia and sloughing to produce an acute ulcer. It is generally self-limiting.

CHRONIC

Comprises spectrum of changes which progress through:

1. Chronic superficial gastritis: lymphocyte infiltrate and minimal gastric atrophy
2. Atrophic gastritis:
   * *Type A*: Associated with parietal cell antibody and affects body of stomach causing pernicious anaemia. Decreased acid and elevated gastrin levels
   * *Type B*: No antibody. Antral involvement with decreased gastrin levels. Associated with HP infection and often called antral gastritis
3. Gastric atrophy: minimal inflammatory infiltrate and marked atrophy with gland loss.

Atrophic gastritis may develop intestinal metaplasia in areas of gland atrophy. Whilst inflammatory changes are reversible, atrophy and metaplasia are irreversible. Fundic gland atrophy leads to hypochlorhydria which allows nitrosating bacteria to proliferate. There is a definite association between atrophic gastritis and gastric cancer. However, 40% of patients over 60 years will have varying degrees of atrophic gastritis.

MÉNÉTRIER'S DISEASE

Uncommon condition also known as hypertrophic gastropathy. There is massive enlargement of rugal folds in the body and fundus of the stomach. Histologically there is an expanded foveolar compartment with elongated and branched gastric pits.

Clinical features

* Epigastric pain, weight loss, anaemia, diarrhoea and oedema
* There is hypochlorhydria and hypoproteinaemia from excessive protein loss.

Treatment

* Aims are to relieve pain and anaemia
* Mainstay is antisecretory drugs
* Some surgeons advocate partial or total gastrectomy to relieve symptoms and eliminate risk of gastric cancer developing.

GASTRIC VOLVULUS

Rare condition, generally in elderly, which, if associated with strangulation, presents as an emergency. Occurs as an organo-axial rotation along the long axis of the stomach or mesentero-axial rotation along the transverse axis. The latter is often associated with a diaphragmatic defect and para-oesophageal hiatus hernia.

Clinical features

* Acute: vomiting/retching, abdominal pain, failure to pass NG tube
* Chronic: post-prandial pain, belching, distension.

Treatment

Acute volvulus is an emergency. Volvulus is reduced, any non-viable stomach is resected and the stomach fixed at the fundus and antrum.

ACUTE GASTRIC DILATATION

Rare and may follow gastric or abdominal surgery, trauma, retroperitoneal haematoma and electrolyte disturbance.

Clinical features

* Tachycardia, hiccups, belching
* Enlarged stomach is visible on abdominal X-ray. Relieved by nasogastric tube and correction of electrolyte loss.

FOREIGN BODIES

Swallowed foreign bodies tend to occur in children under 3 years, psychiatric patients, drug users and convicts. Ninety-nine percent are asymptomatic. Risk is oesophageal impaction and perforation. X-ray will identify location of the majority – a lateral view is required for possible oesophageal foreign bodies to exclude presence in the trachea. If there is still doubt, a contrast study or endoscopy should be performed.

Oesophageal foreign bodies should be removed especially if sharp (e.g. bone) or a disc battery. This can be performed by endoscopy with an overtube to protect the oesophagus and prevent aspiration.

If the foreign body is in the stomach it can be safely left and serial X-ray performed to ensure passage. Surgery is only indicated for perforation or obstruction.

BEZOARS

Concretions of ingested material:

* *Trichobezoar*: composed of hair and most often found in young women

- *Phytobezoar*: composed of vegetable material, particularly fruit fibres, skin and seeds. Most commonly with persimmon, coconut and citrus fruits.

Bezoars result from excessive intake of indigestible fibre or impaired gastric emptying as in diabetic gastroparesis or post-gastrectomy states.

Symptoms only occur when the bezoar has reached a large size and include bloating, abdominal pain, nausea and vomiting. Small bowel obstruction may occur if a fragment of the bezoar breaks off.

Attempts can be made to break down phytobezoars with oral cellulose and endoscopic fragmentation. Surgical removal via a gastrotomy is required if this fails and for trichobezoars.

POST-GASTRIC SURGERY SYNDROMES

PREVIOUS ULCER SURGERY

Recurrent ulceration
Generally occurs within 5 years and most frequently after incomplete vagotomy.

Incidence of recurrent ulceration at 5 years:

HSV	12%
Truncal vagotomy	10%
Partial gastrectomy	4%
Vagotomy and antrectomy	1%

Diagnosis is confirmed by endoscopy and biopsy to exclude cancer. Test for HP. Exclude aspirin, NSAIDs and Z–E syndrome. Treat with PPI.

If refractory, then further surgery is required and the best option is antrectomy and completion vagotomy.

Dumping
Due to rapid and uncontrolled gastric emptying. Occurs most frequently after gastrectomy but also truncal or selective vagotomy.

Early dumping
Rapid emptying of hyperosmolar contents into the small bowel causing large fluid shifts from the vascular compartment into the bowel lumen. This leads to a fall in plasma volume and vasomotor manifestations. Patients complain of faintness, dizziness, palpitations, nausea and vomiting within 15 minutes of a meal. Management is by taking small, frequent meals, low in carbohydrate and with added fibre.

Late dumping
More accurately called reactive hypoglycaemia. Occurs several hours after a meal with similar symptoms but also includes blackouts. There is rapid gastric emptying of a carbohydrate meal

which leads to rapid glucose absorption and excessive insulin release with loss of normal feedback control and thus delayed hypoglycaemia.
    Management is again with dietary advice eating small regular meals low in carbohydrate. The patient is advised to carry glucose.

Surgery
This is only required for intractable symptoms persisting for over 2 years. Results are variable and the best options are revision to a Roux-en-Y drainage or isoperistaltic jejunal interposition.

Diarrhoea

- Occurs most commonly after truncal vagotomy
- Usually episodic with explosive watery diarrhoea and urgency
- Unlike early dumping may be precipitated by a low osmolar meal
- Occasionally secondary to bacterial overgrowth in a blind loop
- Patients should avoid refined carbohydrate and take bulking agents together with loperamide as required.

Enterogastric reflux

- Reflux of alkaline juice and bile into the stomach after pyloroplasty, gastrojejunostomy or partial gastrectomy
- May lead to reflux oesophagitis and bile vomiting
- Presents with persistent dyspepsia and intermittent bile vomiting particularly in the morning
- Management is with mucosal agents such as aluminium hydroxide, altacite or sucralfate and prokinetics such as metoclopramide
- Biliary diversion by Roux-en-Y may be required.

POST-GASTRECTOMY

Small stomach syndrome
Patients complain of early satiety and early post-prandial discomfort. This results from loss of the gastric reservoir although it may be multifactorial and signal early dumping or recurrent ulceration. It may lead to nutritional problems. Patients are advised to eat small, regular meals and are supervised by a dietician to ensure an adequate caloric intake. Various gastric pouch reconstructions have been described but these are rarely used.

Nutritional problems
Malabsorption is a rare cause of malnutrition after gastrectomy unless there is bacterial overgrowth. Most patients regain their postoperative weight loss and should be kept under dietary surveillance. After gastrectomy, carbohydrate absorption is rarely complete, protein absorption is decreased and fat absorption rarely better than 75%.

- Vitamin B_{12}: there is loss of parietal cell intrinsic factor and all patients should receive vitamin B_{12} injections 3-monthly
- Vitamin D: deficiency may occur if there is fat malabsorption. Calcium and ALP should be monitored and, at 5 years, bone densitometry performed. Postmenopausal women and patients over 70 years should receive oral calcium after total gastrectomy
- Iron: the jejunum can usually adjust to absorb iron but occasionally supplements are required.

Gastric cancer risk

Several studies have shown that the relative risk of gastric cancer is increased after partial gastrectomy or truncal vagotomy and drainage. The risk is low with a latent period in excess of 20 years so surveillance is of limited value.

GASTRIC LYMPHOMA

Primary gastric lymphoma represents 5% of gastric malignancies and is the commonest site of extranodal non-Hodgkin's lymphoma. Ninety percent are of B-cell origin. Stomach is normally devoid of lymphoid tissue. Gastric lymphoma shows mucosal infiltration with small centrocytic lymphocytes with the morphological appearance of mucosa-associated lymphoid tissue (MALT).

1. Low-grade MALToma
   - 90% associated with HP infection
   - HP eradication may lead to regression
   - Long latent period to transformation to high-grade tumour
2. High-grade MALToma
   - No clear association with HP
   - Rapidly disseminates.

Clinical features

Similar to adenocarcinoma of stomach. Dyspepsia, anorexia, weight loss, anaemia, nausea.

Investigation

1. OGD and biopsy
   - Subtle changes with enlarged gastric folds, nodules, plaques or ulcers. Biopsies must be deep to reach submucosa
2. Endoluminal ultrasound
   - Useful to determine depth and extent of tumour infiltration and lymph node status
3. CT scan
   - To identify widespread disease.

Treatment

For localised disease, surgery offers the best option with total or near-total gastrectomy. Limited data suggest that combination chemotherapy and radiotherapy may have similar outcome to surgery alone in those unfit for surgery or with unresectable disease. There is no proven role for adjuvant therapy after surgery. The overall 5-year survival is 30%; for resected cases without nodal involvement this increases to 60%.

FURTHER READING

1 Griffin SM, Raines SA 1997 Upper gastrointestinal surgery, WB Saunders
2 Hennessy TPJ, Cushiem A 1992 Surgery of the oesophagus, 2nd edn. Butterworth-Heinemann Ltd.

13. Pancreatic surgery

Mark Vipond

ACUTE PANCREATITIS

Definition (Atlanta 1992)
Acute inflammatory process of the pancreas, usually with rapid onset of pain and tenderness, often accompanied by vomiting and systemic inflammatory responses. Regional tissues and remote organ systems are sometimes involved. Pancreatic enzymes in blood or urine are usually elevated, but not invariably.

Incidence

- Incidence is increasing secondary to alcohol in young patients and gallstones in the elderly
- Currently ≈ 5–30/10⁵ per year; 3% of all cases of abdominal pain admitted to hospital.

Aetiology

- Gallstones   42%
- Alcohol   25%
- Idiopathic   15%
- Post-ERCP   4%
- Rare causes
    — Pancreas divisum
    — Trauma
    — Post-renal transplant
    — Post-cardiac bypass
    — Drugs
    — Viruses
    — Hypercalcaemia
    — Hyperlipidaemia
    — Vascular.

Pathogenesis
Proteases are held in zymogen granules within pancreatic acinar cells. From the acinar cell, proteases are released into the ductal system. Trypsin inhibitors prevent activation of protease until contact with duodenal enterokinase. 'Pancreastasis' leads to loss of intracellular separation of enzymes and intra-acinar activation. There are two main theories to explain this pathological event.

Mechanical obstruction ± hypersecretion
A gallstone obstructs the common channel leading to intrapancreatic bile reflux. Normally pancreatic ductal pressure exceeds bile duct pressure and this back pressure leads to acinar activation of proteases. However, gallstones are usually transitory and sphincterotomy does not lead to pancreatitis. It is suggested that hypersecretion is also required when the gallstone lodges to lead to enzyme activation. This theory also offers an explanation for pancreatitis secondary to intraductal parasites, afferent loop obstruction, choledochal cyst, periampullary carcinoma and pancreas divisum.

Toxic and metabolic causes
Alcohol-induced pancreatitis generally follows longstanding heavy consumption. It is suggested that chronic alcohol abuse induces immaturity and disruption of normal acinar cell separation of lysosymes and proteases leading to activation within the acinar cells. Hypercalcaemia and oxygen free-radicals also affect enzyme partition within acinar cells.

Clinical features

- Epigastric pain: usually severe and constant – may radiate to back or chest and mimic MI
- Nausea and vomiting.

Clinical signs

- Epigastric tenderness and guarding
- Abdominal distension
- Low grade fever
- Mild jaundice
- Hypovolaemic shock: hypotension, tachycardia and oliguria
- Grey–Turner's sign: flank discoloration
- Cullen's sign: periumbilical discoloration.

Diagnosis

1. Serum amylase
   - A level elevated at 4× laboratory normal is regarded as diagnostic
   - The level is highest during the first 24 hours and then decreases rapidly. It is not related to the severity of an attack
   - Conditions such as perforated peptic ulcer, acute cholecystitis and mesenteric infarction may also cause an elevated amylase
2. Urinary amylase
   - Usually remains elevated after serum amylase levels have returned to normal
   - Urinary amylase is normal in macroamylasaemia

3. Serum lipase
   - A level of 2× laboratory normal is diagnostic – sensitivity and specificity > 90%
   - Remains elevated longer than serum amylase and not increased in hyperamylasaemia without pancreatitis.

Initial management

Investigations

1. Blood tests
   - FBC
   - U&E
   - Creatinine
   - Calcium
   - Glucose
   - Blood gases
   - LFT
   - LDH

These also contribute to severity scoring
2. Chest X-ray
   - Shows early pulmonary complications
   - excludes perforated PU
3. Abdominal X-ray
   - May show calcified gallstone or chronic calcific pancreatitis.

Management

1. Analgesia: IM pethidine (PCA or epidural may be required)
2. Intravenous fluids: replace vigorously with crystalloid
3. Nil by mouth and NG tube
4. Supplementary oxygen: required if SaO_2 is reduced
5. Monitoring
   - The disease course is unpredictable for the first 24 hours and HDU is advised for the patient who is shocked on admission or fails to respond to initial management
   - 1-hourly pulse, blood pressure, respiratory rate, urine volume and SaO_2
   - 4-hourly temperature and glucose.

Severity stratification
The initial prediction of the severity of an attack of acute pancreatitis into mild and severe has important implications for management. The most useful multifactor scoring systems are the Ranson or Glasgow systems – the latter have been validated in the UK population (Table 13.1). Three or more positive criteria constitute severe acute pancreatitis.

Blood CRP concentration has independent prognostic value. A level of > 210 mg/ml in the first 4 days or > 120 mg/ml at the end of the first week indicates a severe attack.

Table 13.1   Glasgow (Imrie) scoring system for prediction of severity in acute pancreatitis

Feature	Level
Age	> 55 years
White blood cell count	$> 15 \times 10^9/l$
Glucose	> 10 mmol/l
Urea	> 16 mmol/l
PaO_2	< 60 mmHg (< 8 kPa)
Calcium	< 2 mmol/l
Albumin	< 32 g/l
Lactate dehydrogenase	> 600 units/l
Aspartate/alanine aminotransferase	> 100 units/l

Radiology and other imaging

1. Ultrasound
   * Performed early to detect gallstones and biliary obstruction
   * Used to monitor development of pseudocyst or abscess
2. CT scanning
   * Performed with intravenous contrast which will show enhancement of the normal pancreas
   * Enables CT-guided aspiration for culture
   * The severity of inflammation can be graded (Table 13.2)
3. ERCP
   * Not required to establish diagnosis
   * Used in selected patients to relieve biliary obstruction.

Table 13.2   CT grading system for acute pancreatitis

Grade	Appearance
A	Normal-appearing pancreas
B	Local or diffuse gland enlargement; small intraperitoneal fluid collection
C	Any of above + peripancreatic inflammatory changes and < 30% gland necrosis
D	Any of above + single extrapancreatic fluid collection and 30–50% gland necrosis
E	Any of above + extensive extrapancreatic fluid collection, pancreatic abscess and > 50% gland necrosis

Management of mild acute pancreatitis

* Mild acute pancreatitis accounts for 75% of patients with acute pancreatitis.
* It usually runs an uneventful self-limiting course
* Patients are managed on the general ward with intravenous fluids and analgesia

- Oral fluids and diet are reintroduced after a few days
- Antibiotics are not of proven benefit in mild acute pancreatitis.

Management of severe acute pancreatitis (Fig. 13.1)

- Severe acute pancreatitis comprises 25% of patients and, of these, the mortality is 25%. These patients are managed on the HDU/ITU with full monitoring (CVP, NG tube, urinary catheter) and hourly observations
- With cardiovascular failure a Swan–Ganz catheter may be required
- Regular blood gas analysis is required to detect hypoxia early
- There is some evidence to support the use of antibiotics to prevent the development of local and systemic infective complications, and intravenous cefuroxime is the best option
- Specific therapies, such as aprotinin, somatostatin and FFP, are of no proven value
- Early ERCP and sphincterotomy (within 72 hours) is indicated in patients with severe acute gallstone pancreatitis. There is evidence that overall morbidity is reduced in this subset of patients. Similarly, signs of cholangitis require urgent ERCP
- Severe acute pancreatitis may give rise to local or generalised complications
- In the first few days hypovolaemic shock is the major threat to life; in the first week multisystem organ failure (MOF), and after the first week, sepsis becomes the major threat
- Close monitoring on the HDU/ITU allows identification of systemic problems
- Contrast-enhanced CT scanning should be performed at 1 week to identify local pancreatic complications and performed serially to monitor progress and intervention.

Systemic complications
These range from mild pyrexia to rapidly fatal multi-organ failure. Systemic effects are mediated by inflammatory responses to signals from the damaged pancreas – activation of the systemic inflammatory response sequence (SIRS) by cytokines, free-radicals and other mediators.
Cardiovascular failure   Release of enzymes and vasoactive substances increase capillary permeability and produce oedema in and around the pancreas. Hypovolaemia is indicated by tachycardia, hypotension and decreased systemic vascular resistance. Refractory cardiac shock requires Swan–Ganz monitoring to determine the need for fluids, diuretics, inotropes and vasoconstrictors.
Respiratory failure   Hypoxaemia is common and causes include atelectasis, sputum retention and pulmonary collapse. Regular

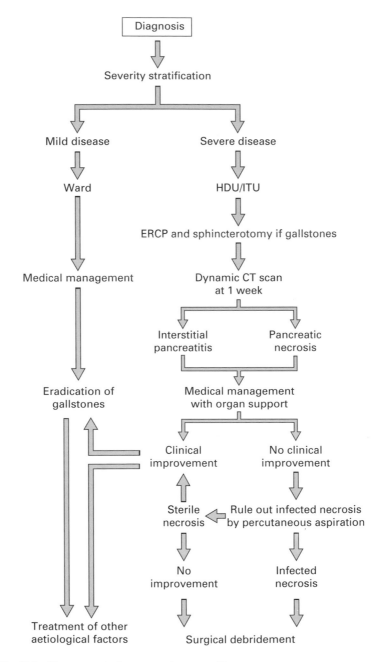

Fig. 13.1 Management of severe acute pancreatitis.

physiotherapy and bronchodilators are required. Pleural effusions may require drainage. Pulmonary capillary injury leads to interstitial oedema and poor compliance with the development of adult respiratory distress syndrome. Management is with early ventilation and PEEP as required.

Renal failure Hypovolaemia, hypoxaemia and endotoxaemia all contribute to tubular dysfunction. The usual cause for persisting oliguria is inadequate fluid replacement. Haemofiltration or dialysis is required if renal failure becomes established.

Disseminated intravascular coagulation The fibrinolytic and coagulation systems become activated in fulminant pancreatitis. Abnormalities should be corrected by the administration of blood products and fibrinolytic inhibitors.

Metabolic problems Hypocalcaemia and hypomagnesaemia may occur. Low calcium often reflects low albumin and only requires calcium infusion if there is tetany or cardiac dysrhythmia. One-third of patients have abnormal glucose tolerance with transient hyperglycaemia which is treated by sliding-scale insulin.

Gastrointestinal complications Vomiting – managed with NG tubes. Gastroparesis persists after ileus because of peripancreatic swelling. GI haemorrhage – increased risk; use prophylactic sucralfate. Starvation – enteral or parenteral nutrition after 5 days.

Hepatobiliary complications Mild jaundice occurs in 15% from decreased clearance of bilirubin and cholestasis. More marked jaundice is likely to be obstructive and requires ERCP.

In fulminant acute pancreatitis the sequence of organ failure is usually respiratory, renal, cardiovascular and DIC. The incidence of one-, two- or three-system failure is 20%, 5%, 2% with a mortality of 20%, 50%, 90% respectively.

INTRA-ABDOMINAL COMPLICATIONS

Acute fluid collection/pseudocyst

Definition
Collection of enzyme-rich fluid in and around the pancreas. Acute fluid collections occur within the first 4 weeks of acute pancreatitis and do not have an enclosing wall of granulation or fibrous tissue. After 4 weeks a mature capsule develops and collections are defined as pseudocysts.

- Arise because of loss of pancreatic duct integrity and leakage
- Present with mass and may cause jaundice or delayed gastric emptying by pressure effect
- Imaged by CT or MRI
- Rupture produces shock and pancreatic ascites; erosion into vessels may cause haemorrhage
- Persistence beyond 6 weeks and size $\geq$ 6 cm means resolution is unlikely

- Percutaneous drainage may lead to infection or fistula
- Surgical drainage is preferred by open or laparoscopic method:
  1. cystgastrostomy
  2. cystjejunostomy
  3. distal pancreatectomy for cyst in tail.

Pancreatic necrosis

- Diagnosed by contrast-enhanced CT scan which shows diffuse or focal areas of non-viable pancreatic parenchyma
- Pancreatic ischaemia leads to sterile necrosis. Infection, by bacterial translocation, may supervene and escalates multiple organ failure
- Initial management of necrosis is by general supportive measures. Serial CT scanning is performed to assess progress and, if infection is suspected, percutaneous aspiration for culture performed
- Infected pancreatic necrosis requires surgical intervention:
  1. Dead and liquefied pancreas is removed and dead retroperitoneal tissue debrided widely to remove all loculi of infection
  2. Peritoneal lavage performed and large drains placed to the pancreatic bed.
- Mortality for necrosectomy, lavage and drainage is 25%.

Pancreatic abscess

- Circumscribed collection of pus adjacent to the pancreas with little or no necrosis
- Arises from liquefaction and infection of small areas of necrosis or secondary to infection of a pseudocyst
- Usually occurs after 4 weeks, as opposed to infected necrosis at 1–2 weeks
- At ≈ 4 weeks patient deteriorates with pain, anorexia, fever, tenderness with or without a mass
- Diagnosis is made by CT scan
- Surgical drainage is preferred as percutaneous drainage does not deal with loculi.

Haemorrhage

- Life-threatening haemorrhage occurs in 2%. Bleeding may occur into the GI tract, pancreas, retroperitoneum or pancreatic duct.

Gastritis, duodenitis, erosions or peptic ulcer

- Prophylactic use of H_2 receptor antagonist and sucralfate reduces incidence
- Diagnosis is made by endoscopy.

Left-sided portal hypertension and varices

- Splenic thrombosis results from pancreatic inflammation and leads to splenomegaly and development of collateral vessels around the greater curvature of the stomach
- Treatment is by splenectomy.

Vascular complications

- Vascular necrosis may develop when proteolytic enzymes and infection affect arteries around the pancreas. This leads to segmental vascular thrombosis and pseudoaneurysm formation (splenic, gastroduodenal or pancreatoduodenal arteries)
- The pseudoaneurysm may rupture with massive bleeding:
  1. intraperitoneal
  2. into pseudocyst
  3. retroperitoneal
  4. into pancreatic duct (haemosuccus pancreaticus)
- Diagnosis is by angiography or demonstrating leakage of contrast on dynamic CT scan
- Management is difficult: embolisation may be feasible or surgery is required with undersewing of affected vessel or pancreatic resection.

Prognosis (Table 13.3)

- Overall mortality from acute pancreatitis is 10%
- 40% of patients dying may only be diagnosed by post-mortem
- Of patients who die, 20% die in first 24 hours and 60% in the first week
- Gallstone pancreatitis has a worse prognosis than alcohol-induced pancreatitis
- Obese patients are at greater risk of necrosis and respiratory complications
- Elderly are at increased risk (> 60 years mortality is 28%).

Table 13.3 Incidence and mortality for acute pancreatitis

	Incidence (%)	Mortality (%)
Mild acute pancreatitis	75	0.3
Severe acute pancreatitis	25	25

PREVENTION OF RECURRENCE

Cause should be identified and removed.

1. Gallstones
   a. Laparoscopic cholecystectomy and bile duct clearance

- If possible in the same admission; 10% of patients will have a further attack within 4 weeks
- Bile duct clearance may be performed by preoperative ERCP or at surgery
- ERCP and sphincterotomy
- Appears to be effective in the elderly and those with high co-morbidity

2. Alcohol
   a. Complete abstention
3. Idiopathic
   a. Search for underlying cause if more than one attack
   b. Endoluminal ultrasound to look for small bile duct stones and bile analysis for microcrystals
   c. Measure calcium and lipids.

CHRONIC PANCREATITIS

Definition
Spectrum of conditions with continuing irreversible pancreatic inflammation characterised by pain of varying severity and ultimately pancreatic atrophy with loss of exocrine and endocrine function.

Incidence

- Overall incidence $\approx 3/10^5$ (UK)
- Peak age is 35–45 years and incidence has increased in last 25 years (fourfold in men and doubled in women).

Aetiology

Alcohol

- Causative agent in 70% and more frequent in men
- Amount of alcohol and years consumption varies greatly, suggesting other co-factors are also important
- Disease may progress despite abstinence from alcohol.

Obstructive pancreatitis
Form of chronic pancreatitis secondary to ductal obstruction. Causes include:

- Traumatic ductal stricture
- Stones
- Pseudocysts
- Tumours
- Pancreas divisum.

Differs from alcoholic pancreatitis in that the obstructed ductal epithelium is usually preserved and the obstructed pancreas shows uniform inflammatory change. Calcification and stone formation is rare.

Tropical pancreatitis

- Thought to be caused by protein malnutrition in impoverished areas of the developing world or by toxic cyanogens in cassava root
- Features are pain, diabetes and steatorrhoea secondary to protein insufficiency
- Characterised by excessive pancreatic calcification.

Hereditary pancreatitis

- Rare; autosomal dominant with incomplete penetrance
- Presents between age 5 and 15 years
- Associated with hyperlipidaemia and aminoaciduria
- Increased risk of pancreatic cancer.

Hypercalcaemia

- Elevated calcium levels secondary to hyperparathyroidism or chronic renal failure can cause both acute and chronic pancreatitis.

Biliary disease

- Rarely causes chronic pancreatitis but chronic pancreatitis may lead to biliary stasis and common bile duct stones.

Idiopathic

- In approximately one-third no aetiological agent is identified.

Others

- Cystic fibrosis and radiotherapy are rare causes.

Pathogenesis
Decreased bicarbonate and water secretion secondary to alcohol toxicity lead to hypersecretion of protein from acinar cells. Protein plugs are formed within ducts and become calcified, by the precipitation of calcium carbonate, forming stones particularly in alcoholic, hereditary and tropical pancreatitis. Alcohol may also impair hepatic detoxification, thus generating toxic free-radicals, which lead to progressive pancreatic damage.

Morphological changes in chronic pancreatitis are extremely variable with oedema, acute inflammation and necrosis superimposed on chronic inflammatory changes with marked fibrosis, loss of acinar cells and ultimately loss of endocrine cells. Ductal system shows variable dilatation and stricture formation. Perineural inflammation and damage may be responsible for chronic pain. Extension of the inflammatory process may lead to CBD obstruction, splenic vein thrombosis and left-sided portal hypertension.

Clinical features

There are few physical signs: evidence of weight loss, epigastric tenderness, rarely a mass.

Pain

- Principal feature often associated with nausea but rarely vomiting
- Localised to epigastric or subcostal area radiating to the back or scapula
- Usually constant with acute exacerbations
- Sometimes helped by leaning forward and may be aggravated by eating
- Addiction to narcotic analgesia is common.

Steatorrhoea

- Occurs with loss of acinar cells or ductal obstruction but is not invariable.

Diabetes

- Occurs late, after exocrine insufficiency
- May progress from diet-controlled through to insulin-dependent.

Weight loss

- Common from malnutrition and also anorexia because of pain
- Exocrine and endocrine insufficiency also contribute.

Investigations

Blood

- No diagnostic serum test
- Serum amylase, lipase or CRP is usually normal unless there is an acute exacerbation
- Thrombocythaemia may be present with hypersplenism
- Blood glucose to exclude diabetes.

Imaging

1. Abdominal X-ray
   - May show pancreatic calcification
2. Ultrasound
   - Excludes gallstones or bile duct dilatation
3. CT scan
   - Investigation of choice with highest sensitivity and specificity for the diagnosis of chronic pancreatitis
   - Shows morphology of the gland and defines the duct
   - Reveals complications such as cyst formation, abscess and necrosis

4. ERCP
   - Complementary to CT and outlines pancreatic duct showing dilatation, stenosis, stones or fistula.

Pancreatic function tests

- Rarely performed now as they provide little diagnostic information
- Measure bicarbonate and enzyme concentration in duodenal juice after a test meal (Lundh test) or secretin-CCK stimulation.

Management
The majority of patients can be managed conservatively for long periods. Surgery does not reverse the loss of exocrine or endocrine function. Principles of management are:

1. Eliminate aetiology
2. Define disease process
   a. Obstruction
   b. Parenchymal.

Conservative

1. Complete abstinence from alcohol
2. Correct metabolic problems
   a. Diabetes
   b. Steatorrhoea: pancreatic enzyme supplements with all meals
   c. Anorexia: vitamin supplements may be required
3. Analgesia
   a. Try to avoid morphine-based drugs to prevent addiction
   b. Use paracetamol or codeine-based drugs
   c. Coeliac plexus block is rarely helpful in long-term management
4. Intestinal rest
   a. Often helps pancreatic pain during acute exacerbations
   b. Provided by TPN, analgesia and H_2 receptor antagonist.

Surgery
The main indications for surgery are obstruction or intractable pain when all conservative measures have failed.
   Biliary tract obstruction   May occur in 30% but is rarely complete. Usually occurs as tapering stricture in the retropancreatic bile duct and caused by oedema or cyst. A temporary endoscopic stent may allow resolution but if the stricture persists surgical bypass by choledochoduodenostomy or Roux-en-Y choledochojejunostomy.
   Pseudocyst   Occurs in 25% and if < 6 cm may be observed by serial scanning. Cysts > 6 cm for more than 6 weeks require drainage.

- Percutaneous drainage leads to recurrence in 70% and may cause fistula
- Endoscopic transgastric stenting is attractive minimally invasive approach but risks other organ injury and bleeding
- Surgical drainage with biopsy of cyst wall for histology
  1. Cystgastrostomy
  2. Cystjejunostomy
  3. Distal pancreatectomy for cyst in tail.

Cyst rupture is a serious complication leading to fistula formation and pancreatic ascites. Immediate management by TPN and somatostatin. ERCP identifies site of leak and a surgical drainage procedure is performed.

Portal hypertension Occurs with splenic vein thrombosis causing left-sided portal hypertension and splenomegaly. This leads to the development of varices and hypersplenism with the risk of acute bleeding. Treatment is by distal pancreatectomy and splenectomy.

Pancreatic duct obstruction Ductal obstruction leads to dilatation and exacerbates pain and exocrine failure. Surgery may offer good relief, by longitudinal pancreato-jejunostomy, provided the pancreatic duct > 7 mm.

Pancreatic resection Indication is intractable pain when all other measures have failed. Resection will not reverse the process of chronic pancreatitis. Best indication is for disease limited to head (Whipple's procedure) or body/tail (distal pancreatectomy). Pain improvement is reported in 75% but symptoms usually return within 5 years. Chronic pancreatitis generally affects the whole gland and extent of resection has to be balanced against development of brittle diabetes and exocrine failure.

Prognosis

- 50% mortality over 25 years. 20% due to complications associated with attack of acute pancreatitis (sepsis, bleeding). Remainder from complications of alcohol, tobacco and malnutrition
- Long-term diabetes in 50%; steatorrhoea in 60%
- Most patients are managed conservatively and successfully.

PANCREATIC CARCINOMA

Incidence and geography

- Increasing incidence in developed countries, now $\approx 10/10^5$ (UK)
- Peak age is 60–80 years and male:female incidence 1.5:1
- Highest incidence is in affluent countries and Asian immigrants to USA exhibit an increased incidence implicating environmental and dietary factors
- Identified risk factors include smoking ($\times 2$), carcinogens (β-naphthelyene, benzidine, ethylene dichloride), black skin and hereditary pancreatitis.

Pathology

- Ductal adenocarcinoma (90%)
- Periampullary carcinoma
- Mucinous/serous cystadenocarcinoma.

Spread

- Direct extension:
  From head to bile duct, duodenum, mesenteric vessels
  From body and tail to retroperitoneum, stomach, spleen
- Lymphatic: to local lymph nodes, porta hepatis and coeliac axis
- Blood-borne: to liver, lungs.

Clinical features

Adenocarcinoma of head

- Obstructive jaundice: 90%; progressive with pruritus
- Weight loss: prominent and secondary to anorexia and malabsorption
- Abdominal pain: 70%; epigastric radiating through to back
- Anorexia
- Nausea.

Adenocarcinoma of body/tail

- Weight loss: insidious onset and asymptomatic early on
- Anorexia
- Back pain
- Mass
- Diabetes.

Diagnosis and investigation

Pancreatic cancer is relatively inaccessible for visualisation and therefore histological confirmation is difficult. The diagnosis is made by a combination of investigations that also serve to stage the disease.

1. Ultrasound
   - First investigation in a patient with obstructive jaundice or epigastric mass
   - May reveal dilated bile duct and hypoechoic lesion in pancreas
   - Overall sensitivity is 70%
2. ERCP
   - Next investigation for obstructive jaundice and dilated bile duct
   - Typically show shouldered stricture of bile and pancreatic duct
   - Brushings may be obtained from the stricture for cytology and biopsy of the papilla to diagnose periampullary carcinoma

- If possible, endoscopic stent should be placed to relieve jaundice
3. CT scan
   - Most useful modality and shows focal mass without evidence of acute or chronic pancreatitis
   - Overall sensitivity is 90%
4. CA 19–9
   - Most useful serum tumour marker with sensitivity of 90%
   - Also elevated in cholecystitis and cholangitis
5. Percutaneous biopsy
   - CT-guided fine-needle aspiration cytology may be helpful
   - However, high rate of false-negative results precludes routine use.

Staging

1. Chest X-ray
   - Lung metastases
2. CT scan
   - Liver metastases
   - Poor for assessment of lymph nodes and resectability
3. Endoluminal ultrasound
   - Best modality for identifying small tumours
   - Assesses resectability, lymph nodes and involvement of mesenteric vessels
4. Laparoscopy
   - Allows inspection of liver and peritoneum for metastases, invasion of mesocolon
   - Combined with laparoscopic ultrasound for nodal and vessel involvement.

Treatment

Surgical resection
Surgical resection offers only hope of cure. Only 20% of tumours in the head, 3% in body or tail, are resectable. Resection is not justified unless macroscopically complete.

Proximal pancreatoduodenectomy (Whipple's procedure)
Removes distal stomach, distal CBD, pancreatic head and duodenum en bloc. Reconstruction by proximal jejunum to pancreas, bile duct and stomach. Procedure of choice for periampullary or pancreatic head tumours. Carries high morbidity (pancreatic fistula, abscess, bile leak) and mortality of 5–10%.

Distal pancreatectomy   Combined with splenectomy for tumours in the body or tail. Adenocarcinoma is rarely resectable but cystadenocarcinoma may be.

Adjuvant therapy
There is no proven benefit from either neo-adjuvant or adjuvant chemotherapy or radiotherapy.

Palliation
Palliative treatment will apply to the majority (80%) of patients.
Aims are to:

* Relieve jaundice
* Relieve or prevent duodenal obstruction
* Control pain.

1. Jaundice
   a. Endoscopic stent
   b. Percutaneous stent (or combined procedure)
   c. Biliary drainage: choledochoduodenostomy or Roux-en-Y
      choledochojejunostomy
      Choice of procedure depends on individual patient and
      co-morbidity. Randomised studies show equally effective relief
      of jaundice by operative or endoscopic methods. Operation
      allows assessment of resectability, combined with
      gastrojejunostomy to prevent duodenal obstruction and longer
      relief of jaundice. However, operation carries a higher 30-day
      mortality and longer recovery.
2. Duodenal obstruction
   * Occurs in 20% of patients
   * Requires gastrojejunostomy, which may be performed
     laparoscopically
3. Pain
   * Extremely common feature
   * Early involvement of palliative care team is important
   * Specific measures include:
     a. Opioid analgesia
     b. Coeliac plexus block
     c. Continuous analgesia by syringe driver
     d. Radiotherapy.

Prognosis (Table 13.4)
Overall 5-year survival is < 2%.

PANCREATIC TRAUMA

Table 13.4   Prognosis of pancreatic adenocarcinoma

	Proportion at presentation (%)	5-year survival (%)	Median survival (months)
Resected	20	10	14
Non-resected	80	–	4

Trauma to the pancreas is rare. It is usually associated with other
injuries which contribute to the high morbidity and are the main
cause of mortality (< 10% of deaths are directly attributable to
pancreatic injury).

- Blunt
  - Usually road traffic accidents and more common in UK
  - Most injuries are anterior and mid-body as the pancreas is compressed against the vertebral column
- Penetrating
  - Secondary to knife or gunshot; seen most frequently in USA
  - Any part of the gland may be involved.

Investigations

1. CT scan
   - With intravenous contrast to assess pancreatic and ductal integrity
   - May need to be repeated at 48 hours as signs develop
2. ERCP
   - Useful in stable patient to identify ductal injury.

Classification

I   Superficial contusion without ductal injury (80%)
II   Partial or complete pancreatic duct transection in body or tail
III Pancreatic duct injury in head or injury of intrapancreatic CBD
IV   Combined pancreato-duodenal injury.

Management

- 75% of patients dying with a pancreatic injury do so within the first 48 hours from associated injuries
- Management is directed to immediate resuscitation and then correction and treatment of immediate life-threatening injuries
- Specific treatment is governed by the type of pancreatic injury:
  - I   Conservative management only is required
  - II   With no duct damage drainage only is required. Duct damage to the left of the superior mesenteric vessels is treated by distal pancreatectomy and drainage
  - III On-table pancreatogram to assess duct integrity. If the duct is intact a drain is placed. Isolated duct injury is managed by onlay pancreato-jejunostomy
  - IV   Primary repair of duodenum.
       Roux-en-Y duodenojejunostomy and pancreatojejunostomy
       Duodenal diversion
       Whipple procedure.

CONGENITAL ANOMALIES OF THE PANCREAS

ANNULAR PANCREAS

- Encirclement of duodenum by pancreatic tissue
- Incidence $5/10^5$
- May cause duodenal obstruction in infants; abdominal pain or duodenal ulcer in adults
- Treatment is by duodenoduodenostomy or duodenojejunostomy.

HETEROTOPIC PANCREAS

- Pancreatic tissue has been described in a number of sites including jejunum, Meckel's diverticulum and stomach
- Usually small (< 0.5 cm) and in submucosal layer
- Rarely causes clinical symptoms and is found incidentally.

PANCREAS DIVISUM

- In 5% of people the ducts of Santorini and Wirsung do not communicate within the pancreas. The duct of Santorini then drains the dorsal pancreas, and the majority of pancreatic juice, through the minor papilla
- Majority of patients are asymptomatic but the condition may cause pancreatic pain or pancreatitis
- Treatment is by sphincterotomy of the minor papilla or stenting.

ENDOCRINE TUMOURS OF THE PANCREAS
(Table 13.5)

- Rare: annual incidence $4/10^6$
- May be functioning (75%) or non-functioning (25%)
- Cell of origin is unclear as some produce hormone not normally found in the pancreas or multiple hormones
- May be part of MEN 1 (Wermer's syndrome) – associated with hyperparathyroidism but without medullary cell carcinoma or phaeochromocytoma.

Table 13.5   Pancreatic endocrine tumours (PET)

Tumour syndrome	Incidence (cases/10^6/year)	Primary symptoms	Rate of malignancy	Hormone
Functional PET				
Gastrinoma (Z–E syndrome)	0.5–1.5	Abdominal pain 75% Diarrhoea 65% Dysphagia	60–90%	Gastrin
Insulinoma	1–2	Hypoglycaemia	< 10%	Insulin
VIPoma (Verner–Morrison syndrome)	0.05–0.2	Diarrhoea 100% Flushing 20%	> 60%	VIP
Glucagonoma	0.01–0.1	Dermatitis 80% Weight loss 80% Diarrhoea 15%	50–80%	Glucagon
Somatostatinoma	Rare	Diarrhoea 50%	> 70%	Somatostatin
Non-functional PET				
PPoma	1–2	–	> 60%	Pancreatic polypeptide
Other	1–2	–	> 60%	No

Diagnosis

- Key to making diagnosis is to suspect the syndrome
- Measure serum peptide concentration
- For insulinoma measure C-peptide and pro-insulin – both are elevated in insulinoma but decreased with the use of exogenous insulin.

  Localise by:

- CT scan
  - Size-dependent and will miss small tumours (sensitivity < 70%)
  - Detects metastatic disease
- Angiography
  - Most are hypervascular
- Selective venous sampling
- Endoluminal ultrasound
- Intra-operative ultrasound.

Treatment

- Resection for solitary functioning tumour
- If tumour is metastatic, unresectable or non-detectable then octreotide is the most useful drug for control of symptoms.

FURTHER READING

Trede M, Carter DC 1997 Surgery of the pancreas, 2nd edn.

14. Hepato-biliary surgery

Adam Widdison

HEPATO-BILIARY ASSESSMENT

The liver is the largest solid organ in the body. It is vital for gluconeogenesis, protein synthesis (principally albumin), manufacturing clotting factors, bile production, detoxification and as part of the reticulo-endothelial system. Hepato-biliary disease frequently affects these functions early so they must be assessed both clinically and through investigations.

The assessment of most patients with hepato-biliary disease is straightforward. On occasions, however, the presentation is atypical and a detailed and careful assessment is required. An accurate history and examination are vital to ensure the most appropriate of the many available investigations are used to make the diagnosis and treatment is tailored to suit the patient.

HISTORY – GENERAL

Most patients with hepato-biliary disease present with abdominal pain, jaundice or a mass, or a combination of these. A few present with vague symptoms of being unwell, with weight loss, the effects of portal hypertension (varices, ascites) or of liver failure (oedema, coagulopathy, hypoglycaemia, sepsis). Rarely, asymptomatic derangements in liver function are detected during screening investigations.

Pain

The liver and biliary tree are foregut structures innervated by vagal and T 7–9 sympathetic afferents. Pain is usually localised to the right hypochondrium or presents as an upper abdominal pain worse on the right than the left. Localisation is better when inflammation irritates the overlying somatically innervated parietal peritoneum, as occurs in acute cholecystitis. Pain may be referred to the right subscapular region or to the shoulder when the diaphragm is irritated.

Hepato-biliary pain may be caused by

- Gallstones in biliary colic
- Cholecystitis
- Choledocholithiasis
- Cholangitis

- Hepatitis
- Choledochal cyst.

Differential diagnosis

- Appendicitis
- Acute pancreatitis
- Peptic ulcer
- Shingles
- Pleurisy
- Pneumonia
- Ischaemic heart disease.

Malignant obstructive jaundice, liver cysts, liver cancer and liver secondaries are usually relatively painless.

Infrequently, acute cholecystitis, necrotising cholecystitis, empyema of the gallbladder, and biliary peritonitis from a perforated gallbladder present with generalised peritonitis. Clinically it may be impossible to distinguish these from more common causes of peritonitis such as perforated appendicitis, perforated peptic ulcer, acute pancreatitis, intestinal perforation, ischaemic bowel or acute colitis.

Jaundice
A full history and careful examination will usually discriminate between 'medical' (for example hepatitis, cirrhosis) and 'surgical' causes of jaundice but further investigations are always required (Fig. 14.1).

A full history is vital in directing the clinician to the correct diagnosis and should include:

- Race (Far East)
- Occupation (e.g. exposure to industrial solvents)
- Diet (aflatoxin)
- Foreign travel (e.g. to hepatitis endemic areas)
- Recent transfusion of blood products (hepatitis)
- Medication (including ethanol or intravenous drug abuse)
- Sexual history (hepatitis)
- Co-morbidity (e.g. Crohn's or ulcerative colitis)
- Family history (e.g. infective and auto-immune hepatitis, metabolic liver disease).

Surgical causes are usually associated with obstructive jaundice which presents with pruritus, dark orange or murky brown urine and pale grey stools.

Mass
Occasionally, patients present with an abdominal mass. These are usually of a large size with a persistent aching discomfort in the right upper quadrant. Malignant masses are associated with

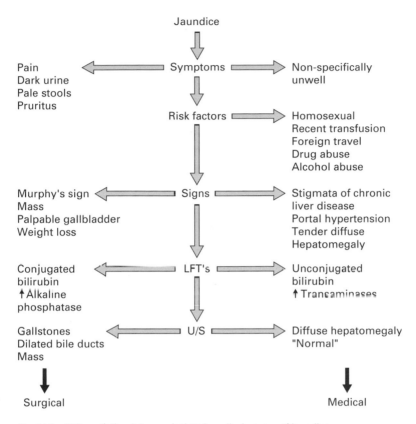

Fig. 14.1 Differentiation into surgical and medical causes of jaundice.

weight loss and cachexia. The causes of hepatomegaly are presented in Table 14.1.

EXAMINATION

General
Liver disease usually makes patients look ill and, if chronic, lose weight whether it is due to malignant secondaries, hepatitis or cirrhosis. Cholecystitis, cholangitis, liver abscesses and hepatitis cause a fever.

Specific
- It is unusual to clinically detect jaundice if the bilirubin is less than 40
- In obstructive jaundice, pruritus may be manifest as excoriation

Table 14.1   Differential diagnosis of 'hepatomegaly'

	Solitary	Diffuse	Multinodular
Congenital	Riedel's lobe	–	Polycystic liver disease
Inflammatory	Liver abscess	Hepatitis	–
Parasitic	Hydatid, amoebic	–	–
Neoplastic	Hepatocellular cancer Metastasis	Metastasis	Metastasis
Drugs	Pill tumour	Alcohol	Alcohol
Haemopoietic		Lymphoma Polycythaemia Myelodysplasia	
Metabolic		Haemochromatosis Wilson's disease Amyloidosis	
Gallbladder	Mucocoele Empyema Courvoisier's sign Cancer		
Bile duct	Choledochal cyst		

- The following suggest chronic liver cirrhosis and, although a hepatocellular carcinoma may present as a dominant mass, this is infrequent in Western countries:
  — Palmar erythema
  — Liver flap
  — Bruising
  — Spider naevi
  — Portal hypertension (Caput medusae)
  — Ascites
  — Gynaecomastia
  — Testicular atrophy
- On palpation, liver secondaries appear as an irregular liver surface. It is usually impossible to feel above a solitary liver mass. A mucocoele or empyema of the gallbladder may be palpated as low as the right lower quadrant. A palpable gallbladder in the jaundiced patient is unlikely to be caused by obstructing choledocholithiasis (Courvoisier's law).

NON-INVASIVE ASSESSMENT

Further investigations are required in all patients with hepato-biliary disease to confirm the diagnosis and assess liver function.

Liver function tests
The basic tests of liver function include assessment of anabolic processes by measuring:

1. Serum total protein
2. Albumin

3. Glucose
4. Prothrombin time (a measure of the extrinsic pathway of the coagulation cascade).

Prothrombin time is usually compared with a normal value and reported as international normalised ratio (INR). The prothrombin time is increased if the vitamin K and calcium-dependent factor VII is deficient. Serum bilirubin gives an insight into excretory function and serum levels of cellular enzymes, alkaline phosphatase and the serum transaminases reflect cellular damage.

Bilirubin is a breakdown product of the porphyrin component of haem from effete erythrocytes. It is bound to albumin in the blood and transported to the liver where it is conjugated with glucuronic acid to make it water-soluble. The normal production of 300 mg/day is greatly increased in haemolytic disorders (sickle cell disease, hereditary spherocytosis).

Haemolytic and most hepatocellular causes of jaundice are characterised by unconjugated hyperbilirubinaemia. Unconjugated hyperbilirubinaemia, in the absence of deranged liver function or haemolysis, occurs in Gilbert's syndrome. This benign condition affects 1–2% of females and 3–7% of males who are congenitally deficient in liver glucuronyl transferase. Elevated conjugated bilirubin is diagnostic of obstructive jaundice which is usually post-hepatic. Non-mechanical causes of obstructive jaundice (cholestatic) can be caused by drugs (for example oestrogens, anabolic steroids, chlorpromazine or methyldopa), pregnancy or inflammatory bowel disease.

Alkaline phosphatase is a membrane-bound enzyme localised to the bile canalicular pole of hepatocytes. During intra- or extrahepatic biliary obstruction, synthesis is increased and the enzyme is released into the blood. Serum alkaline phosphatase also arises from bone, small intestine or placenta. Other enzymes of the intrahepatic bile canaliculi elevated in the serum in biliary jaundice include gamma-glutamyl transferase, 5'-nucleotidase and leucine aminopeptidase.

The serum alanine (ALT) and aspartate (AST) aminotransferases are vital enzymes present in most cells to convert amino acids to the corresponding alpha keto acids. They are, however, particularly abundant in the liver and are released when hepatocytes are damaged. Marked elevation of these is characteristic of the acute and chronic forms of infectious, drug, metabolic, auto-immune, biliary and genetic liver diseases and occur to a lesser degree in obstructive jaundice. Lactate dehydrogenase is similarly abundant in many cells but elevations occur in many diseases and it is less specific for liver disease.

Patterns of abnormality in the liver function tests will suggest the nature of the liver damage and give an insight into severity (Table 14.2).

Table 14.2   Interpretation of serum liver function tests (+ = elevated, +++ = very high)

Onset	Type of jaundice	Alkaline phosphatase	Serum transaminase	Prothrombin time	Serum albumin
Acute					
	Obstructive	+++	+	+	Normal
	Hepatocellular	+	+++	++	Normal
Chronic					
	Obstructive	+++	+	+	Low
	Hepatocellular	+	+++	++	Very low

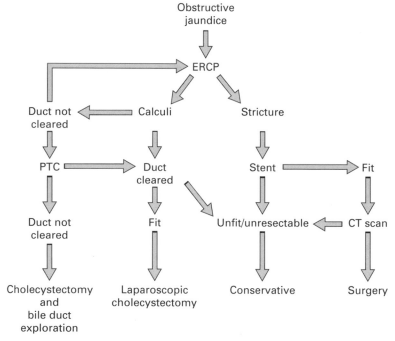

Fig. 14.2   Algorithm for the post-ultrasound management of obstructive jaundice.

An algorithm for the management of a patient with obstructive jaundice is illustrated in Figure 14.2.

Viral markers

The hepatotrophic viruses hepatitis A, B, C, and more recently G, are all associated with liver disease. At-risk groups include:

- Male homosexuals
- Intravenous drug abusers

- Haemophiliacs
- Recipients of blood transfusions
- Recent travellers to Africa or the Far East.

These patients, and those presenting with features atypical for obstructive jaundice, should be screened for viral infections by measuring viral antigens and immunological responses in the blood.

Antibody tests

- Immune tests are important in discriminating simple cysts shown on radiological tests from hydatid disease
- The intradermal Casoni test is inaccurate and no longer used
- Currently the most useful tests are the hydatid immunoelectrophoresis (IEP) and enzyme-linked immunosorbent assay (ELISA). IEP is useful to check that treatment has been successful and to screen for disease recurrence
- Antimitochondrial antibody is usually raised in primary biliary cirrhosis.

Other tests

- Alpha fetoprotein is elevated in hepatocellular cancer
- Alpha-1 antitrypsin deficiency is a cause of cirrhosis
- Caeruloplasmin is low in Wilson's disease
- Serum iron and total iron binding capacity are high in haemochromatosis.

Abdominal radiograph

- These are infrequently useful in hepatobiliary disease
- Less than 10% of gallstones are seen on plain abdominal radiographs
- Gas may be seen within the biliary tree in gallstone ileus, clostridial cholangitis, or after sphincterotomy, a biliary enteric anastomosis or stenting
- Gas seen within the liver suggests either an abscess or chlostridial cholangitis.

Ultrasound (US)

Application of an alternating voltage across a piezo-electric crystal causes high frequency vibration (0.5–20 Mhz). The higher the frequency, the greater the resolution but penetration is reduced. US waves are partially reflected from naturally occurring boundaries between different tissues within the body. Waves are almost totally reflected by calcification (gallstones) or gas/soft tissue interface. Reflected waves can be detected and the echo amplitude displayed as shades of black or white.

- US examination of the liver and biliary tree is simple and quick to perform, readily available and false-positives are rare

- It has become a first-line investigation in all patients suspected of hepato-biliary disease
- It is simple to perform, inexpensive and non-invasive
- There are no contraindications but its efficacy is dependent on the skill of the operator, the quality of the machine, obesity and gastrointestinal gas.

Oral cholecystogram
With the widespread availability of US, oral cholecystograms are rarely indicated. It may still be required if the US is not diagnostic or to assess gallbladder function prior to a trial of oral dissolution therapy for gallstones.

- Radio-opaque contrast (for example calcium iopodate) taken orally is excreted by the liver and concentrated by a functioning gallbladder
- Radiographs taken 12–18 hours after oral ingestion and fasting should show an opacified gallbladder
- Gallstones may be visualised as mobile filling defects and failure to opacify suggests a diseased gallbladder. Gallbladder emptying can then be observed in response to a fatty meal, or typical pain may be reproduced on gallbladder emptying
- The test is dependent on the contrast tablets being taken, normal liver function and the absence of diarrhoea.

Intravenous cholangiogram (IVC)
In the laparoscopic era there is a resurgence of interest in IVC for screening for choledocholithiasis in an attempt to reduce the number of ERCPs performed. The technique has the advantage of being a non-invasive method of screening the biliary tree in patients suspected of choledocholithiasis.

- It is contraindicated in patients with iodine or contrast sensitivity and is dependent on normal liver function
- A bolus intravenous injection of contrast is rapidly concentrated by the liver and excreted into bile
- Tomograms image the bile ducts
- The technique gives poorly defined images of the bile duct and small calculi may be missed.

Computed tomography (CT) scan
The CT scanner uses multiple circumferential fine collimated beams of X-rays and computer reconstruction to produce high definition radiographs of the body in transverse slices.

- The sensitivity and specificity depends on the quality of the machine, the distance between slices (usually 10 mm), the cooperation of the patient in breath holding and staying still and interference from foreign bodies such as stents or metal clips

- The disadvantages are that there is a high radiation exposure, oral and intravenous contrast are usually required, patients need to lie still and breath hold on demand, and the morbidly obese will break the machine
- Helical CT scans acquire data during a single breath hold and at increments as small as 0.5 cm with overlapping reconstruction
- Three-dimensional (3D) rendering of biliary and vascular structures can facilitate preoperative assessment and surgical planning, particularly in patients with cholangiocarcinoma or pancreatic cancer
- Contrast-enhanced CT scan is more sensitive than US scan in detecting liver lesions or a mass but is less useful in diagnosing gallstones and choledocholithiasis. Helical or spiral CT scans and 3D reconstruction software are, however, greatly improving resolution, diagnostic and anatomic accuracy
- In the future, increased sensitivity in the detection of choledocholithiasis may make it important in preoperative screening for choledocholithiasis.

Magnetic resonance imaging (MRI)

MRI produces multiplanar images with excellent tissue differentiation without using ionising radiation. MRI uses strong magnetic fields first to align tissue protons. The application of a radiofrequency pulse at 90° to this magnetic field causes the protons to change their alignment or resonance. Following the radiofrequency pulse the protons relax back to their previous state emitting characteristic radiofrequency waves which can be measured. The energy of this signal depends on the proton density. The time this relaxation takes also varies. Protons initially relax in phase with each other (T2 relaxation time or spin echo). Thereafter, because of the different proton densities and interactions between protons they relax out of phase until they return to their original positions of equilibrium within the magnetic field. The total time taken to reach equilibrium is the T1 relaxation time (inversion-recovery time). By measuring the initial size of the relaxation signal and its relaxation times the nuclear magnetic resonance parameters of a tissue can be recorded. Different initial radiofrequency pulse sequences will produce signals weighted to different proton density or degrees of T1 or T2 relaxation times.

- MRI is likely to become an important investigation of the liver with the increasing availability of rapid sequence MRI and the development of improved techniques and new contrast agents
- Liver MRI should be performed with a fast spin echo sequence and consist of both T1- and T2-weighted images with respiratory compensation or phase ordering
- Typically a stack of images can be acquired through the liver within 15 seconds but image quality is compromised by respiratory, muscle and bowel movement

- Intravenous contrast agents such as the gadolinium chelates improve diagnostic accuracy
- Novel MRI contrast agents are being developed which target specific cell types, for example super paramagnetic iron oxide particles which accumulate within Kupffer cells, or manganese chloride which targets the biliary tract
- Modern MRI may be more sensitive than contrast-enhanced CT scans in the detection of liver metastasis
- MRI may be particularly useful in diagnosing focal nodular hyperplasia with its central fibrous scar, distinguishing liver haemangiomata from metastasis, and regenerating nodules or adenomata from hepatocellular carcinoma.

Nuclear medicine

A gamma ray emitting radiopharmaceutical is administered intravenously. After allowing time for tissue distribution, gamma rays emitted cause sodium iodide crystals to liberate photons of light which are converted into a pulse of electricity or recorded on film. The number of photons is proportional to the concentration of radioactivity. The radiopharmaceutical used for hepato-biliary scintiscans is usually a technetium-99m-labelled derivative of ethyl hydroxyiminodiacetic acid (HIDA) which is rapidly concentrated in the liver and excreted into the bile. The isotope is further concentrated in the normal healthy gallbladder.

- In acute cholecystitis there is failure to concentrate HIDA. If the gallbladder is imaged contractility can also be assessed
- The definition of biliary anatomy is poor but a HIDA scan may be useful to assess biliary drainage, the patency of a biliary-enteric anastomosis or demonstrate a bile leak
- Other radiopharmaceuticals currently used include iodine (if thyroid metastases are suspected), somatostatin (if endocrine secondaries are suspected) and carcinoembryonic antigen (CEA) (to screen for colorectal secondaries)
- With increasing availability of specific radiopharmaceuticals, isotope scans may become more important.

Provocation tests

The gallbladder contracts upon stimulation by the hormone cholecystokinin-pancreozymin (CCK-PZ) released from the small intestine when exposed to fat. Exogenous CCK-PZ (1 unit/kg body weight infused over 5 minutes) similarly stimulates the gallbladder and may reproduce the patient's symptoms. The hormones' effects are not, however, confined to the gallbladder and the test is notoriously unreliable with false-positives in patients with irritable bowel and false-negatives in gallbladder disease.

INVASIVE INVESTIGATIONS

Endoscopic retrograde cholangiogram (ERC) or pancreatogram (ERP)

A side-viewing endoscope with at least one instrument channel is passed per orum into the duodenum. Withdrawal and rotation of the endoscope brings the ampulla of Vater into view. This can then be intubated under direct vision and contrast injected to delineate either the lumen of the biliary (ERC) or pancreatic ducts (ERP) using an X-ray image intensifier and coned X-ray films (Fig. 14.3).

- Brush cytology, biopsy of ampullary lesions, or bile collection for microscopy or cytology may be undertaken
- If calculi are imaged a sphincterotomy is performed and they can be removed using either a Dormia basket or balloon

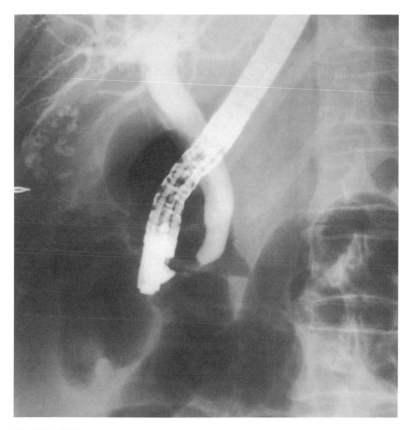

Fig. 14.3 ERC.

- Large stones may be crushed, or fragmented with a hydraulic or laser lithotriptor
- Cotton-Leung stents can be placed across strictures or if calculi cannot be removed
- Concerns about late strictures after performing sphincterotomy in young patients have not so far been realised.

ERC may be used for both diagnosis and therapy. Indications include:

- The investigation of atypical upper abdominal pain
- Suspected choledocholithiasis or choledochal cyst
- Obstructive jaundice
- Biliary acute pancreatitis
- Sclerosing cholangitis
- Investigating bile duct trauma or a cystic duct leak.

For toleration of intravenous sedo-analgesia patients need a combination of an opiate (for example fentanyl) and a benzodiazepine (for example midazolam). Clotting abnormalities are corrected beforehand and a group and save sent. Prophylactic antibiotics (for example oral ciprofloxacin) are required. ERC is technically difficult when large diverticula hide the ampulla of Vater and impossible if the second part of the duodenum cannot be accessed (for example duodenal obstruction or after a Polya gastrectomy).

ERC is successful in imaging the ducts in 90–95% of attempts depending on the expertise of the operator. When intubation of the ampulla is unsuccessful a guidewire may be inserted percutaneously transhepatically by a radiologist or at operation through the cystic duct. This can then be used by the endoscopist.

Complications occur in up to 5% of patients and include:

- Bleeding (usually only after a sphincterotomy)
- Acute pancreatitis (particularly if a pancreatogram is performed or repeated cannulations of the ampulla are required)
- Cholangitis
- Perforation.

Endoluminal endoscopic or laparoscopic US

Endoscopic endoluminal or laparoscopic US use a B mode linear or radial contact US probe on the end of an endoscope or laparoscope. A high frequency probe gives high resolution, and the close proximity to the areas of interest reduces the need for penetration. Endoluminal US is performed in a similar way to an upper GIT endoscopy. The endoscope is passed into the stomach or duodenum and a balloon inflated with water. This provides the medium through which the ultrasound waves pass. It is easier and simpler to perform and has fewer complications than ERCP. Laparoscopic US is performed through a standard 10 mm port and can be used throughout the abdomen as a contact US probe.

The indications for endoluminal US include patients suspected of distal bile duct calculi, and cystic or solid lesions in the head of the pancreas or porta hepatis. Endoluminal ultrasound is likely to become more widely used in the future. With increased availability and expertise it may reduce the number of diagnostic ERCPs required by screening the distal bile duct, a section poorly visualised by standard US methods. It may also aid in discriminating between chronic pancreatitis and carcinoma of the head of the pancreas, and in the staging of cholangiocarcinoma and pancreatic cancer.

Percutaneous cholangiogram (PTC)

Percutaneous imaging of the biliary tree is used when ERC is unavailable or unsuccessful or to assist endoscopic intubation. The indications are the same as those for ERCP. A catheter is inserted into a peripheral bile duct using a Seldinger technique under either US or CT control. The bile duct can then be imaged by taking X-rays after injection of contrast. In patients with a bile duct stricture the biliary tree can be decompressed with an internal-external biliary drain and a stent placed across the stricture.

Percutaneous access to the Roux loop of a hepaticodocho-jejunostomy can also be used to diagnose and treat anastomotic strictures. This can be facilitated by apposing part of the Roux loop to the abdominal wall laterally and marking the position with metal clips or steel wire.

Liver biopsy

Improved laboratory investigations and radiologic techniques have reduced the need for liver biopsies. It is still necessary, however, in many patients with hepatitis, cirrhosis, after liver transplantation or when a histological diagnosis of a solid liver lesion is required. If resection of a liver tumour is contemplated a liver biopsy risks seeding the track and is rarely performed.

Diagnostic laparoscopy

Diagnostic laparoscopy complements other techniques particularly if combined with laparoscopic ultrasound or biopsy. It is particularly useful for staging malignant disease or diagnosing carcinomatosis peritonei when this is suspected clinically but cannot be demonstrated by radiological techniques. It does, however, require a general anaesthetic with muscle relaxation and risks dissemination of malignant disease and port site recurrence. With the use of low insufflation pressures and smaller (2 mm) telescopes and instruments it may become possible to perform under local anaesthesia.

Open

There is really no place for open surgery for diagnosis in the laparoscopic era.

THERAPY – GENERAL

The aims of therapy need to be clearly defined and tailored to suit both the patient and the abnormality. On the one hand liver cancer can be cured with hemihepatectomy, on the other multiple liver secondaries frequently need symptomatic palliative care. In this section non-invasive supportive measures are discussed. Specific treatments will be discussed in the next section.

Antibiotics

Bactobilia is frequently associated with gallstones, bile duct obstruction and an endoprosthesis, and cholangio-venous reflux can cause bacteraemias. Therefore, any biliary intervention requires prophylactic antibiotics. Antibiotics, however, are not indicated for the treatment of biliary colic or obstructive jaundice per se.

* Most biliary infections are caused by Gram-negative enteric aerobes (Table 14.3)
* Acute cholecystitis usually responds to a cephalosporin such as cephradine or cefuroxime. More serious infections, such as ascending cholangitis, are treated with third-generation cephalosporins (for example cefotaxime), pipericillin or ciprofloxacin
* *Streptococcus faecalis* is a common biliary pathogen which is resistant to many penicillins and cephalosporins, and aminoglycosides reach poor levels in bile
* Rarely, gas-forming *Clostridia* and anaerobes cause necrotising cholecystitis or cholangitis. High-dose broad-spectrum cover is required.

It is a fundamental surgical principle that infection is rarely eliminated while a duct remains obstructed or if devitalised tissue is infected. Therefore, in ascending cholangitis, necrotising cholecystitis, an empyema of the gallbladder, or a liver abscess, antibiotics are used in conjunction with either drainage or cholecystectomy.

Table 14.3 Principal bacterial isolates from bile (NB isolates are frequently polymicrobial)

	Ascending cholangitis (%)	*Uncomplicated cholelithiasis (%)*
Klebsiella	41	11
E. coli	36	38
Enterococci	38	15
Enterobacter	16	5
Proteus	< 5	6
Staphylococci	< 5	5
Anaerobes	< 5	10

Fluid balance

- Patients admitted with obstructive jaundice are at risk of developing renal failure. This is largely caused by hypovolaemia but other factors such as atrial naturetic peptide and endotoxaemia may be important
- Renal failure can be prevented by restoring and maintaining circulating volume to ensure more than 30 ml/min urine output. Most patients drink enough normally and it is therefore necessary only to monitor the urine output
- For patients with profound jaundice and oliguria, intravenous rehydration and hourly monitoring of urine output are required
- The role of mannitol is controversial. It was traditional practice to give a rapid infusion of 10% mannitol (1 g/kg body weight) to 'flush out' the endotoxins and 'kick start' the kidneys. The resulting diuresis can, however, give a false sense of security causing intracellular dehydration and aggravating the hypovolaemia
- In patients with significantly compromised liver function, fluid and salt restriction is necessary with careful monitoring of fluid balance.

Analgesia

- Biliary pain usually responds to non-steroidal analgesics (for example diclofenac) given orally or rectally
- The intramuscular route should be avoided if clotting is abnormal
- If a stronger analgesic is required, pethidine is preferred because it does not significantly increase the tone of the sphincter of Oddi
- Opiates and drugs metabolised by the liver should be used with caution in patients with liver failure. On the other hand, terminally ill patients often require large doses of opiates
- Acute liver swelling from multiple liver secondaries may be helped by dexamethasone.

Coagulation

- Vitamin K is fat-soluble requiring intestinal bile and micelle formation to be absorbed. It is vital for the hepatic synthesis of clotting factors II, VII, IX, X
- All jaundiced patients and patients with liver failure are coagulopathic with a tendency to bruise and bleed. Haematologically they have a prolonged prothrombin time (increased INR)
- Derangement of the coagulation abnormalities can be corrected by Vitamin K (10 mg intravenously per day). This usually takes at least 24 hours to work
- In emergencies, rapid intravenous infusion of fresh frozen plasma will temporarily restore INR to normal.

Protein

- In liver failure, hypoalbuminaemia may cause sequestration of fluid in the extravascular compartment. This usually corrects with treatment of liver failure
- Intravenous salt poor albumin may be required.

Pruritus

- This merits treatment if severe
- Antihistamines (for example chlorphenyramine), topical creams or cholestyramine may provide some relief until definitive therapy relieves the jaundice.

GALLSTONES

Gallstones are stones that arise from the gallbladder. They may remain in the gallbladder or migrate into the main bile duct through the cystic duct. Rarely, calculi form de novo in the bile duct itself.

Presentation

Most gallstones are asymptomatic. The remainder present with biliary colic, cholecystitis (Table 14.4), or a complication such as acute pancreatitis or obstructive jaundice (Fig. 14.4).

Pathogenesis

- Most gallstones are composed of alternating layers of cholesterol crystals and mucin glycoproteins with protein, bilirubin and calcium salts intermixed
- Less frequent are the black pigment stones associated with chronic haemolytic disorders (which consist of polymers of bilirubin and mucin glycoproteins), and the brown pigment stones associated with bactobilia (made of calcium salts of unconjugated bilirubin)

Table 14.4   Differential diagnosis of biliary colic

	Biliary colic	Cholecystitis
Onset	Rapid	Gradual
Nature	Colic	Constant
Pyrexia	Absent	Present
Peritonism	Absent	Present
Murphy's sign	Weak	Positive
Mass	Absent	Present in empyema
Leucocyte count	Normal	Elevated
Liver function	Normal	May be abnormal
Gallbladder on ultrasound	Thin-walled	Thick-walled, pericystic fluid
HIDA scan	Normal	Non-functioning gallbladder

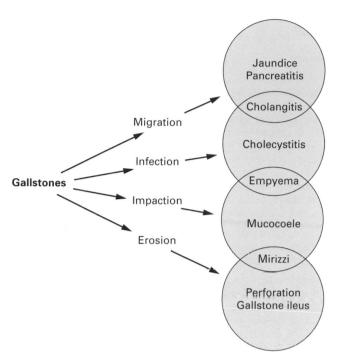

Fig. 14.4 Complications of gallstones.

- In its crudest sense, gallstones form when the cholesterol concentration in bile exceeds the available bile acids and phospholipids required for solubility in the form of micelles
- Stone formation in supersaturated bile is then dependent on the balance between nucleating or stone forming factors such as mucin, glycoprotein, desquamated cells and bacteria and antinucleating factors such as lipid vesicles and apolipoproteins, and the duration of stasis.

Epidemiology

- 17% of adults will develop gallstones of which only about one-third become symptomatic
- Females are affected more frequently than males and prevalence increases with age and obesity so that 30% of women over 80 years of age have gallstones
- Gallbladder sludge, the precursor of gallstones, frequently occurs with pregnancy, prolonged total parenteral nutrition, starvation or rapid weight loss
- Other risk factors for gallstones include decreased serum high-density lipoprotein cholesterol and increased triglyceride,

disease of the terminal ileum (disrupts the entero-hepatic circulation of bile salts) and oestrogen treatment.

Assessment

- Most patients admitted to hospital with biliary colic or cholecystitis require basic haematological and biochemical investigations and non-invasive monitoring of their vital signs
- Patients with severe acute cholecystitis, ascending cholangitis, empyema, necrotising cholecystitis or biliary peritonitis require invasive monitoring in a high-dependency or intensive care unit
- Liver function tests and an US scan are performed on all patients
- An algorithm for the management of patients with biliary pain is illustrated in Figure 14.5 and for the management of jaundice in Figure 14.2.

The vast majority of gallstones are diagnosed by their characteristic appearance and acoustic shadow on US. Further information from the US scan is helpful in planning management:

- Are there multiple stones or a single large impacted stone?
- How thick and inflamed is the gallbladder wall, or is it a mucocoele or empyema?
- Could gallbladder cancer be present?
- What is the diameter of the main bile duct and can bile duct stones be imaged?

In the laparoscopic era it is important to make a preoperative diagnosis of Mirizzi's syndrome. Type I Mirizzi's syndrome occurs when a large gallstone is impacted in Hartmann's pouch and is eroding into the main bile duct. Type II is found when the calculus has eroded through causing a cholecyst-hepatic fistula. The clinical features, deranged LFTs and US appearance will usually suggest the diagnosis which is then confirmed on ERC.

Rarely the symptoms suggest biliary colic but the US scan is normal. If, in a patient with typical biliary pain, a repeat US scan is still inconclusive, an oral cholecystogram, HIDA scan or provocation test may provide further information. Pain arising from sphincter of Oddi spasm or irritable bowel syndrome can mimic biliary colic.

Therapy

Surgery

Indications   Cholecystectomy is the treatment of choice for symptomatic gallstones to treat pain and prevent complications. Within 1 year, one-third of patients with biliary colic will get severe biliary pain and one-fifth acute cholecystitis or another serious complication if left untreated. Asymptomatic gallstones do not usually require treatment. Only 18% go on to develop biliary colic

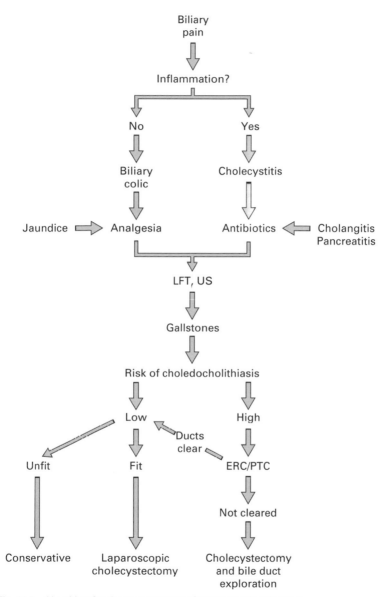

Fig. 14.5 Algorithm for the management of symptomatic gallstones.

over 20 years and the mortality from the operation is greater than from the condition. Exceptions include children, sickle cell disease, and 'porcelain' gallbladder (premalignant). Incidental cholecystectomies are performed as part of a Whipple's procedure, bile duct resection or hemi-hepatectomy. It is rarely indicated if gallstones are found incidentally while performing a laparotomy for another procedure.

Contraindications Patients need to be fit for a general anaesthetic and to withstand upper abdominal surgery.

There are no absolute contraindications to laparoscopic cholecystectomy. The relative contraindications include choledocholithiasis, intra-abdominal adhesions and intra-abdominal cancer. In obese patients, laparoscopic surgery is easier to perform than open surgery. The conversion rate to an open procedure is increased if the operation is performed as an emergency and in patients with a history of recurrent cholecystitis or who have had previous surgery.

Assessment Patients need to be fit for a general anaesthetic. Specific preoperative investigations depend on the availability of local facilities and expertise. In many centres patients are screened for choledocholithiasis preoperatively (Table 14.5). Choledocholithiasis is present in about 15% of patients with gallstones, of which about half become symptomatic over 10 years.

Patients at risk of choledocholithiasis require cholangiography (endoscopic, intravenous or operative). The advantages and disadvantages of selective preoperative ERC compared with routine cholangiography are presented in Table 14.6.

Cholecystectomy The principle of the operation are the same whether it is performed laparoscopically, through a small (< 10 cm) incision (mini-cholecystectomy), or by the open approach (Table 14.7).

There are essentially 3 parts to the operation:

1. Expose the gallbladder
   a. At open surgery a transverse subcostal or upper midline incision are used
   b. For laparoscopic surgery a pneumoperitoneum is created using either a Veres needle or by placement of an operating port (e.g. a Hassan cannula) under direct vision

Table 14.5   Risk factors for choledocholithiasis

Risk factors	Risk of choledocholithiasis (%)
Biliary colic (no risk factors)	< 1
History of jaundice	40
Jaundiced	90
Acute pancreatitis – urgent cholangiogram	50
– late cholangiogram	10
Abnormal LFTs	40
Dilated main bile duct	40

NB 5–10% of patients with bile duct calculi have a non-dilated bile duct.

Table 14.6 Advantages and disadvantages of preoperative ERC or routine cholangiography

Criteria	ERC	Operative cholangiogram
Number of patients	Selective (< 40%)	90%
Successful cholangiogram	90%	90%
Successful duct clearance	90%	90%
False-positives	5%	5%
False-negatives	5%	5%
In-hospital stay	1 day extra	No extra time
Operating list planning	Good	Uncertainty
Operative time	No extra time	Variable (> 10 min)
Demonstration of biliary anatomy	Good	Good
Complications	Acute pancreatitis	Perforation
	Bleeding	
	Perforation	

Table 14.7 Advantages and disadvantages of the different surgical approaches

	Laparoscopic	Mini	Open
Supervision	Easy	Difficult	Relatively difficult
Training	Well structured	Unstructured	Unstructured
Conversion to open	5–10%	5%	–
Mortality	< 0.5%	?	0.5%
Bile duct injury	0.5%	< 0.5%	< 0.5%
Chest infection	< 5%	< 5%	> 5%
Wound infection	< 5%	< 5%	> 5%
DVT	< 1%	?	< 5%
Hospital stay	1–2 days	2–4 days	4–10 days
Return to full activity	4–6 weeks	4–6 weeks	> 6 weeks
Cosmesis	Excellent	Good	Poor
Incisional herniae rate	Very low	Low	High

   c. Adhesions are then removed to reveal Hartmann's pouch and the region of Calot's triangle

2. Demonstrate the anatomy
   a. There must be no doubt about the anatomy before any structures are divided
   b. Variations in the anatomy of Calot's triangle are so frequent that the cystic duct and artery must be 'proven beyond all reasonable doubt' before division (Fig. 14.6)
   c. If there is doubt about the anatomy then further dissection, or a cholangiogram, is indicated or a laparoscopic approach converted to an open operation

3. Removal of the gallbladder from the liver bed.

Variations in surgical technique A tense gallbladder is easier to manipulate if it is decompressed first. The 'fundus first' technique

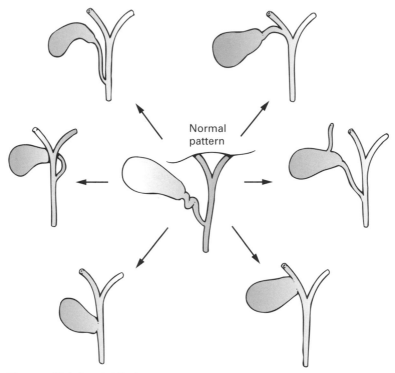

Fig. 14.6   Variations in bile duct anatomy.

may be the method of choice when severe inflammation makes dissection of Calot's triangle hazardous. Occasionally the neck of the gallbladder needs to be incised to displace a stone impacted in Hartmann's pouch. Rarely a sub-total cholecystectomy with removal of as much of the gallbladder as possible, extraction of all gallstones and ablation of any functioning gallbladder mucosa may be the safest option. Operative trans-cystic duct cholangiograms are used by many surgeons to both screen for choledocholithiasis and define the biliary anatomy.

Indications for conversion from a laparoscopic approach to an open operation include:

1. Major vascular or intestinal injury
2. Intolerance of carbon dioxide pneumoperitoneum
3. Dense adhesions
4. Uncontrolled bleeding
5. Anatomical uncertainty
6. Cancer of the gallbladder.

Type I Mirizzi's syndrome may be treated by laparoscopic sub-total cholecystectomy with placement of a T tube after preoperative ERC, extraction of bile duct calculi and stenting. This is technically very demanding and open sub-total cholecystectomy is usually indicated.

Type II Mirizzi's syndrome usually requires cholecystectomy and hepaticodocho-jejunostomy Roux-en-Y. For these reasons laparoscopic cholecystectomy should only be performed by those trained to perform open surgery.

Complications   The advantages of laparoscopic cholecystectomy include reduced mortality, chest and wound infections, reduced blood loss, earlier discharge from hospital and return to full and normal activity, and smaller wounds. It is likely that in the long term the incidence of incision herniae and adhesional obstruction will also be reduced. Laparoscopic cholecystectomy is, however, associated with a higher rate of bile duct injury, particularly during 'the learning curve'.

A postoperative bile leak should be suspected in any patient who does not recover from a laparoscopic cholecystectomy within 48 hours. It may be manifest as diffuse abdominal pain, nausea, a prolonged ileus, abdominal distension, and/or urinary retention. The serum bilirubin is usually slightly raised without associated enzyme changes. An ultrasound scan and ascitic fluid aspiration, ERC or HIDA scan will reveal the diagnosis.

Bile duct leaks may be either minor or major. Minor leaks arise from small cholecyst-hepatic ducts, from a cystic duct or after a sub-total cholecystectomy. Cystic duct leaks occur when a ligaclip is displaced because it is incorrectly placed, dislodged, sloughs off or is 'blown off' by biliary hypertension. These bile leaks usually resolve if drained percutaneously and an internal biliary stent placed to secure preferential drainage into the duodenum. Laparotomy is indicated if biliary peritonitis supervenes.

Major bile leaks are more serious and may be recognised at the time of surgery or become manifest in the early postoperative period. When they are recognised at the time of surgery a cholangiogram is required to define the anatomy. A clean transverse division of up to 50% of the diameter of a main bile duct may be primarily repaired over a T tube if seen at the time of surgery. If diagnosed postoperatively a stent should be placed across the site of the duct injury and the bile drained percutaneously. Complete division of a main bile duct, and diathermy injuries require hepaticodocho-jejunostomy Roux-en-Y. Attempts at primary repair are unlikely to succeed because most of the blood supply to the bile duct arises from distally and the proximal stump is relatively avascular.

Bile duct occlusion may occur as a result of misapplication of a ligaclip, clipping a tented main bile duct, or confusion about the anatomy. Patients develop progressive postoperative jaundice. The obstruction needs to be surgically relieved and a hepaticodocho-jejunostomy Roux-en-Y may be required. Bile duct strictures may present as a late complication months or years after the initial operation. These are usually ischaemic being caused by diathermy injury. They may respond to endoscopic dilatation and stenting but if intractable require a hepaticodocho-jejunostomy Roux-en-Y.

Medical
With the improved safety of surgery dissolution therapy is rarely used. Attempts to dissolve gallstones rely on the premise that gallstones remain only while bile is supersaturated with cholesterol. Increasing the concentration of bile salts in bile (ursodeoxycholic acid, the principal bile acid in bears) or decreasing biliary output of cholesterol (chenodeoxycholic acid) increase the solubility of cholesterol causing dissolution of gallstones. Oral ursodeoxycholic acid treatment alone reduces the diameter of a stone linearly with time at a rate of about 1 mm each month. Combined urso- and chenodeoxycholic acid appears to dissolve stones more quickly.

- Oral dissolution therapy has limited use clinically. It is only successful in non-calcified cholesterol stones within a functioning gallbladder and a patent cystic duct. This needs to be confirmed with an oral cholecystogram
- Treatment is expensive and stones frequently recur once treatment is stopped
- Dissolution therapy also has a limited role during extracorporeal shock wave gallstone lithotripsy (ESWL), in preventing the formation of gallstones during rapid weight loss, or maintaining patency of biliary stents
- More rapid dissolution, within 24 hours, can be achieved by percutaneous transhepatic or naso-biliary or naso-cholecystic infusion of methyl *tert*-butyl ether or *n*-propyl acetate
- Methyl *tert*-butyl ether causes severe mucosal irritation if it enters the duodenum. It therefore needs repeated instillation and drainage to be safely used.

EMPYEMA

This rarely responds to antibiotic treatment alone. An experienced surgeon can perform a laparoscopic cholecystectomy in the fit patient. Some patients with an empyema are seriously ill or unfit for surgical treatment. Percutaneous cholecystostomy can be performed to drain the gallbladder while systemic antibiotics eradicate infection. This does not remove the underlying problem of gallstones in an inflamed gallbladder but will provide temporary relief. At a later stage the patient may be fit for a cholecystectomy or it may be necessary to remove the gallstones either percutaneously or via an open cholecystostomy under local anaesthetic.

ACALCULOUS CHOLECYSTITIS

This occurs in critically ill patients and is associated with trauma, surgery, burns, acquired immune deficiency syndrome and prolonged intravenous nutrition. The symptoms and signs are those of acute cholecystitis. Patients who develop it are, however, receiving intensive support for multiple organ failure and a high index of suspicion is therefore required. Localised peritonitis with a palpable gallbladder are suggestive. US, CT scans, or HIDA scans are diagnostic.

Acalculous cholecystitis is a serious condition which may lead to gallbladder necrosis. Cholecystectomy is associated with up to 66% mortality. Less invasive treatments include percutaneous cholecystostomy and endoscopic transpapillary placement of a naso-cholecystic drain.

CHOLEDOCHOLITHIASIS

Presentation

• Bile duct calculi may be asymptomatic, or cause deranged liver function tests, acute pancreatitis, obstructive jaundice or cholangitis
• Most symptomatic patients present with painful obstructive jaundice
• There is often a history of previous attacks of biliary colic
• If cholangitis supervenes patients are ill, jaundiced, with rigors, sweats and fever
• Acute pancreatitis presents as a sudden onset of severe epigastric pain.

Epidemiology

• In young patients (< 50 years) less than 5% of patients with symptomatic gallstones have choledocholithiasis. This increases to 20% in the over 70-year-olds.

Assessment

• Patients with gallstones and abnormal liver function tests, bile duct dilatation on US or a past history of acute pancreatitis or jaundice are at increased risk of having choledocholithiasis (Table 14.5)
• The diagnosis can be confirmed on external, endoscopic or laparoscopic US scans, or on endoscopic, percutaneous, intravenous or operative cholangiograms.

Therapy

Indications   Small calculi (less than 5 mm in size) may pass spontaneously. Indeed, it is likely that biliary acute pancreatitis is precipitated by the passage of small calculi. Larger calculi remaining within the bile duct causing jaundice or cholangitis are removed by urgent ERC or PTC. When these are unsuccessful, surgical drainage is required.

Bile duct calculi should be removed if found during a diagnostic ERC, PTC or at operation. Choledocholithiasis, diagnosed during laparoscopic cholangiography, can be treated by laparoscopic or open duct exploration, or by ERC postoperatively. This may be facilitated by placing a fine catheter within the bile duct via the cystic duct for insertion of a guidewire at a later stage.

If preoperative endoscopic or percutaneous treatment of choledocholithiasis is unsuccessful then cholecystectomy and bile duct exploration can be performed laparoscopically or at open surgery.

Treatment

ERC

- Emergency or urgent ERC and re-establishment of adequate bile duct drainage is mandatory in patients presenting with ascending cholangitis or obstructive jaundice
- It is usually possible to remove bile duct calculi at the time of the procedure, although a biliary stent may be necessary in some patients
- Elective ERC is indicated in the preoperative management of patients at risk of choledocholithiasis
- In elderly patients or those with significant co-morbidity this may be all that is required.

Percutaneous treatment

- An internal–external percutaneous transhepatic biliary drain is an alternative to an ERC or may be used when endoscopic treatment is not possible. This will provide emergency relief from obstruction and enable planned stone removal or stenting either percutaneously or as a combined procedure with an endoscopist.

Extracorporeal shock wave gallstone lithotripsy (ESWL)

- High amplitude shock waves are focused through water at US or fluoroscopically localised stones. These waves pass through soft tissues to create stresses that fragment stones. Fragments may then pass into the duodenum or respond to oral dissolution therapy
- ESWL is rarely clinically indicated and cannot be used in 25–30% of patients for technical reasons
- Contraindications include heavily calcified stones, multiple stones and a non-functioning gallbladder

- Fragmentation occurs in 40–50%, and gallstones are cleared within 6 months in 21% when adjuvant oral dissolution therapy is taken
- In 10% of patients gallstones recur within 1 year
- Complications include pain, biliary colic, acute pancreatitis and obstructive jaundice.

Laparoscopic bile duct exploration

- Small (< 1 cm in diameter) calculi in the common bile duct can be removed by trawling with a balloon or Dormia basket after dilatation of the cystic duct
- Larger calculi or calculi proximal to the insertion of the cystic duct are removed via a longitudinal choledochotomy
- Clearance is checked by choledochoscopy and cholangiography.

Open bile duct exploration

- The common bile duct is explored through a longitudinal choledochotomy
- Calculi are removed using Desjardins forceps and irrigation
- Clearance is checked by choledochoscopy and cholangiography
- A T-tube catheter is usually positioned.

BILIARY STRICTURES

In the West most extra-hepatic biliary strictures are caused by pancreatic carcinoma or cholangiocarcinoma. Benign strictures are rare.

Presentation

- Biliary strictures usually present with obstructive jaundice or cholangitis
- Patients with malignant bile duct stricture usually have a slow onset of painless jaundice and weight loss
- A persistent dull ache in the back, between the shoulder blades may, however, be present. It is important to exclude early gastric outlet obstruction as this will influence management
- If untreated, hepato-renal failure will cause death.

Risk factors

- Benign strictures are associated with choledocholithiasis, chronic pancreatitis and sclerosing cholangitis, or may be iatrogenic
- The increased incidence of cholangiocarcinoma in Asia is associated with liver fluke (Clonorchis) infestation
- In the West it is associated with sclerosing cholangitis and choledochal cysts.

Epidemiology

- Cholangiocarcinoma accounts for 3% of cancer deaths.

Assessment

- Liver function tests and an abdominal US are the first-line investigations. These will usually confirm extrahepatic biliary obstruction but will not usually reveal the cause
- An ERC or PTC is usually diagnostic and shows both the location and length of a stricture
- If a malignant stricture is suspected brushings are sent for cytology
- With the exception of iatrogenic strictures a biliary stricture should be presumed to be malignant until there is histological proof to the contrary
- Pancreatic carcinomas or large cholangiocarcinomas are readily apparent on CT scans but peri-ampullary tumours or small cholangiocarcinomas may not be imaged even with helical CT scans and overlapping reconstruction.

Treatment

Medical

- Patients unfit for surgery or with advanced malignant disease are best treated with an endoscopic or percutaneously placed biliary endoprosthesis. These stents tend to occlude after 3 months
- Expanding metal stents have a longer life expectancy but are more expensive and cannot be removed
- Cholangiocarcinomas are not radio- or chemosensitive.

Surgical

- Surgical bypass is the treatment of choice for patients with unresectable malignancy and a life expectancy of more than 3 months, or benign bile duct strictures
- An end-to-side hepaticodocho-jejunostomy is preferred to a cholecyst-jejunostomy to bypass malignant disease because of concern about cystic duct obstruction with disease progression
- If duodenal obstruction is present or likely a gastro-jejunostomy will relieve gastric outlet obstruction
- Benign strictures can be bypassed by either a side-to-side hepaticodocho-jejunostomy or an end-to-side hepaticodocho-jejunostomy.
- The treatment of cholangiocarcinomas depends on their site and length
- Most (50–75%) are located in the upper third of the extra-hepatic biliary tree or are diffuse
- Resection and end-to-side hepaticodocho-jeunostomy is indicated for middle and lower third cancers

- Less than one-third of hilar cholangiocarcinomas are resectable because of vascular involvement.

Prognosis

- Less than half of patients with cholangiocarcinoma survive 1 year and less than 10% are alive after 5 years.

PRIMARY BILIARY CIRRHOSIS (PBC) AND PRIMARY SCLEROSING CHOLANGITIS (PSC)

Elevated serum anti-mitochondrial antibody is the hallmark of PBC and beading on ERC is diagnostic for sclerosing cholangitis. Liver biopsy may be indicated for diagnosis and to assess liver damage. Asymptomatic patients with a normal serum bilirubin are simply observed. Most patients are middle-aged with jaundice, pruritus and fatigue. Ursodeoxycholic acid leads to a rapid fall in all of the biochemical markers of cholestasis, gives symptomatic relief, slows disease progression and delays the time to liver failure. Cholestyramine, antihistamines or rifampicin help the pruritus. Parenteral vitamin A, D, E and K and oral calcium supplements are required. Immunosuppression with cyclosporin A treatment may have a role in PBC. In PSC, dominant extra-hepatic strictures can be stented. Transplantation may be indicated for end-stage disease, cholangiocarcinoma or intractable symptoms.

CHOLEDOCHAL CYSTS

As in the cardiovascular system the biliary tract is afflicted by both occlusive disease and aneurysmal disease. Combined wall weakness and increased luminal pressure possibly caused by pancreatico-biliary reflux may cause choledochal cyst formation.

Presentation

- Three-quarters present in infancy but the remainder are diagnosed in adults
- The features are typically intermittent but progressive
- The classic triad of abdominal pain, jaundice and an abdominal mass is uncommon
- Most patients present as children with intermittent abdominal pain, occasionally with jaundice and cholangitis. A few have a palpable mass
- US is the first-line investigation followed by ERCP
- The pancreatogram may show an abnormal pancreatic duct and a long common channel
- Some patients present with cholecystolithiasis or choledocholithiasis, cholangitis, secondary biliary cirrhosis, liver abscesses, and a few develop cholangiocarcinoma reflecting prolonged stasis and chronic infection.

Epidemiology

- Choledochal cysts are rare, occurring every 100 000–150 000 live births
- They are up to 4 times more common in females.

Classification

- Type I cysts, the most frequent, are solitary extra-hepatic cysts
- Type II consist of a supraduodenal diverticulum
- Type III is a choledochocoele
- Type IVa are extra- and intra-hepatic cysts
- Type IVb are multiple extra-hepatic cysts
- Type V is Caroli's disease.

Treatment

Surgery
Cyst excision and Roux-en-Y hepaticodocho-jejunostomy is the operation of choice for extra-hepatic cysts in view of the risk of malignancy. In the presence of severe inflammation or significant portal hypertension the posterior cyst wall can be left. Intra-hepatic dilatation may improve with excision of the extra-hepatic cystic component. Internal drainage is associated with late onset of cancer and stricture formation.

LIVER CANCER

Liver cancers may be primary or secondary, single or multiple.

Presentation

- Most liver cancers present in elderly patients with a painful mass, weight loss or, in patients with pre-existing cirrhosis, as a deterioration in their condition
- The fibrolamellar variant of HCC occurs in younger patients (mean age 25 years)
- Liver secondaries may be the first presentation of an occult cancer or arise in a patient known to have cancer. An increasing number of liver metastases are found during cancer surveillance
- Jaundice suggests extensive liver infiltration, hilar obstruction or pre-existing cirrhosis
- A few patients may present with shock or peritonitis from intra-peritoneal haemorrhage or with a para-neoplastic syndrome (for example thrombophlebitis migrans, polycythaemia, hypoglycaemia).

LIVER METASTASIS

In Western countries most liver tumours are metastatic (Table 14.8).

Table 14.8   Common primary tumours metastasising to the liver

Primary	Histology	Serum marker
Colon	Adenocarcinoma	CEA
Gastric	Adenocarcinoma	–
Exocrine pancreas	Adenocarcinoma	–
Endocrine pancreas	Gastrinoma, etc.	Hormone
Small bowel	Carcinoid	5 HIAA
Skin	Melanoma	–
Breast	Adenocarcinoma	–
Thyroid	Follicular cancer	Thyroglobulin
Prostate	Adenocarcinoma	PSA
Ovary	Adenocarcinoma	CA125
Kidney	Renal cell carcinoma	–

Treatment

Medical
Most patients do not have hormone or chemosensitive metastasis or they are unfit for chemotherapy. Colorectal, breast and ovarian secondaries are chemosensitive and usually respond for a short time to chemotherapy. There is no place for radiotherapy. Breast and prostate metastasis may respond to hormone manipulation. Functioning endocrine tumours may respond to sandostatin, and Zollinger–Ellison syndrome from metastatic gastrinoma may be treated by high-dose proton pump inhibitors. Thyroid cancers may be ablated with radioactive iodine.

Surgical
Localised or solitary secondaries from a treated colonic primary may be resected, with a 25% 5-year survival.

Prognosis

- The mean overall survival is 6 months depending on the response to chemotherapy
- Endocrine metastases are usually slow-growing.

HEPATOCELLULAR CARCINOMA

Risk factors

- In high-risk areas, 90% of patients with hepatocellular carcinoma (HCC) are carriers of hepatitis B virus which is endemic and often acquired in utero
- In Western countries HCC is associated with alcoholic liver cirrhosis
- There is increasing recognition of an association with hepatitis C infection

- Other risk factors include aflatoxin B1 exposure (the toxic metabolite of the fungus *Aspergillus flavus* found in poorly stored nuts and grain) and some hereditary conditions (haemochromatosis, alpha-1 antitrypsin deficiency and hereditary tyrosinaemia)
- The fibrolamellar variant of HCC is associated with the oral contraceptive pill
- Ingestion of thoratrast, arsenic or vinyl chloride are associated with hepatic angiosarcoma.

Epidemiology
HCC is one of the most common cancers in the world.

- In Africa and South East Asia, the incidence is 100 per 100 000 per year
- In the West, HCC, the principal primary liver cancer, has an incidence of only 2 per 100 000 per year.

Assessment

- Further investigations are indicated in all patients with a liver mass (Fig. 14.7). These will determine whether it is solid or cystic, single or multiple, its location, size, and the involvement of vital structures
- Liver function tests, hepatitis screen, serum alpha fetoprotein levels and an US scan are performed in all patients.

Treatment

Medical
HCC is not radio- or chemosensitive. Numerous treatment strategies are being explored in an attempt to improve prognosis for irresectable HCC. These include:

- Neoadjuvant chemotherapy
- Transarterial chemo-embolisation
- Cryotherapy
- Percutaneous brachytherapy

The efficacy of these treatments remains uncertain.

Surgical

Assessment   Preoperative investigations are required to confirm the tumour is resectable and liver function will withstand an operation prior to regeneration. A CT scan and angiography are indicated if resection is planned. Diagnostic uncertainty may indicate the need for a liver biopsy.

Anatomy   Assessment of resectability and surgery are based on a thorough understanding of the anatomy. The liver, enclosed in the tough Glissons's capsule, is divided into two functional halves by the main fissure, an invisible line running from the middle of

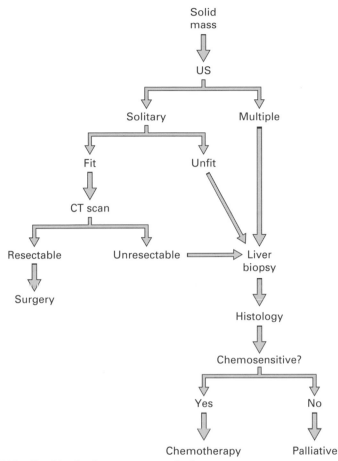

Fig. 14.7 Algorithm for the management of a liver mass.

the gallbladder notch through the gallbladder bed to the middle hepatic vein. The hepatic artery, common hepatic duct and portal vein (portal triad) divide at the porta hepatis upon entering their respective lobes.

The branches of the three components of the portal triad are bundled together within the liver parenchyma as they pass to each of the eight liver segments.

- Segment I, the caudate lobe, is inferior
- Segment II forms the left lateral corner
- Segment IV, the quadrate lobe, is bounded by the falciform ligament on the left and the gallbladder on the right
- Segment VI is the right lateral liver edge

- The middle hepatic vein drains blood from both functional lobes, the right hepatic vein from the right lobe and the left hepatic vein from segments II and III of the left lobe
- The caudate lobe drains directly into the vena cava.

Resection   Liver resections are usually right or left hemi-hepatectomy (with preservation of the caudate lobe), extended right hemi-hepatectomy (leaving segments I, II and III) or segmentectomies in cirrhotic patients with reduced functional reserve.

The principles of liver surgery are now well established:

- Adequate exposure is achieved through a midline or bilateral subcostal incision
- After assessing resectability and stage the main hepatic pedicle is controlled with a sling (Pringle's manoeuvre)
- The hepatic veins are dissected sufficiently to apply a vascular clamp if necessary
- The liver and gallbladder are mobilised and the right and left hepatic pedicles secured with slings
- The pedicle on the side to be removed is clamped to mark the line of demarcation
- The liver substance is divided 1 cm within line of demarcation ('finger-fracture', clip and cut, or an ultrasound dissector)
- The hepatic vein is divided and oversewn within the liver substance
- Ensure haemostasis (diathermy, suture ligation, argon diathermy, fibrin glue) before closing.

Prognosis

- Irresectable cancer survival is usually less than 6 months
- Operative mortality is 5% with a 25–50% 5-year survival.

GALLBLADDER CANCER

Most (90%) are associated with gallstones and arise in the elderly with a peak age incidence of 75 years. Gallbladder cancer is found in less than 1% of cholecystectomies. The risk is increased in porcelain gallbladder.

Presentation

- Most patients present with an abdominal mass and pain; some are found incidentally.

Treatment

Medical

- Obstructive jaundice is palliated with a stent
- Chemotherapy and radiotherapy do not alter disease progression.

Surgical

- Curative resection may be attempted if local extension is limited to the liver bed
- Cholecystectomy with excision of the liver bed and radical lymphadenopathy or extended right hemi-hepatectomy may be indicated.

Prognosis

- Cancer confined to the mucosa is associated with a 50% 5-year survival
- With local invasion the survival is less than 1 year.

LIVER CYSTS

Liver cysts are divided into true cysts and pseudocysts. Pseudocysts lack an epithelial lining and are either post-traumatic or neoplastic. True cysts may be parasitic, usually hydatid and non-parasitic.

Presentation

- Most liver cysts are asymptomatic incidental findings on abdominal US or CT scan
- Large cysts may give rise to upper abdominal pain or discomfort, an abdominal mass and rarely jaundice if sited near the porta hepatis
- A few cysts present with a complication such as bacterial infection (when there is communication with the biliary tree), bleeding, rupture or malignancy.

Assessment (Fig. 14.8)

- Cysts are readily imaged on abdominal or laparoscopic US or CT scan
- Hydatid must be suspected in patients from, or who have recently visited, areas where Echinococcus is endemic. In which case immunological tests (hydatid immuno-electrophoresis or enzyme-linked immunosorbent assay) should be performed to distinguish simple cysts from hydatid disease.

HYDATID DISEASE

This is a zoonosis caused by the cestode (tapeworm) *Echinococcus granulosus* (Unilocular cysts) or *E. alveolaris* (multilocular cysts). Hydatid is endemic in grassland regions of Africa, South America and Australia. The adult tapeworm lives in the gut of carnivores (usually dogs) and sheds eggs into the faeces. These are ingested by a grazing animal (sheep, for example), the intermediate host, where the larvae hatch and grow. The cycle is completed, or spread

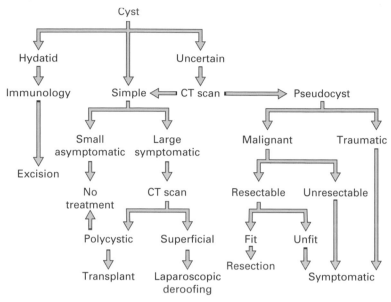

Fig. 14.8 Algorithm for the management of a liver cyst.

to humans occurs, when the herbivore is eaten. Spread to the liver is via the portal vein. Hydatid cysts may also form in the lung, bones or other organs and immune complex disease may cause mesangial proliferative glomerulonephritis.

Treatment
Hepatic hydatid is usually resistant to eradication by even prolonged (8-week) courses of a benzimidol (albendazole or mebendazole). Surgical drainage, excision and sterilisation is usually the only effective treatment and is recommended for both symptomatic and asymptomatic patients.

There are strict principles governing hydatid surgery which prevent dissemination and reduce complications such as postoperative bile leak:

1. The hydatid cyst needs to be isolated to prevent spillage before opening using either an Aaron's suction cone or scolicide-soaked packs
2. The cyst is opened between stay sutures and the contents and daughter cysts are sucked out
3. The lining hydatid membrane is gently peeled, leaving the tough outer inflammatory pseudocyst. The cavity is then sterilised by soaking with scolicide for 5 minutes (1% cetrimide solution or fresh 0.5% silver nitrate)

4. The cavity is carefully inspected and all bile duct communications suture ligated
6. Evidence of cyst spread into the bile duct necessitates bile duct exploration and removal of cysts.

SIMPLE LIVER CYST

Epidemiology

- Liver cysts are found in 5% of the population, with an increasing incidence in old age. These are probably formed by cystic dilatation of embryological remnants of aberrant bile ducts
- Polycystic liver disease is genetic.

Treatment

Medical
Simple percutaneous aspiration is associated with a high recurrence rate and may lead to infection. Unfit patients with uncomplicated simple cysts without bile duct communication may be treated by percutaneous aspiration followed by ethanol or minocycline sclerotherapy.

Surgical
Most symptomatic liver cysts are treated surgically by deroofing (fenestration), which is usually performed laparoscopically. The cyst lining needs to be carefully inspected for communication with the biliary tree or malignancy. Cystadenoma, cystadenocarcinoma or squamous cell carcinoma may present as a liver 'cyst' and may be suitable for liver resection. Carefully selected patients developing liver failure from polycystic liver disease may be suitable for liver transplantation.

LIVER INJURY

Presentation

- Upper abdominal or shoulder tip pain will indicate the possibility of liver trauma
- Patients may be in shock or this may develop later
- A high index of suspicion is required in all patients with lower thoracic or upper abdominal trauma and the possibility of liver injury should be excluded if it is considered possible.

Epidemiology

- In Western countries, blunt liver trauma from road traffic accidents or sporting injuries is more common than penetrating injuries such as stab wounds or gunshot wounds.

Pathogenesis

- Blunt liver trauma causes bursting or deceleration injuries with hepatic parenchymal damage, areas of devitalised tissue and bleeding. If the liver capsule remains intact the haematoma is contained and blood loss minimal. These patients are at risk of developing reactive haemorrhage or late infection particularly if the biliary tree is also disrupted
- It is unusual for blunt liver trauma to be isolated; it is frequently associated with other intra-abdominal injuries, chest, head and musculoskeletal trauma and consequently has a higher mortality
- The severity of the injury in stab wounds is dependent on whether or not major blood vessels or bile ducts have been divided. If not then the prognosis is usually good
- Gunshot wounds, especially if high velocity, always cause extensive parenchymal and vascular damage.

Assessment

- A liver US or CT scan will usually reveal significant liver damage
- If US is not available more than 100 000 erythrocytes/ml of peritoneal lavage fluid suggests clinically significant intra-abdominal haemorrhage which may arise from liver injury
- Contrast-enhanced CT scans should be reserved for the haemodynamically stable patient.

Treatment

Medical
Control of the airway and breathing with vigorous volume replacement and invasive monitoring is required in all shocked patients. Subcapsular haematomas and closed intrahepatic haematomas may be closely watched with frequent CT scans and angiography. Aneurysms, infection or an increase in size can then be detected early.

Surgical
An emergency laparotomy through a full midline incision should be performed on all haemodynamically unstable patients or patients continuing to bleed. The first priority to control bleeding is achieved by packing and applying a Pringle's manoeuvre (placing an atraumatic clamp across the lesser omentum). Once bleeding is controlled liver damage and associated injuries can be assessed. Dead and devitalised liver parenchyma is debrided or formal hepatic resection performed. If an experienced liver surgeon is not available, packing alone will stabilise the patient to allow immediate transfer to a specialist centre.

Prognosis

- Overall mortality is 13%
- Blunt trauma is associated with a higher mortality at 30% compared with gunshot wounds, 10% and stab wounds 1%.

LIVER TRANSPLANTATION

About 300 liver transplants are performed annually in the UK. There is demand for more but a shortage of donors. Liver transplantation is indicated for acute and chronic liver failure (alcohol, primary biliary cirrhosis and various metabolic disorders). Brain-dead, ventilated, heart-beating victims of spontaneous intracranial haemorrhage or severe head injuries are the usual donors.

The excised liver is flushed with cool, hypertonic fluid, such as the University of Wisconsin preservation solution, to enable transfer with a 12–15-hour preservation time. Traditionally, blood group ABO compatibility was all that was required and HLA matching was considered unnecessary. With improved long-term survival the role of HLA compatibility and chronic rejection is being further investigated. Cyclosporin and prednisolone remain the principal immunosuppression drugs. The clinical and biochemical parameters of acute rejection are so variable that a liver biopsy is required to make the diagnosis. Chronic rejection is manifest as increasing jaundice due to destruction of small biliary radicles. Other complications include recurrence of hepatitis or cancer and viral infection (CMV is the most common).

'MEDICAL' LIVER DISEASE

Surgeons treat many patients with liver disease and need to have a working knowledge of management. Essential surgical management concerns the identification of these patients from others presenting with jaundice or liver disease. The diagnosis and treatment of these patients has advanced considerably with the development of complex and expensive investigations and novel treatments requiring management by an experienced hepatologist.

Presentation

- Patients may present non-specifically unwell, with jaundice, weight loss, or with a complication such as haematemesis from oesophageal varices
- Acute hepatitis presents with anorexia, fever, weight loss, jaundice and tender hepatomegaly
- Early liver failure is manifest by jaundice, palmar erythema, spider naevi, hepatomegaly, ascites, gynaecomastia, gonadal atrophy, bruising and nose bleeds

- In decompensated liver failure these signs are gross with clinically significant coagulopathy and portal hypertension, and encephalopathy
- Chronic metabolic derangements, such as haemochromatosis and Wilson's disease, are associated with large joint arthropathy, skin pigmentation and cardiac dysfunction.

Risk factors

- In all patients it is important to take a history of
  — occupation (possible exposure to industrial solvents)
  — chronic alcohol abuse
  — foreign travel (to hepatitis endemic areas)
  — recent transfusions of blood products
  — oral and intravenous drug use and abuse
  — male homosexuality
  — family medical history
- Chronic auto-immune hepatitis and primary biliary cirrhosis are associated with polyarthritis, thyroiditis, Sjögren's syndrome, vasculitis, etc.
- Sclerosing cholangitis is associated with inflammatory bowel disease.

Assessment

- A full battery of liver function tests is required
- Blood should be sent for hepatitis A, B and C serology, and an auto-immune antibody screen (including serum anti-mitochondrial and alpha-1 antitrypsin)
- ERC is diagnostic for sclerosing cholangitis
- Serum ferritin, copper and caeruloplasmin will exclude haemochromatosis or Wilson's disease
- Liver biopsy is indicated in most patients for diagnosis and to assess liver damage.

FURTHER READING

Lannois B, Jamieson GG 1993 Modern operative techniques in liver surgery. Churchill Livingstone, London
Toouli J 1993 Surgery of the biliary tract. Churchill Livingstone, London
Watt PCH, Spence RAJ 1993 Pathology for surgeons. Wright Bristol

15. Colorectal surgery

Terry O'Kelly

COLORECTAL CANCER

Colorectal cancer is the second most common malignancy in the UK after lung cancer. Each year approximately 20 000 patients die from the condition and there has been little improvement in mortality during the last 40 years with the overall 5-year survival rate less than 40%. Colorectal cancer affects men and women equally although carcinoma of the rectum is more common in men. The peak incidence is in the seventh decade.

Aetiology

Genetic predisposition

Two broad groups are recognised both of which are inherited in an autosomal dominant manner.

- Conditions which predispose to a large number of adenomatous polyps, each of which has a degree of malignant potential. Examples include familial adenomatous polyposis (FAP) and Gardiner's syndrome. Both result from mutations occurring in the APC gene which is contained within the long arm of chromosome 5. FAP is characterised by the development of hundreds to thousands of adenomatous polyps in the colon and rectum from the second decade of life. Left untreated, polyps increase both in size and number and colorectal cancers develop within the 4th and 5th decade of life. Extracolonic manifestations also occur, most notably congenital hypertrophy of the retinal pigment epithelium (CHRPE) and gastroduodenal polyps. Duodenal and peri-ampullary adenomas have a malignant potential and patients with FAP have been estimated to have a 100 times greater risk of developing upper gastrointestinal malignancy than the normal population. Desmoid tumours are also common (affecting 10–15% of FAP patients) and occur in the abdominal wall, retroperitoneum and small bowel mesentery. Although they are benign they can have serious and even fatal consequences due to their physical presence which can lead to compression of vital structures. The findings in Gardiner's syndrome are similar to those in FAP except that epidermoid cysts, osteomas (especially of the mandible) and dermoid tumours are common
- Conditions which are not associated with the presence of large numbers of adenomatous polyps but each of the adenomas that does occur has an increased malignant potential.

Hereditary non-polyposis colon cancer (HNPCC)

1. The peak incidence of cancer development is in the 5th decade and two-thirds of colorectal tumours are located proximal to the splenic flexure. There is an increased incidence of metachronous tumours, both within and without the large bowel. The precise genetic abnormality responsible for HNPCC has not yet been determined, but most patients appear to have mutation of a gene contained within the short arm of chromosome 2. As with FAP this is a tumour suppressor gene that has two sub-divisions:
   a. Families where affected individuals only develop colorectal cancer, known as Lynch syndrome 1
   b. Families in whom extracolonic tumours can also occur, within endometrial, gastric, ovarian, renal and the small bowel, known as Lynch syndrome 2
2. Other patients also have an inherited susceptibility to colorectal cancer, but the pattern of inheritance is less clear cut and environmental factors also play an important role. Patients with one or more first-degree relatives affected by colorectal cancer have an increased risk of developing the disease themselves. **The risk is 12% if the relative was diagnosed before the age of 45 years and 7.5% if the diagnosis was made before 54 years**. It might be that a genetic predisposition coupled to exposure to a dietary carcinogen leads to the production of colorectal cancer in these patients. Current opinion favours a common mechanism for cancer development which is known as the *adenoma carcinoma sequence*. It is believed that colorectal cancers develop from a pre-existing adenoma and these themselves arise from normal mucosa. A sequence of mutations has been proposed by Fearon and Vogelstein as a possible genetic pathway for the development of colorectal cancer in normal mucosa.

Acquired factors in the development of colorectal cancer
Apart from genetic predisposition, the following have been implicated in the production of colorectal cancer: diet, inflammatory bowel disease, surgical procedures, irradiation, smoking.
   Diet   Observational studies consistently show an inverse association between consumption of vegetables and fruit and colorectal cancer. In addition there appears to be a direct relationship between colorectal cancer and consumption of dietary fat and total protein intake. It should be noted, however, that diets rich in vegetables and fruit commonly have a low fat and total protein content. *Note that available evidence is inadequate to make recommendations regarding specific nutrients.*

- Dietary factors might explain why the incidence of colorectal cancer varies in different regions and cultural groups within the same country

Table 15.1 Probability of developing a carcinoma in chronic total colitis

3% at 15 years from the onset of symptoms
5–7% at 20 years from the onset of symptoms
10% at 25 years from the onset of symptoms

- Colon cancer is more prevalent in urban compared to non-urban environments
- More prevalent in Scotland than England, and in the northern USA compared with the southern USA
- Colorectal cancer is also more common amongst white South Africans and New Zealanders when compared to black South Africans and Maoris
- Migrants moving from a low- to a high-risk environment adopt the cancer incidence of the latter within one generation.

Inflammatory bowel disease Ulcerative colitis *and* Crohn's disease are associated with an increased incidence of colorectal cancer. The link is most clearly established in the case of ulcerative colitis but the risk may be of similar magnitude with Crohn's colitis.

Patients suffering chronic total colitis with the onset a severe attack in childhood are at greatest risk (Table 15.1). Mucosal dysplasia appears to be a pre-cancerous stage, colonoscopic surveillance programmes assess dysplasia to determine the need for colectomy.

Very few, if any, cancers develop before a 10-year history of colitis. Those with mild distal colitis are probably not at any greater risk of developing colorectal cancer than the normal population.

Surgical procedures Ureterosigmoidoscopy is associated with the development of colon cancer at or near the ureterocolic anastomosis. It may result from the presence of phenols and other hydrocarbons excreted in the urine as a consequence of cigarette smoking.

Gastrectomy and cholecystectomy have also been implicated as causative factors in the production of colon cancer, perhaps because both increase the delivery of bile acids to, and hence the concentration of, secondary bile acids in the colon. Lithocholic and deoxycholic acid are both secondary bile acids and are powerful tumour promoters.

Clinical features
The mode of presentation and the findings at examination are determined by the site of the primary tumour and the presence or otherwise of metastatic disease.

- The nature of stool in the colon changes from fluid in the caecum to semi-solid as the stool passes the splenic flexure, to solid in the sigmoid colon and rectum. This is in part responsible for the varying presentation of colon cancers

- Right-sided lesions usually present with anaemia, but may also have a mass in the right iliac fossa. Beware the elderly patient, taking iron sulphate for anaemia that has not been investigated
- Transverse colon tumours may present with abdominal pain and episodes of subacute obstruction and anaemia
- Approximately 75% of colorectal cancers are situated distal to the splenic flexure. Obstruction is more likely and up to 15% of patients with colorectal cancer present with acute large bowel obstruction
- The ileocaecal valve remains competent in 50–60% of cases, the caecum is therefore at risk of perforation. Perforation of a tumour occurs in 5% of patients
- Stage for stage the prognosis in those presenting with either obstruction or perforation is worse than in those patients who present electively
- Blood loss per rectum, change in bowel habit and tenesmus are important symptoms, especially in rectal carcinomas.

Investigations
Investigations are used to confirm the diagnosis, stage the disease and demonstrate synchronous tumours.

- In patients presenting electively the entire colorectal mucosa should be imaged, either directly by colonoscopy or by double-contrast barium enema combined with sigmoidoscopy
- Water-soluble contrast enemas should be performed prior to surgery in all patients presenting with large bowel obstruction except where there is sign of free intraperitoneal perforation
- In elective cases the presence or otherwise of liver metastases should also be determined and this is best achieved by ultrasound
- The *gold standard* in imaging rectal cancers is transrectal ultrasound (TRUSS) to determine local extent of the tumour
- Those tumours which have invaded beyond the rectal wall by more than 5 mm are classified as locally extensive and are associated with a high incidence of mesorectal and pelvic side wall lymph node metastases
- Neither MRI nor CT scans are as accurate as TRUSS
- Currently there is not a non-invasive technique to precisely determine the presence or not of lymph node metastases.

Surgical treatment
Surgery offers the best chance of a permanent cure. Wherever possible the primary tumour should be resected to prevent local complications and alleviate symptoms. Each patient must, however, be assessed on their own merits and surgical intervention may be inappropriate in very elderly, the infirm and in those with advanced disease.

Preoperative preparation

- All patients should give informed consent. This should include stoma formation (i.e. with low rectal cancers)
- All patients should receive thrombo-embolic prophylaxis. Heparin ± thrombo-embolic stockings ± mechanical measures according to risk
- Prophylactic antibiotics should be administered in the perioperative period and single-dose prophylaxis just prior to surgery is as effective as more prolonged administration, however a second dose of antibiotics may be required perioperatively for procedures taking more than 2 hours
- Mechanical bowel preparation is not essential prior to elective colorectal surgery but is favoured by most surgeons
- Concern has been expressed that blood transfusion may increase the likelihood of recurrence in colorectal cancer but this has not been confirmed by recent prospective studies and therefore blood should not be withheld if there is a clinical indication to give it.

Principles of surgery

Colorectal cancer spreads in a predictable fashion and survival is directly related to the stage of the disease, e.g. depth of penetration through the bowel wall and the presence of dissemination at the time of surgery. Locoregional control is best achieved by surgery and is essential for a satisfactory outcome. Unlike with solid tumours of other organs radical as opposed to localised resection appears to play a crucial role in determining survival. En bloc resection is advised if a colorectal cancer is invading surrounding structures such as the uterus, bladder or small bowel.

If the primary tumour is fixed and resection is not feasible then the tumour should be bypassed or the distal segment defunctioned by formation of a proximal stoma (i.e. rectal cancers). No-touch and high-tie techniques have not been shown to be of benefit in randomised controlled trials. No difference has been demonstrated between stapled and hand-sutured anastomoses in randomised trials; however, there is some evidence that in the management of rectal cancer stapled anastomosis might be associated with a lower incidence of recurrence, albeit at an increased risk of anastomotic stenosis. Although it has not been subjected to prospective randomised controlled trials, consensus of opinion suggests that patients with middle and lower third rectal cancers should undergo total mesorectal excision as this appears to be associated with the lowest incidence of locoregional recurrence. Distal spread of tumour within the rectal wall is present in less than 10% of patients with rectal cancer and in these cases the tumour is invariably poorly differentiated. For well and moderately differentiated tumours, therefore, a macroscopic distal resection margin of 2 cm or so is ample and will not compromise local control or survival. Sphincter-saving surgery is feasible in all but the lowest rectal cancers. Formation of a colonic pouch, followed by pouch-anal anastomosis, is associated with a more superior functional outcome than straight colo-anal anastomosis. Lateral pelvic lymph node dissection is advocated by some surgeons but is associated with a high incidence of morbidity, including pelvic nerve damage, and is not recommended until it has been shown to be of additional value in prospective randomised trials. Small, superficial, well differentiated rectal cancers can be satisfactorily managed by local per anal excision with a surrounding cuff of normal rectum. Transanal endoscopic microsurgery combined with transrectal ultrasound permits precise management of such problems. Electrocoagulation and laser are alternative treatment modalities but these do not provide tissue for histological analysis. In advanced rectal cancer, symptoms can be palliated satisfactorily by endoscopic resection, using apparatus similar to that for resection of bladder tumours. Laser therapy also has a role and can be administered endoscopically where the tumour lies more proximally. Placement of endolumenal stents may have a useful role in colonic cancers which cause obstructive symptoms and which are not suitable for resection.

Outcome of surgery
Stage remains the most important determinant of prognosis. If the tumour is localised to the mucosa or muscularis propria and is adequately treated by surgery, then the expectation for survival is little different from that of an otherwise healthy individual of a similar age in the same population. If the tumour has spread through to the serosa, however, there is only a 40–60% chance that the patient will survive 5 years. With lymph node metastases the 5-year survival drops to 30%, although it is rather higher for those with metastatic deposits confined to nodes adjacent to tumour (up to 60% 5-year survival rate). Few patients survive 5 years with hepatic metastases, indeed 85% of patients will be dead within 1 year.

Tumour stage is determined by time to presentation rather than time to diagnosis or treatment. Many tumours are of an advanced nature when first encountered, with 45% being locally extensive and 25% exhibiting evidence of distal metastases. The overall resection rate is approximately 70–80% of which 50–60% are regarded as curative procedures. Fifteen to 20% of patients undergo a palliative diversion only, and the remainder either have no surgical treatment or undergo laparotomy alone. In those undergoing apparently curative resection, half will be dead within 5 years and it is now apparent that approximately 25% who are thought to undergo curative surgery harbour occult hepatic metastases, which are almost certainly present for many months prior to initial presentation.

Surgeons also have a profound effect upon the outcome of colorectal cancer and significant variations have been consistently demonstrated in local recurrence and survival rates between operators following resection of similar stage tumours. Tumour present at resection margins (longitudinal and circumferential), perforation of tumour during mobilisation and anastomotic dehiscence are all associated with a high rate of local recurrence and are potentially all surgeon-dependent variables which, if they occur, are associated with a poor outcome.

ROLE OF CHEMOTHERAPY IN THE MANAGEMENT OF COLORECTAL CANCER

Adjuvant chemotherapy

There is now good evidence that adjuvant chemotherapy confers a survival advantage on patients who undergo curative resections and are found to have no metastases in the surgical specimen. Trials so far have shown a statistically significant decrease in the risk of death from cancer in the medium term (3–5 years) when chemotherapeutic regimens based on 5-fluorouracil are administered. The activity of this agent is commonly modulated either by addition of folinic acid or levamasol. Trials are currently being carried out to determine which combination of agents is best and how they should be administered. It is not yet clear if the 20–30% survival advantage at 3–5 years is associated with an increase in cure rate or whether there is only a significant delay in death. It has been suggested that the increased cure rate will be in the order of 5–10% but this may be significant in view of the large numbers of patients affected. Whether treatment is cost-effective has also not been established. Currently, however, it is recommended that patients with Dukes' stage C colorectal cancer should receive adjuvant chemotherapy. The role of chemotherapy with Dukes' stage B tumours has not been established and they should only receive treatment within the confines of randomised trials. The use of systemic adjuvant chemotherapy in patients with Dukes' stage A colorectal cancer is not recommended.

Chemotherapy for advanced disease

The intention of chemotherapy in advanced disease is to provide palliation and current evidence suggests that, when compared with best supportive care, chemotherapy confers a worthwhile significant prolongation in survival (5–9 months versus 11–14 months) as well as a significant increase in symptom-free survival time (2 months versus 10 months). All patients with advanced or metastatic colorectal cancer should therefore be considered for palliative chemotherapy. As with adjuvant chemotherapy, regimens are based on 5-fluorouracil and trials are currently running to determine the most beneficial therapeutic option.

ROLE OF RADIATION IN THE MANAGEMENT OF COLORECTAL CANCER

Patients with locally extensive rectal cancer are at risk of developing locoregional recurrence even if surgery is thought to be curative and the patient undergoes total mesorectal excision. It is suggested that metastases in pelvic lymph nodes are responsible and current data demonstrate that radiotherapy significantly reduces the incidence of local recurrence and confer a survival advantage on these patients. Preoperative pelvic irradiation (neo-adjuvant radiotherapy) is favoured because it is associated with less morbidity than radiotherapy administered in the postoperative period. The presence of a locally extensive tumour can be defined by transrectal ultrasound (extension outwith the rectal wall by more than 5 mm) or it can be judged clinically by either fixity or tethering of the neoplasm. Primary radical radiotherapy can be administered as an alternative treatment to surgery in patients who are medically unfit or refuse operation. Symptom control can also be achieved in some patients who present with locally advanced unresectable tumours or who return with pelvic recurrence following surgery.

PATIENT FOLLOW-UP

The aims of follow-up are to provide information for audit and clinical trials, to provide patient support, to detect and treat metachronous tumours, and to detect locoregional or distant recurrent disease. Patients who have had either palliative or curative treatment but are not fit for further intervention should be spared intensive follow-up regimens. Once it is established that the colon is tumour-free patients should undergo surveillance colonoscopy every 3–5 years. This significantly decreases the incidence of future colorectal cancer and there is no evidence that shorter surveillance intervals have any additional impact. Liver metastases and pelvic recurrence after excision of rectal cancers might be amenable to further curative treatment (i.e. by surgery) and should therefore undergo 6-monthly hepatic ultrasound and pelvic examinations for 2–3 years. Routine monitoring of CEA has not been demonstrated to be of survival advantage and may in fact be of negative benefit in that patients experience impaired quality of life once they know their CEA level has risen.

MANAGEMENT OF MALIGNANT LARGE BOWEL OBSTRUCTION

Colorectal cancer accounts for 70% of cases of large bowel obstruction (LBO). Ten to 15% of colorectal cancers present with LBO.

Patients affected are commonly elderly, dehydrated, hypovolaemic and oliguric, *therefore* fluid resuscitation to restore circulating volume and establish an adequate urine output is the first priority. If there are signs of peritoneal irritation or radiological evidence that the ileocaecal valve is competent then further investigation and decompression is urgent. Gastrografin enemas to exclude acute colonic pseudo-obstruction and to confirm mechanical obstruction is mandatory, with the exception of evidence of colonic perforation. The site of the obstruction is also shown in the majority of cases, however synchronous tumours are not excluded with this limited technique. Flexible sigmoidoscopy or colonoscopy can be performed in the absence of an enema but an expert endoscopist is required in such circumstances. The rectum should be examined digitally and sigmoidoscopically to exclude synchronous neoplasms because radiological imaging is weak here.

Principles of surgical treatment
These are essentially the same as those for the surgical treatment of colorectal cancer in the elective setting. It must be recognised that surgery offers the patient the only chance of cure and can effect the best palliation in more advanced cases. Stage for stage, obstructing lesions have been shown to have a poorer outcome in terms of survival than non-obstructing tumours but there seems no reason this should be so if established oncological principles are adhered to. If resection is not possible then a tumour may be bypassed or defunctioned by raising a proximal stoma. If there is gross disparity between bowel ends then an end-to-end anastomosis can be fashioned by making an anti-mesenteric cut along the narrower diameter intestine. An alternative is to fashion either an end-to-side or side-to-side anastomosis.

Right and transverse colon
These should be managed by standard right or extended right hemicolectomy wherever possible. If the caecum is very tense then it can be decompressed either by passing a catheter through the ileocaecal valve from the ileum or by inserting a needle tangentially into the bowel lumen along a taenia.

Left-sided colonic obstruction
This is an area of controversy and can be managed in three, two or one stage.

- Three-stage management: First the obstructed colon is decompressed by formation of a proximal loop stoma then the obstructing carcinoma is resected, and finally the stoma is closed
- Two-stage management: This is known as the Hartmann's procedure and involves primary resection with formation of a

proximal end stoma and closure of the distal loop. At a subsequent laparotomy intestinal continuity is restored
• One-stage management: Here the obstructing carcinoma is resected and a primary anastomosis is fashioned, usually following on-table, antegrade colonic lavage.

There is little prospective randomised data available to draw firm conclusions as to which of these is best, but the last seems most advantageous because it only involves one operation, it is associated with the shortest hospitalisation time, it is not associated with increased morbidity and mortality when compared with the others (the cumulative mortality rate is approximately 10% for each) and it avoids the patient acquiring a stoma. In both the three- and two-stage procedures a substantial proportion of patients fail to complete the management cycle and are left with a permanent stoma. When one-stage management is instituted intestinal continuity can be restored, either by segmental resection combined with on-table, antegrade colonic lavage, or sub-total colectomy can be performed followed by ileocolic or ileorectal anastomosis. Recent prospective randomised data suggest that the former offers the best functional outcome and is thus preferred.

VOLVULUS

The caecum, transverse and sigmoid colons can undergo volvulus, the latter accounting for the vast majority of cases. Volvulus accounts for 30% of intestinal obstruction in adults in developing world communities where there is a high consumption of vegetable material. In Western societies, where the diet is more refined, volvulus is uncommon and principally seems to affect those who are institutionalised. Factors which are thought to predispose to volvulus are:

• Intestinal dysmotility
• Narrow sigmoid mesocolon
• Distal obstruction (volvulus of transverse colon and caecum)
• Previous surgery
• Incomplete mid-gut rotation (caecal volvulus)
• Pregnancy (transverse colon and caecum).

Clinical features

• Pain, constipation and marked abdominal distension are common
• If colonic gangrene has occurred there are signs of sepsis and peritonitis.

Radiology

• With sigmoid volvulus there is massive gaseous distension of the sigmoid loop which loses its haustrations and appears as an

inverted U, extending from the pelvis to its apex in the right upper quadrant. If a contrast study is performed then the proximal end of the column of contrast will have a beaked appearance
- With caecal volvulus the coma-shaped caecal shadow will be seen lying remote from the right iliac fossa which will be filled with loops of small bowel
- Transverse colon volvulus has a similar appearance to sigmoid colon volvulus and will require contrast imaging to make a definite diagnosis. This is seldom achieved preoperatively.

Treatment

Sigmoid volvulus

- If gangrene is not suspected then the sigmoid loop should be decompressed either by rigid sigmoidoscopy and insertion of a flatus tube or by colonoscopy. The latter is preferred as it allows completion of the procedure under direct vision and permits thorough inspection of the mucosa to determine if ischaemia is present
- Following decompression there is a high incidence of recurrence (approximately 60%) and the overall mortality is high (approximately 15%). For this reason definitive corrective surgery is advocated following decompression and bowel preparation.
- Primary resection and anastomosis is the best option in ideal circumstances, but sigmoidopexy and suturplasty of the mesentery are also reported
- In the emergency situation all cases must be considered on their own merits
- Resection of ischaemic/gangrenous bowel is vital for survival
- Restoration of continuity may be possible but a Hartmann's procedure may be required if circumstances make anastomosis ill-advised
- A double-barrel divided stoma (Paul-Miculicz type) might also be considered.

Caecal volvulus
There is little place for colonoscopic decompression here.

- If gangrene is present then treatment is by right hemicolectomy
- If it is not then patients can be treated in a similar fashion or by caecopexy/insertion of caecostomy.

Transverse colon

- This is seldom discovered preoperatively so colonoscopic decompression is inappropriate
- If gangrene is present then treatment is by extended right hemicolectomy. This is also suitable in non-gangrenous cases

- Suture of the sides of the transverse colon to the adjacent ascending and descending colons has also been described.

ACUTE COLONIC PSEUDO-OBSTRUCTION

In this condition there are symptoms, signs and radiological features of large bowel obstruction, but a mechanical cause is absent. In the vast majority of cases this occurs in patients who have significant co-existing problems most notably trauma, pelvic surgery and electrolyte imbalance (hypernatraemia, hyperkalaemia and hypocalcaemia). Drugs are also commonly associated with pseudo-obstruction, particularly opiates and those with an anticholinergic action. The precise cause of colonic pseudo-obstruction has not been ascertained, but it is almost certainly multifactorial and arises from a dysmotile segment of the large bowel which does not allow coordinated peristalsis. Abnormal activity of the autonomic nervous system has been implicated but whether this involves the sympathetic, parasympathetic or enteric nervous systems is unknown.

Clinical features

- Acute colonic pseudo-obstruction is often indistinguishable on clinical grounds from mechanical large bowel obstruction and plain abdominal radiographs may be of little additional benefit
- Pseudo-obstruction should be considered in all patients presenting with large bowel obstruction and particularly those with co-existing problems (see above). For this reason a water-soluble contrast enema should be carried out in all cases.

Treatment

Non-operative treatment

- *Correction of the underlying cause if possible (i.e. stop narcotic and anticholinergic drugs, correct electrolyte imbalance).* If the colon is moderately distended (i.e. less than 9 cm diameter) then this alone may be sufficient but obstruction may take several days to resolve
- *Colonic decompression.* This should be considered when the colonic diameter is greater than 9 cm and is urgently required when the diameter exceeds 12 cm. Decompression is best achieved by colonoscopy. Minimal insufflation should be used and the instrument should be passed as far round the colon as possible. The procedure can be repeated if colonic distension recurs
- *Pharmacological manipulation.* Neostigmine (administered with glycopyrrolate to prevent cardiac complications) can lead to rapid resolution of pseudo-obstruction and might be considered in recalcitrant cases.

Operative management

- This is required when conservative measures fail, or when there are signs of peritonitis
- Caecostomy fashioned through a right iliac fossa laparotomy is the procedure of choice either when the caecum is viable or when there is only a patch of necrotic tissue present
- If more extensive caecal necrosis is found then right hemicolectomy or ileostomy and mucous fistula are required.

ULCERATIVE COLITIS

Ulcerative colitis is an inflammatory condition of unknown origin which is confined to the large bowel mucosa. Ulcerative colitis affects the rectum and extends proximally in confluent fashion for a variable distance; in *pancolitis* the entire colorectal mucosa is involved. Pseudopolyps occur where oedematous mucosa is retained but is surrounded by denuded/ulcerated mucosa. In severe acute colitis inflammation may extend to affect the full thickness of the bowel which can undergo toxic dilatation. The microscopic features include mucosal inflammation/ulceration, goblet cell depletion and crypt abscess formation. Granulomata are not seen. The aetiology of ulcerative colitis is unknown but genetic and acquired factors have been implicated.

Clinical features
A spectrum of presentation is seen ranging from severe acute colitis to mild intermittent proctitis.

Severe acute colitis

- This is characterised by passage of more than six loose, bloody motions each day combined with signs of systemic upset (malaise, fever, tachycardia, raised WBC, raised ESR and hypoalbuminaemia)
- If untreated it can progress to toxic dilatation with perforation and prior to effective treatment with steroids the mortality was 30%.

Chronic

- Episodes of relapse interspersed with periods of remission is the norm
- Frequent and severe relapses can significantly impair quality of life and jeopardise employment
- Drugs may not control symptoms and can produce unwanted side-effects (especially steroids).

Chronic illness and risk of carcinoma

- Previously the risk was thought to be 10% at 10 years from onset of disease but is now recognised to be lower (see above)

- Screening programmes have been established for chronic colitics to detect dysplasia but the benefit of such programmes has been questioned and is currently under evaluation.

Extra-intestinal manifestations

- Ankylosing spondylitis
- Uveitis/iritis
- Pyoderma gangrenosum
- Erythema nodosum
- Sclerosing cholangitis.

Severe uveitis/iritis and pyoderma gangrenosum are rare indications for surgery.

Differential diagnosis

- Other causes of colorectal inflammation should be excluded, particularly infection
- Differentiation from Crohn's colitis can be difficult and doubt may exist even after colectomy
- Clinical impression *and* pathology should be taken into account.

Treatment

Medical

- In severe acute colitis the '5-day' regimen is instituted: intravenous (i.v.) and rectal steroids, i.v. fluids as required, sips only by mouth and regular review by the gastrointestinal team
- Surgery is indicated if the patient fails to settle or deteriorates during this time
- Toxic dilatation (maximum normal colonic diameter 5 cm) can be treated medically but rapid resolution must be ensured
- Steroids and non-steroidal anti-inflammatory agents given orally or rectally are the mainstay of treatment in chronic illness
- Azathioprine can have a steroid-sparing action.

Surgical
The traditional approach has been challenged over the last 10–15 years by introduction of restorative proctocolectomy with ileal pouch-anal anastomosis. This is perhaps now the 'gold-standard' treatment but other options are available (most notably panproctocolectomy with ileostomy formation) and many patients opt for these in view of significant morbidity associated with pouch procedures. All patients contemplating pouch surgery should be realistically counselled about potential morbidity and long-term failure and must realise that restorative proctocolectomy is not a return to normality.

Surgical options

Panproctocolectomy and formation of Brooke ileostomy comprises the following:

- Well tried and usually uncomplicated
- Removes all diseased tissue and so cancer risk
- Potential social and psychosexual consequences from stoma
- At least 30% of patients in many UK centres opt for this procedure.

Colectomy with formation of Koch continent ileostomy has the following features:

- Retains advantages of above but replaces Brooke ileostomy with a flush, continent stoma
- 'Continent' nipple valve difficult to construct
- Could be considered in a patient who has already undergone complete proctocolectomy and who wishes to be rid of a stoma.

Colectomy with ileorectal anastomosis This has the following qualities:

- Attractive because it is relatively straightforward and avoids stoma but it remains controversial because, by leaving behind the rectum, it is associated with an ever present risk of carcinoma
- It might be considered in a young patient with a compliant rectum which is relatively spared from disease. The patient must be reliable as follow-up will be lifelong
- Co-existing sclerosing cholangitis or portal hypertension, where rectal dissection would be hazardous, also favour this option.

Restorative proctocolectomy This is the procedure of choice for elective treatment of ulcerative colitis. It is *not* indicated in Crohn's disease or with a lower third rectal cancer or poor anal sphincter function. Current operations involve the creation of an ileal reservoir of various designs followed by its anastomosis to the anal canal. The commonest configuration is the 'J' pouch.

Emergency surgery for severe acute colitis Sub-total colectomy, with formation of a Brooke ileostomy, is the procedure of choice. The best way to manage the rectal stump remains undecided but it is clear that pelvic dissection should be avoided as this will make a subsequent restorative procedure technically difficult. A 'long' stump can be left within the peritoneal cavity or it can be delivered as a mucous fistula. More unconventionally, it can be closed and placed subcutaneously at the lower end of the laparotomy wound to avoid a second stoma.

RESTORATIVE PROCTOCOLECTOMY

The original operation was pioneered by the late Sir Alan Parks and colleagues at St Mark's Hospital in London in 1976 and it has undergone considerable modification since then. The following are important issues:

The plane of rectal dissection

This can be conducted either in the perimuscular or mesorectal plane. Many patients suffering from ulcerative colitis are sexually active and great care is required to preserve the pelvic nerves and in particular the nervi erigentes.

Pouch design

The pouch originally described by Parks was a triple loop S pouch; however, two-loop J pouch, four-loop W pouch and lateral isoperistaltic or H pouch have also been described. These pouches can be hand sewn or stapled and use approximately 40–50 cm of terminal ileum.

The ileal pouch-anal anastomosis

Excision of the rectal mucosa down to the dentate line achieves the aim of excising all potentially diseased epithelium but *also* removes the anal transition zone which has a rich sensory nerve supply and is thought to play an important role in sensory discrimination as well as continence. The functional results are better if the anal transition zone is preserved but there is a long-term risk from leaving behind potentially diseased mucosa. Based on the current balance of information mucosectomy should be avoided in the absence of rectal mucosal dysplasia but is required if rectal dysplasia is diagnosed preoperatively or is found on subsequent histological examination of the surgical specimen. The ileo-anal anastomosis can be either hand sewn or stapled and although there is no solid evidence to favour either, most surgeons use a stapling device because it is quicker and technically easier. Under ideal circumstances a temporary ileostomy is not required.

Postoperative management and course

- If a defunctioning ileostomy is formed, then this is closed at 6–8 weeks. If an ileostomy is omitted, then the pouch may be intubated with a wide-bore balloon catheter for 7 days to divert the faecal stream. The perianal region should be protected by barrier cream and a careful record kept of fluid balance. Patients can be allowed home at 10–14 days postoperatively if well and confident. Early review is sensible in order to monitor and advise on pouch function. Constipating medication will reduce stool frequency in the first few months
- Very few deaths have been reported after restorative proctocolectomy but there is appreciable morbidity and approximately 20–25% of patients will experience a serious complication which requires further surgery. Abdominal/pelvic sepsis (with and without anastomotic breakdown), adhesional

obstruction, haemorrhage, pouch ischaemia, fistula formation and anastomotic strictures are the main complications here.

The functional results

- Most patients will defaecate spontaneously about 4–6 times per 24 hours and will not experience urgency. Few patients suffer frank incontinence but minor imperfections such as spotting or soiling can occur
- Some 20–30% of patients use codeine phosphate or loperamide hydrochloride
- The best clinical results are associated with a large capacity, compliant pouch which empties completely and which sits above normal anal sphincters. It is recognised that the pouch functions in part by modifying terminal ileal motility but the relationship between this, capacity and compliance remains unexplained
- Outright failure which requires pouch excision occurs in only 5–10% of patients and is caused by persistent pelvic sepsis, undiagnosed Crohn's disease or unacceptable stool frequency.

Long-term mucosal changes

- Colonic metaplasia of the ileal pouch epithelium is noted on histological examination and is supported by histochemical and immuno-reactivity studies
- Chronic inflammation as well as villous atrophy are also seen. The cause of these changes is not known but probably involves bacteriological and immunological agents
- The risk of future dysplasia and even frank malignancy cannot be ignored but to date no such occurrence has been reported in either a pelvic or a Koch pouch. More acute inflammatory changes also occur and can produce 'pouchitis' in up to 30% of cases
- Pouchitis is characterised by diarrhoea in the presence of endoscopic and histological features of acute inflammation. It is more common in patients who had extensive disease than in those whose colitis was left-sided or distal. The pathogenesis of pouchitis is not known and is almost certainly multi-factorial
- Contact between the pouch mucosa and ileal contents is an essential feature as are stasis and bacterial overgrowth within the pouch
- The importance of genetic predisposition, specific bacterial strains, epithelial defects and immunological abnormalities is uncertain but they have all been implicated as causative agents
- Outlet obstruction, pouch ischaemia and Crohn's disease are important differential diagnoses which should be excluded
- Treatment of pouchitis is empirical
- Metronidazole is probably the most commonly used agent and is often combined with steroid enemas

- *Rarely*, pouchitis is intractable and necessitates the formation of a defunctioning ileostomy or even pouch excision.

CROHN'S DISEASE OF THE COLON, RECTUM AND ANAL CANAL

Crohn's disease can affect any part of the large bowel but tends to do so in recognised patterns:

- The caecum and ascending colon as part of ileocolonic Crohn's disease
- Segmental colitis. Here discontinuous disease occurs with areas of macroscopically unaffected bowel in between
- Diffuse Crohn's colitis
- Peri-anal disease.

Clinical features
These are determined by the mode of presentation.

- Patients with diffuse colitis can have symptoms similar to those experienced with ulcerative colitis
- Healing by fibrosis can lead to stricture formation and hence obstructive symptoms
- Ileocolonic and segmental disease can lead to the formation of an inflammatory mass
- Fistula formation is not uncommon and perforation can occur in the absence of toxic megacolon
- Fissures are common with peri-anal disease and may be painless
- More penetrating sepsis can lead to abscess formation and fistula-in-ano
- Fistulous tracts can be complex, can extend above the levators and can be multiple
- Investigation of any patient with Crohn's disease should concentrate upon establishing diagnosis, the extent of the gut involved, together with severity of the involvement (the large and small bowel should be imaged), and the nutritional consequences of the disease
- It is not uncommon that patients with severe Crohn's disease are malnourished and require resuscitation/nutritional support prior to treatment.

Principles of treatment
In severe acute diffuse Crohn's colitis the indications for surgery are similar to those with severe acute ulcerative colitis.

- Surgery is commonly required in the presence of abscess formation, fistula and obstruction
- Chronic debility and unwanted drug side-effects may also be indications for surgery

- Minimal access treatment may be considered in certain instances, i.e. endoluminal balloon dilatation of a colonic stricture, but it is essential that this is only performed where the diagnosis is certain (i.e. colonic obstruction in Crohn's disease may be due to fibrosis, but can also occur secondary to carcinoma)
- As with surgery for Crohn's disease, elsewhere it is important to preserve gut if possible
- Limited resections are permissible for segmental disease, and sub-total colectomy with ileorectal anastomosis is reasonable where there is colonic disease but rectal sparing
- Where both the colon and rectum are affected then panproctocolectomy with ileostomy formation is best; however, in the emergency treatment of panproctocolitis, resection should be limited to the colon only with formation of the ileostomy and either formation of a mucous fistula or closure of the rectal stump (intraperitoneal), depending upon the degree of rectal involvement
- In some selected cases, faecal diversion by formation of a loop ileostomy can facilitate resolution of large bowel disease sufficient to allow restoration of continuity in approximately 30% of cases
- In the management of peri-anal disease, sepsis must be drained promptly and adequately but in all other respects it is important to pursue a conservative path
- Fissures should not be treated unless they are symptomatic and GTN paste should be used prior to any consideration of sphincterotomy
- Fistulae should be explored to ensure adequate drainage and then managed by insertion of loose setons
- Sphincter muscle should not be cut due to possible future consequences of this upon continence.

DIVERTICULAR DISEASE

This is a common condition in Western societies whose prevalence increases with age such that it affects over 60% of 70-year-olds. The left colon and in particular the sigmoid colon are most frequently affected although right-side diverticulae are seen.

Aetiology and pathophysiology

- This is an acquired condition which is believed to occur secondary to high intra-luminal pressure within the colon. Lack of dietary fibre is thought to be the cause although abnormalities of colonic wall connective tissue and sedentary lifestyle have also been implicated
- Diverticulae consist of mucosa and serosa only and protrude at weak points in the colonic wall where arterial branches penetrate circular smooth muscle adjacent to taenia

- Diverticulitis occurs following obstruction of the neck of a diverticulum and proliferation of bacteria within the sealed space. Surrounding tissue becomes inflamed leading to the formation of a phlegmon (inflammatory mass). The outcome depends upon how well the sepsis is localised and is determined by site, speed of progression and degree of contamination
- Peritonitis can complicate diverticulitis. A widespread inflammatory exudate can occur with a phegmon. Purulent peritonitis usually results from rupture of a previously localised abscess and faecal peritonitis occurs when there is free communication between the peritoneal cavity and the colonic lumen
- Resolution of sepsis can result in chronic inflammation, fibrosis and stricture formation
- Bleeding from a diverticulum is an important cause of major lower gastrointestinal haemorrhage in the elderly.

Clinical features

Elective presentation
Diverticular disease is commonly found in those investigated for left iliac fossa pain, alteration in bowel habit and bleeding per rectum. Few of these patients come to resection and in those that do, symptom relief is not invariable.

Emergency presentation
This can result from the following:

- Acute diverticulitis
- Abscess formation
- Fistula
- Haemorrhage
- Obstruction.

The causal diagnosis might not be apparent and therefore these conditions should be managed on their own merits with appropriate investigation and treatment. For instance, carcinoma and Crohn's disease can cause fistulae and colonic obstruction.

ACUTE DIVERTICULITIS

Patients can present with either localised or generalised peritonitis and time taken obtaining a careful history and examination can be invaluable in determining the underlying cause of mischief. Patients should be reassessed following resuscitation and analgesia as an apparently diffuse process usually becomes more localised. A decision to perform emergency surgery is made in the septic patient with generalised peritonitis and evidence of free perforation. All other patients should receive a trial of conservative treatment (fluid resuscitation, broad spectrum antibiotics, analgesia, gut rest and frequent reassessment). This should be continued where there is clinical improvement.

Investigation

- Sigmoidoscopy should be avoided in the acute setting but is mandatory following resolution or if the patient proceeds to surgery to exclude anorectal pathology
- Plain abdominal radiographs may show free gas or signs of soft tissue inflammation (thickened bowel wall or an extra-luminal mass)
- Contrast enema, CT (with contrast) and ultrasound are useful in the acute setting to establish diagnosis, demonstrate complications and they can direct treatment. Water-soluble contrast enemas may demonstrate diverticulae, tissue thickening, mucosal irregularity and perforation. The latter makes recourse to surgery more likely but not inevitable. Water-soluble contrast should be used in the emergency situation, to avoid the formation of barium granulomata should a perforation or spillage occur. Contrast-enhanced CT is favoured in many centres and can also demonstrate extra-luminal changes such as abscess formation. The clinical utility of these modalities is similar, whereas ultrasound is heavily operator-dependent and is less often used except when abscess formation is suspected
- The presence of synchronous colorectal pathology should be determined following an acute attack or if surgery is required (intra-operative colonoscopy).

Treatment

- Most episodes of acute diverticulitis settle with conservative measures, even if there is evidence of perforation
- Surgery is required infrequently but is necessary in the septic patient with generalised peritonitis where the diagnosis is unclear and when conservative measures fail
- Resection of the diverticular affected segment combined with copious peritoneal lavage is the lynch-pin of surgical treatment as it removes sepsis and its source. This is most commonly achieved as part of a Hartmann's procedure (sigmoid resection, oversewing of the rectal stump and formation of left iliac fossa colostomy)
- Resection with primary anastomosis is seldom advisable under these circumstances
- Defunctioning the affected bowel by formation of a proximal stoma does not remove the source of sepsis and is associated with a higher degree of morbidity and mortality
- If non-perforated diverticulitis is discovered at the time of laparotomy then the patient is best served by peritoneal lavage and institution of conservative measures only. Resection or formation of a proximal stoma is not required

- Following resolution of an acute episode, consideration should be given to elective resection. Each patient should be assessed individually. It is suggested that those less than 50 years of age are at high risk of developing a further serious complication and thus should proceed to surgery after the first acute episode. This, however, has not been appraised scientifically.

PSEUDOMEMBRANOUS COLITIS

This is a diarrhoeal illness which derives its name from yellowish-white plaques of an acute inflammatory exudate which are found throughout the large bowel in the severe form of the disease.

Aetiology

- Pseudomembranous colitis (PMC) is caused by a cytotoxin produced by *Clostridium difficile*, a Gram-positive, anaerobic, spore-forming bacillus. The bacteria is not normally present in the colon and infection only occurs when there is diminished resistance to colonisation
- PMC most commonly occurs as a complication of broad-spectrum antibiotic treatment.

Clinical features

- Watery diarrhoea and a low-grade fever are common and occur from 2 days to 3 weeks after antibiotic treatment
- Colicky abdominal pain, bloody diarrhoea and toxic megacolon are recognised, but infrequent, complications
- Sigmoidoscopy will usually reveal rectal plaques in severe cases. The mucosa between plaques appears normal
- Diagnosis is established by demonstrating the presence of *C. difficile* toxin in the stools or biopsy from rectum/sigmoid colon of symptomatic individuals
- In the absence of measurable toxin an alternative diagnosis should be considered even if the organism is present.

Treatment

- The mainstay of treatment is antibiotic therapy – oral metronidazole 250 mg or vancomycin 125 mg every 6 hours. Other antibiotics should be withdrawn
- Clinical improvement should be noted within 48 hours but relapse may occur either because of re-infection or the failure to eradicate the bacteria
- Barrier nursing is required to prevent spread of the organism to other patients.

ISCHAEMIC COLITIS

Ischaemic colitis is an inflammatory condition produced by interruption of the blood supply to the colon which is insufficient to cause full thickness tissue death. It most commonly affects those in the sixth to the eighth decades of life.

Aetiology

Ischaemic colitis can be caused by:

- Occlusion of a major artery
- Small vessel disease
- Venous obstruction
- 'Low flow' states
- Intestinal obstruction.

The mucosa and sub-mucosa are predominantly affected. Ischaemia reduces the integrity of the mucosa and allows invasion by pathogenic organisms which produce inflammation with mucosal ulceration. The splenic flexure is particularly susceptible to ischaemic injury because it is the site of the watershed between the superior mesenteric artery (SMA) and the inferior mesenteric artery (IMA). These vessels are linked by a marginal artery, but this is frequently absent or poorly developed at the splenic flexure. Occlusion of either major artery or their branches can therefore result in ischaemia. Resolution is the usual outcome but healing by fibrosis and subsequent stricture formation can occur. Necrotising colitis is a rare complication.

Varying degrees of ischaemic colitis can occur after abdominal aortic aneurysm repair, as the IMA is usually sacrificed. Surgical technique advises that the IMA is oversewn from within the aneurysm sac to preserve collateral circulation.

Clinical features

History

- The typical patient is 50 years of age or more and complains of left-sided abdominal pain. They may pass loose stools which characteristically contain **dark blood** as well as clots
- A history of previous episodes, peripheral or cardiovascular disease, or collagen vascular disease should be noted.

Examination

- There may be a low-grade pyrexia and tachycardia
- On abdominal examination, the affected colon is tender and may be palpable
- Dark blood will be present per rectum
- Signs of peripheral vascular disease or other associated conditions should be sought

- It is important to first establish the diagnosis and then determine the presence of any treatable aetiological factors.

Radiological investigations

- A plain abdominal radiograph and a contrast enema are the most useful investigations in the initial stages
- 'Thumb-printing' is seen early on, particularly at the splenic flexure and is diagnostic. Later, mucosal ulceration and irregularity may develop and these can resemble the findings present in ulcerative colitis or Crohn's disease
- Stricture formation, if it occurs, causes further diagnostic problems
- Ischaemic strictures are often long, uniform and have smooth, gradual beginnings and ends, an appearance called 'funnelling'. These findings do not, however, exclude carcinoma and this diagnosis should be uppermost if only a short segment of colon is affected
- The role of angiography is not established. Although it can be valuable in isolated cases where significant, symptomatic occlusive lesions are revealed, there is generally no correlation between the appearance of vessels at angiography and the integrity of the colonic blood supply.

Direct visualisation

- Ischaemic lesions are usually beyond the reach of the rigid sigmoidoscope
- Colonoscopy can be used to visualise and biopsy affected colon
- In the early stages of ischaemia, the mucosa will be heaped up, oedematous and bluish purple (the 'thumb-prints' seen radiologically)
- Later, ulceration as well as strictures may be seen.

Differential diagnosis
This includes the following:

- Inflammatory bowel disease
- Ulcerative colitis
- Crohn's colitis
- Pseudomembranous colitis
- Amoebic dysentry
- Bacillary dysentry
- Others, i.e. campylobacter
- Carcinoma
- Diverticular disease
- Pancreatitis.

Treatment

- Conservative management is the mainstay for those seen with acute symptoms. The patient is given intravenous fluids

- Broad-spectrum antibiotics are often administered although there is no hard evidence that they influence outcome
- There is no place for anticoagulation or steroid administration unless this is indicated by an underlying disorder such as vasculitis
- It is very rare for ischaemic colitis to progress to frank colonic gangrene but clearly frequent, careful review is required
- If the injury is transient then resolution occurs after a few days. More severe insults lead to stricture formation
- These require investigation and treatment if they produce symptoms or if there is another diagnosis
- Excision followed by end-to-end anastomosis is safe, although it is essential to ensure the viability and vascularity of the resection margins.

MASSIVE COLONIC BLEEDING

Acute massive lower gastrointestinal bleeding accounts for 20% of acute gastrointestinal haemorrhage and can be defined as blood loss from a source distal to the ligament of Treitz which has a transfusion requirement of more than two units. Bleeding from the small bowel and Meckel's diverticulum are included here but these are uncommon and represent only 1% of acute gastrointestinal haemorrhages. The incidence of acute massive colonic bleeding increases with age.

Aetiology
The causes of massive colorectal bleeding are:

- Diverticular disease
- Angiodysplasia
- Ischaemic colitis
- Others:
  - Colorectal neoplasms
  - Irradiation proctocolitis
  - Inflammatory bowel disease
  - Haemorrhoids
  - Haemangiomas.

Diverticular disease
In many series this is the most common cause of massive colorectal bleeding. Bleeding is thought to emanate from erosion or rupture of arterial branches at the neck or dome of diverticula. Larger right-sided lesions are more commonly affected than those on the left, perhaps reflecting the greater length of vessel exposed to possible injury.

Angiodysplasia
Angiodysplasia (or vascular ectasia) is thought to result from intermittent, incomplete low-pressure obstruction of submucosal

veins which leads to arteriovenous shunts. It occurs in approximately 25% of those over 60 years. This has been increasingly recognised as a cause of bleeding during the last two decades. Bleeding is characteristically intermittent and can cease spontaneously although re-bleeding is common. Right-sided colonic lesions predominate although the left colon can also be affected. In the acute setting angiodysplasia is diagnosed at angiography which reveals early filling of tortuous arteries, vascular lakes in the capillary phase and early filling of dilated veins. Extravasation of contrast is seldom seen. Dilated tortuous vessels and 'cherry-red' areas are seen at colonoscopy but these are only visible following thorough bowel preparation.

Clinical features

Initial assessment
All patients should have their haemodynamic status determined on admission and appropriate resuscitative measures should be instituted. Elderly patients are intolerant of major blood loss and fluid replacement should start early to avoid hypotension. There should be a low threshold for invasive monitoring (urinary catheterisation and CVP monitoring) in this group. Procto-sigmoidoscopy is an important part of the initial assessment and upper gastrointestinal endoscopy is mandatory in massive haemorrhage to exclude a proximal source of blood loss. If blood loss is less than 4 units in 24 hours then it will almost certainly stop spontaneously but if more than 4 units is lost then there is a greater than 50% chance that this will not occur and surgery will be required.

Investigation
The aim of investigation is to define the site of bleeding and so allow 'targeted' segmental colonic resection if surgery is required.
   Colonoscopy   This can be performed following resuscitation (early), intra-operatively or electively once bleeding has ceased (late), and has the advantage that it can facilitate both diagnosis and treatment. When the bowel is unprepared colonoscopy can be technically demanding and considerable expertise is required to complete an examination satisfactorily. It is crucial that demonstration of an abnormality is supported by recognition of stigmata of recent haemorrhage before a definitive diagnosis of the source of blood loss is made. Intra-operative colonoscopy, combined with antegrade colonic lavage, is recommended when the source of bleeding has not been defined previously and has been shown to have a high degree of diagnostic accuracy. Prior mobilisation of both the right and left colons makes the examination technically easier.
   Angiography   Selective angiography of the splanchnic circulation can be very helpful, particularly if extravasation of

contrast into the bowel lumen is seen (a rate of blood loss of 1–1.5 ml/min is required). All patients must be adequately resuscitated and must be carefully monitored throughout. Angiography also provides the opportunity for treatment either by infusion of vasopressin or embolisation of the bleeding vessel. The latter is particularly useful in haemorrhage from the rectum but can produce colonic infarction when used more proximally.

Radio-nuclide scanning 99m Technetium-labelled red cell scanning can detect rates of blood loss down to 0.1 ml/min and can be repeated at intervals over a 24-hour period. It can therefore be helpful in cases of intermittent haemorrhage but due to rapid movement of blood in the gut it frequently fails to localise the source of blood loss. Its precise role in the management of massive colorectal bleeding is not yet established.

Operative treatment

- The need for surgery and its urgency is dictated by the rate of blood loss. If the source of bleeding can be confidently diagnosed then segmental resection with primary anastomosis (± antegrade colonic lavage) should be the aim
- When more than one possible source is identified (for instance right-sided colonic angiodysplasia in a patient with co-existing left-sided diverticular) and neither shows stigmata of recent haemorrhage, then sub-total colectomy is recommended
- In such circumstances, however, great care must be taken to exclude a small bowel or rectal source of bleeding. On-table enteroscopy can be helpful here.

CHRONIC CONSTIPATION IN ADULTS

Two groups of patients can be identified:

- Those with normal propulsion but who are unable to expel stool from the rectum. This has been called obstructed defaecation or anismus
- Those with abnormal colonic propulsion.

OBSTRUCTED DEFAECATION

Careful assessment will reveal a characteristic history of evacuatory difficulties including prolonged straining, manipulation of the anal margin and perineum, and even self-digitation to effect a bowel action. The investigation of choice is defaecating proctography which will reveal rectal architectural abnormalities (for instance prolapse) if these are present.

Treatment should be conservative with careful explanation of the problem to the patient and reassurance that digital manipulation is unlikely to cause problems. Biofeedback can teach patients to relax their pelvic floor and anal sphincter muscles and this can be helpful in approximately 50% of patients.

Attempts at surgical treatment have proved disappointing. Correction of rectal prolapse by rectopexy, lateral division of puborectalis, and myectomy of the internal anal sphincter and rectal smooth muscle have been tried as treatments, but have given poor results.

ABNORMAL COLORECTAL PROPULSION

When colonic propulsion is abnormal patients can be differentiated into those who have a normal calibre colon and those who have a dilated colon. Idiopathic slow transit constipation is the cause of the former. Adult Hirschsprung's disease and idiopathic megacolon/ megarectum account for the latter. In chronic idiopathic intestinal pseudo-obstruction both the large and small bowels are dilated.

Investigation

- These conditions are usefully differentiated by barium enema which defines colonic diameter and if this is increased then adult Hirschsprung's disease can be excluded by anorectal physiology if the recto-anal inhibitory reflex is unequivocally present
- A diagnosis of idiopathic megarectum and megacolon can be made once Hirschsprung's disease and secondary causes of colonic dilatation are excluded
- In adult Hirschsprung's disease the diagnosis should be confirmed by demonstration of absence of ganglia in a full thickness rectal biopsy
- Tracer studies using radio-opaque markers or radio-isotope 'stool' will confirm slow transit.

Treatment

- Adult Hirschsprung's disease is best treated by Duhamel's operation in which normally ganglionated colon is anastomosed to the posterior wall of the aganglionic rectum. Care is required to ensure that the colon anastomosed to the rectum is normally ganglionated and frozen sections taken at the time of surgery are required to confirm this
- Idiopathic megarectum and megacolon might be treated satisfactorily by conservative measures (laxatives, enemas and suppositories) but many patients require surgery. It is unclear which procedure is best
- If there is only moderate dilatation of the large bowel then colectomy with ileorectal anastomosis can be helpful, but in many instances either Duhamel's operation or resection and either colo-anal or ileal pouch-anal anastomosis are required
- If constipation remains a persistent problem then a permanent stoma may be needed

- In severe idiopathic slow transit constipation, full conservative measures should be instituted in the first instance and the patient encouraged to persist with these in an effort to achieve some benefit. If this is unsuccessful then surgical intervention might be considered and the most successful procedure appears to be colectomy with ileorectal anastomosis
- Unfortunately some patients continue to experience untoward symptoms such as abdominal pain in spite of the fact that their defaecatory habit is improved.

ANORECTAL INCONTINENCE

This can be defined as the inability to prevent inadvertent discharge from the anal canal. Both the type (flatus, fluid or solid) and the amount of leakage can vary but even small amounts can cause embarrassment and social disability. Prevalence increases with age such that 1.1% of men and 1.3% of women over 65 years are affected. In some groups, notably long stay geriatric and psychogeriatric patients, the prevalence is even higher with up to 25% leaking faeces each day.

MECHANISM OF NORMAL ANORECTAL CONTINENCE

Anorectal continence is determined by a number of factors which are illustrated in Figure 15.1. Of these, the smooth muscle internal

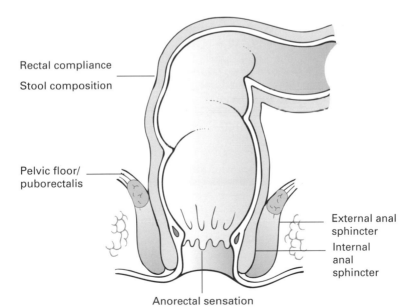

Rectal compliance

Stool composition

Pelvic floor/ puborectalis

External anal sphincter

Internal anal sphincter

Anorectal sensation

Fig. 15.1 Factors which play an important role in anorectal continence.

anal (IAS) and striated muscle external anal (EAS) sphincters are of prime importance.

Causes of anorectal incontinence

Anorectal incontinence can occur when any facet of the normal continence mechanism is defective. The causes of such abnormalities are:

1. *Incontinence with abnormal sphincters*
   - Direct sphincter injury (trauma, surgery)
   - Sphincter neuropathy (upper/lower MNL)
   - Congenital abnormalities
   - Rectal prolapse
   - Ageing
2. *Incontinence with normal sphincters*
   - Severe diarrhoea (infection, IBD)
   - Faecal impaction
   - Fistula
   - Dementia or mental retardation
   - Anorectal carcinoma.

Idiopathic anorectal incontinence

This is the most common cause of primary anorectal incontinence seen in adult surgical practice and it particularly affects middle-aged women. Histological and electrophysiological examination of the striated muscle components of the continence mechanism indicate the presence of a denervation/re-innervation injury which is probably caused by stretching of the pudendal and pelvic nerves. Such stretch injuries may occur first during childbirth and are then compounded by subsequent, chronic straining at stool. As well as striated muscle weakness, affected patients may have diminished anal sensation and abnormal internal and sphincter function.

Clinical features

History

- All patients attending coloproctology or gastroenterology clinics should be asked directly about anorectal incontinence as this may be a hidden symptom
- The character of the leakage and its frequency of occurrence should be determined and careful attention paid to defaecatory, previous medical and obstetric histories
- Neurological symptoms must be documented.

Examination

- Examine the patient as a whole because incontinence can be a manifestation of disease outside the anorectum

- The integrity of perineal innervation should be determined by testing pin-prick sensation and the ano-cutaneous reflex
- Digital anorectal examination allows qualitative assessment of sphincter pressures
- All patients should undergo proctoscopy and sigmoidoscopy.

Investigations
A thorough clinical assessment will usually reveal a diagnosis without recourse to specialist investigations. They may, however, be required.

Anorectal imaging In most instances it is wise to assess the entire large bowel to exclude a proximal contributory lesion such as an unsuspected carcinoma. High-resolution images of both sphincters can be obtained by anal ultrasonography. Magnetic resonance imaging (MRI) is of great value in assessing patients with congenital anorectal anomalies.

Tests of anorectal function These are useful because they aid diagnosis and objectively measure abnormalities but, as yet, they do not have a more extended role in management. Many have been used to assess the effects of treatment in clinical research, but they do not predict outcome in individual patients. Manometry quantifies anal canal pressures which reflects sphincter function (maximum resting proooure – IAS, resting sphincter length and maximum squeeze pressure – EAS). Anorectal sensation can be measured, for instance, by anal mucosa electrosensitivity and is reduced in some patients with anorectal incontinence. Anorectal electromyography (EMG) can demonstrate delayed pudendal nerve latency (idiopathic anorectal incontinence) and areas of electrical silence (direct sphincter injuries) but it is seldom utilised outside the research arena.

Treatment

Conservative measures

- These should be tried in all patients except when the clinical features and results of investigations suggest an underlying pathology such as inflammatory bowel disease, carcinoma or prolapse which requires alternative appropriate treatment
- Patients should be counselled and given advice with the aim of producing a solid stool once each day
- Codeine phosphate or loperamide may be helpful and a low fibre diet is recommended
- A successful outcome can be expected in up to 40% of patients treated by diet and drugs alone
- Other non-operative therapies include pelvic floor physiotherapy, biofeedback conditioning and electrical stimulation
- Promising early results have been reported but they have not yet been shown to be of long-term benefit.

Surgery in anorectal incontinence
This should be considered if conservative measures fail to ameliorate the problem. Patients undoubtedly fear the prospect of a permanent stoma and this should only be considered as a last resort.

Direct sphincter injuries   These should be explored through an incision in the area of the previously defined defect. The abrupted ends of the external sphincter are isolated and overlapping repair is fashioned so that an anal canal of adequate length can be reconstructed. Following the repair of a direct sphincter injury, 70–90% of patients can expect to have full continence restored with less than 10% achieving no benefit at all.

Postanal repair   This is the most commonly performed operation in cases where there is pelvic floor and external sphincter weakness due to neuropathy. Here the muscles are approximated in turn and the external sphincter is imbricated to recreate acute anorectal angulation. Although most patients gain some benefit from postanal repair, the quality of continence achieved is often imperfect and declines with time.

Novel treatments   These are listed as:

• Gracilis neosphincter
• Artificial sphincter
• Sacral nerve stimulation.

Gracilis transposition has been combined with prolonged neurostimulation with the effect of converting it from a fast twitch to a slow twitch muscle. These techniques are still in their evolutionary phases but hold promise for the future.

HAEMORRHOIDS (DISRUPTED ANAL CUSHIONS)

Pathophysiology

• Anal cushions are found within the submucosa of the anal canal and have the gross appearance of 'cavernosal' tissue. They consist of a sacculated venous plexus with a rich arterial supply supported by fibromuscular connective tissue. The arterial supply is derived from the superior middle and inferior rectal arteries and this communicates with the venous system, not only through capillaries but also by direct arteriovenous shunts. Anal cushions are found in surprisingly constant positions within the anal canal (3, 7 and 11 o'clock positions) and their volume increases and decreases to fine tune closure of the anal lumen. (It has been calculated that the sphincter muscles by themselves are incapable of achieving this.) When anal cushions are disrupted they become haemorrhoids, or piles
• The precise mechanism responsible for disruption is uncertain, although straining at stool and hard stool consistency are almost certainly responsible. The former leads to engorgement

of the cushions and passage of the latter produces shearing forces which lead to fragmentation of the supporting fibromuscular matrix. Any factor therefore which promotes straining or leads to hard stools will predispose to anal cushion disruption and hence piles

- Blood loss from haemorrhoids is characteristically bright red. It is separate from the motion and it may be present just on the lavatory paper. When haemorrhoids prolapse they may reduce spontaneously, they may require manual reduction, or they may be irreducible. Prolapsing mucosa becomes inflamed and may result in serous/blood-stained discharge from the anal canal. Pruritus ani and defaecatory disturbance can be attributed to haemorrhoids but other sources should be sought. Indeed, it is important to exclude other more significant diagnoses prior to ascribing any symptom just to haemorrhoids.

Differential diagnoses

- Anal skin tags
- Fibrous anal polyp
- Sentinel pile
- Fissure
- Peri-anal haematoma
- Rectal prolapse
- Anal or rectal tumour
- Dermatological condition.

Treatment

- Appropriate dietary and defaecatory advice should be given to prevent the patient straining at stool and producing hard motions
- A number of therapeutic modalities are available to treat the disrupted cushions themselves (injection sclerotherapy, elastic band ligation, infra-red photocoagulation, cryotherapy and haemorrhoidectomy)
- Anal dilatation was once recommended as a mode of treatment but is now of historical interest only
- The precise form of treatment used will depend upon local prejudices and facilities. It should be borne in mind that anal cushions are dynamic structures and minimal symptoms may require no intervention apart from manipulation of dietary and defaecatory habits
- Treatments apart from haemorrhoidectomy produce fibrosis which replaces support once provided by fibromuscular tissue
- Sclerotherapy is suitable for haemorrhoids which bleed but do not prolapse. If prolapse does occur then it is best treated by elastic band ligation
- Haemorrhoidectomy should be reserved for irreducible prolapse and where other treatments have failed.

ANORECTAL ABSCESS

The anal canal and rectum are surrounded by a number of potential tissue spaces and anorectal abscesses are classified according to which of these they occupy.

- Submucosal
- Peri-anal
- Intersphincteric
- Ischiorectal
- Peri-rectal.

Peri-anal and ischiorectal abscesses are encountered most frequently (80% of the total) whilst intersphincteric and peri-rectal abscesses occur much less commonly.

Aetiology

- In 20% of patients there is a predisposing cause such as inflammatory bowel disease (especially Crohn's disease), anorectal cancer, anal fissure, complicated haemorrhoids and local trauma
- Peri-rectal abscesses can occur secondary to infection of another pelvic structure
- In 70–80% there is no obvious cause and here sepsis is thought to arise in an anal gland (cryptoglandular sepsis)
- There are 6–10 such glands distributed around the anal canal which drain into the base of the anal crypts. Glands commonly ramify into the internal anal sphincter and can extend as far as the intersphincteric plane. Peri-anal infection may develop when a gland fails to drain adequately. If this results in abscess formation, then communication with the anal canal and involvement of either the internal anal sphincter or the intersphincteric plane (or both) is expected
- Organisms which invade from the peri-anal skin and those which enter from a distant site by haematogenous spread are a further source
- Pus from an anorectal abscess will generally reveal either skin derived or constituents of gut flora. The former are rarely associated with a communication between the abscess and the gastrointestinal tract, whilst the latter makes such a communication more likely.

Clinical features

History
Pain is prominent with peri-anal and superficial ischiorectal abscesses, followed by local signs of inflammation. These are less evident with deep collections, which tend to develop insidiously with pyrexia and systemic upset.

Examination
Superficial lesions produce obvious signs of localised acute
inflammation but these are more diffuse with ischiorectal sepsis.
Skin necrosis and crepitus (if a gas-forming organism is present)
may be present. Deeper infections produce less obvious
abnormalities which are only apparent on digital rectal
examination, for instance a tender mass or an area of induration.
The position of such lesions with respect to the pelvic floor should
be determined.

Investigation

* In most instances diagnosis is clear but examination under
  anaesthesia is required to establish the full picture
* Endoluminal ultrasound, CT and MRI may be helpful in more
  complicated cases
* Predisposing conditions should be investigated on their own
  merits.

Treatment
The principles of treatment are:

* *Relief of symptoms and prevention of further tissue damage.*
  This is achieved by incision of the abscess to facilitate adequate
  drainage
* *Investigation of an underlying cause.* Gentle examination might
  reveal a communication between the abscess and the
  gastrointestinal tract. If a fistulous communication is obvious
  then it can either be laid open if it is very low, or it can be
  marked with a seton for subsequent definitive treatment. A
  specimen of pus should be sent for microbiological examination
* *Action when a fistula is not found at the first operation.* If the
  presence of a fistula is suspected (clinical impression, recurrent
  abscess or presence of gut flora in pus) then endo-anal
  ultrasound with infusion of hydrogen peroxide into the resolving
  abscess cavity is recommended as this is likely to demonstrate
  the presence of a tract if one exists.

FISTULA-IN-ANO

By definition a fistula is an abnormal communication between two
epithelial-lined surfaces. With fistula-in-ano a communication can
exist between the peri-anal skin and either the anal canal or rectum.
The aetiology is the same as that described for anorectal abscess.

Classification
Fistulae can be classified as:

* Superficial
* Intersphincteric

- Trans-sphincteric
- Suprasphincteric
- Extrasphincteric.

Superficial, inter- and trans-sphincteric tracts account for the vast majority of fistulae encountered.

Clinical features

The aim of management is to define and eradicate sepsis whilst preserving anal function. The crucial steps are:

- Definition of anatomy
- Effective drainage of sepsis (abscess and tracts)
- Eradication of the source of sepsis (for instance from an anal gland)
- Preservation of sphincter function
- Care of the wound.

Definition of anatomy

This relies on careful clinical examination with the patient awake and under anaesthesia. The site of internal and external openings is defined together with the distribution of induration which reflects the distribution of fistula tracts. Lockhart Mummery probes are particularly helpful for exploring tracts. Goodsall's law states that if an external opening lies anterior to a transverse line which bisects the anal opening, its tract will pass directly into the anal canal, whereas if the opening lies posterior to the line then it will enter the anal canal in the midline posteriorly. Sepsis can horseshoe around the anal canal either in the intersphincteric plane or outside the external anal sphincter. Endo-anal ultrasound (with hydrogen peroxide infusion) and MRI can be helpful in defining tracts when they are obscure or form part of a complex fistula.

Treatment

- When the tract is low (it only traverses the most distal fibres of the sphincters or none at all – superficial, low inter- and trans-sphincteric fistula) then the tract is laid open, granulations are curetted, a simple dressing is applied (packing is not required) and the patient is instructed to take regular baths
- When more of the sphincter apparatus is involved and by dividing it continence would be endangered, it is best to insert a seton first to drain sepsis. (A seton is a thread or suture which is passed along a fistula tract. Tied loosely it acts as an effective drain or it can be tied tightly and so will slowly cut through tissues enclosed. Caustic setons are also described but are little used in the West.) The seton can subsequently be tightened to slowly cut through the enclosed sphincter muscle (cutting seton) or the external part of the fistula can be excised and the internal opening can be closed by advancement of a mucosal flap

- If a fistula complicates Crohn's disease the management is directed at ensuring that sepsis is drained but tissue is preserved and in particular sphincter muscle is not divided
- Defunctioning stomas are seldom required in the management of fistulae.

FURTHER READING

Goligher C J 1984 Surgery of the anus, rectum and colon. Harcourt Brace, London
Keighley M R B, Pemberton J H, Parc R, Fazio V 1996 Atlas of colorectal surgery. Churchill Livingstone, New York

16. Intensive care

Neil Bugg

Intensive care has evolved from the respiratory care units of the 1940–1950s. These started with 'iron lungs' developed for use during polio epidemics. Alongside developments in ventilator technology, intensive care has expanded to manage failure of multiple organ systems.

ADMISSION CRITERIA

- Organ failure: usually cardiovascular or respiratory, often combined with other system failure
- Postoperative monitoring. e.g. post cardiac/neurosurgery
- Intensive monitoring in severe disease, e.g. trauma, burns
- Condition should be potentially reversible.

Outcome in critical illness is determined by the nature and severity of the underlying disease, previous health and response to interventions.

SYSTEMS FOR RELATING SEVERITY OF ILLNESS TO OUTCOME

- Specific: accurate for one disease state: Glasgow Coma Score for head injuries, Ranson criteria for pancreatitis
- General: scoring of physiological variables to predict outcome regardless of disease.

For example:

Acute Physiology and Chronic Health Evaluation (APACHE 2)

- Numerical value is assigned to twelve physiological variables proportional to deviation from the norm and evaluation of chronic health
- Scores are weighted according to illness
- Evaluations within 24 hours of ICU admission may predict outcome
- Regular scoring is used to assess interventions.

Mortality Prediction Models (MPM)

- Yes or no answers relating to eleven admission variables
- Weighed according to their contribution to mortality
- APACHE 2 is a better outcome predictor in the UK.

Therapeutic Intervention Scoring System (TISS)

- Used to classify illness according to interventions
- Provides accurate assessment of care/workload
- Individual physician-dependent.

PROBLEMS ENCOUNTERED

- Management of the underlying condition
- Management of related complications, e.g. ARDS, renal failure
- Infection
- Adequate nutrition and fluid balance
- Prevention of stress ulceration
- DVT prophylaxis
- Sedation.

SEDATION AND ANALGESIA

Uses

- Reduce pain and distress
- Aid tolerance of endotracheal tube, ventilation, suction and physiotherapy.

Desired end point

- Peaceful, cooperative patient, responsive to commands
- Scores used to grade sedation.

Routes of administration

- Inhalational, e.g. isoflurane
- Intravenous, e.g. bolus or infusion.

Opioid analgesics

- Usually first-line, e.g. morphine, fentanyl, produce analgesia, euphoria and sedation
- Also cause respiratory depression, ileus
- Metabolites accumulate in renal failure.

Benzodiazepines

- Used in conjunction with opioids, e.g. midazolam, diazepam
- Produce sedation, hypnosis, amnesia

- Metabolites accumulate in renal failure
- May produce cardiorespiratory depression.

Propofol by infusion

- Rapid metabolism, sedation easily controlled
- Expensive to use
- Not licensed for use in children.

Neuromuscular blocking drugs

- Risk of awareness
- Used infrequently – with reduced chest wall compliance and raised intracranial pressure.

RESPIRATORY FAILURE AND SUPPORT

Defined as hypoxaemia with or without hypercarbia due to inadequate gas exchange.

Type one – pneumonia, asthma, left ventricular failure, ARDS

- Due to ventilation – perfusion mismatch
- Picture of hypoxia, hypocapnia, small tidal volume and tachypnoea.

Type two – spinal cord damage, Guillain–Barré, polio, motor neurone disease, myasthenia gravis

- Ventilatory failure
- Blunted response to rising P_aCO_2.

The two types are frequently combined. Type one deteriorates to a mixed picture with exhaustion.

Management

- Oxygen: for type one and mixed picture (beware blue bloaters) – face mask, facial CPAP, ventilation
- Reduce ventilatory load: treat pyrexia
- Optimise ventilatory capacity: drain pleural effusions, manage distended abdomen, posture, physiotherapy
- Adequate hydration, humidification of gases
- Treat cause, e.g. asthma, pneumonia.

Intubation and ventilation
Indications

- Respiratory failure refractory to the above
- Tiring patient

- Secretion retention
- Airway protection.

Intubation complications

Early

- Trauma (teeth, tongue, pharynx, larynx)
- Hypertensive response, arrhythmias
- Laryngospasm, vagal events
- Gastric aspiration, oesophageal intubation
- Tube obstruction.

Late

- Laryngeal nerve damage
- Tracheal stenosis
- Ulceration (nose, mouth, cords)
- Cord granuloma
- Sinusitis (nasal intubation).

Mechanical ventilation

Advantages

- Control of ventilation
- Secretion clearance
- Decreased afterload (LVF).

Disadvantages

- Disconnection, failure of gas or power supply
- Increased pulmonary vascular resistance, decreased venous return, decreased cardiac output
- Loss of normal ventilation perfusion matching
- Barotrauma leading to pneumothorax, pneumomediastinum, subcutaneous emphysema
- Volutrauma – normal tidal volumes are inappropriate in diseased lung
- Nosocomial pneumonia: 30% incidence at 30 days ventilation
- Hepatic dysfunction
- Renal impairment with salt and water retention.

Patterns of ventilation

Intermittent positive pressure ventilation (IPPV)   Two types:

1. Volume-controlled: delivery of a fixed volume, peak pressures vary according to lung compliance
2. Pressure-controlled: lungs are inflated to a preset pressure, tidal volumes vary with compliance.

Variations added to IPPV:

- Degree of oxygenation is proportional to mean airway pressure. Reverse I:E ratio ventilation allows higher than normal mean pressures with lower peaks
- Positive end expiratory pressure (PEEP). Allows alveolar recruitment by splinting open small airways at end expiration.

Both variations exacerbate the effects of IPPV. Pressure-controlled ventilation and reverse I:E ratio are frequently combined in patients with poor compliance.

High frequency ventilation   Small breaths delivered at high frequency to reduce the risk of barotrauma.

- High-frequency positive pressure ventilation (HFPPV): Rate of 60–150 cycles per minute and tidal volumes of 100–400 ml
- High-frequency jet ventilation (HFJV): 60–600 cycles per minute via cannula in ETT tube or cricothyroid membrane. Tidal volumes up to 150 ml/min
- High-frequency oscillation (HFO): 500–3000 cycles per minute. Mechanism of action unclear.

Weaning criteria

General

- Nutritional state: muscle weakness, electrolyte disturbances – phosphate, potassium
- Level of consciousness and residual drug effects
- Cardiovascular stability: especially cardiac failure
- Anaemia corrected
- Mechanical factors: distended abdomen, pleural effusions.

Pulmonary

- Gas exchange: $PO_2 > 8$ KPa, at FiO_2 0.4
- Vital capacity: 10–15 ml/Kg
- $P_{imax} > -20$ cm H_2O
- Respiratory frequency: tidal volume ratio of < 105 ml/min/L.

Modes of weaning
Traditionally a trial of spontaneous respiration on a T-piece. The patient is re-ventilated if tachypnoea, tachycardia, hypertension or desaturation beyond preset limits occurs. More recently 'gentle' weaning techniques have been employed:

- Synchronised Intermittent Mandatory Ventilation (SIMV): ventilatory breaths are synchronised with the patient's own efforts. Weaning is by gradual reduction in set rate
- Pressure Support (PS): inspiration triggers gas flow to a pre-set inspiratory pressure

- Continuous positive airways pressure: similar to PEEP but used in spontaneous respiration. Reduces work of breathing via a T-piece.

ADULT RESPIRATORY DISTRESS SYNDROME (ARDS)

First described in 1967 as non-cardiogenic pulmonary oedema secondary to conditions not directly affecting the lungs.

Features

- Diffuse pulmonary infiltrates
- Arterial hypoxaemia
- Stiff lungs
- PCWP < 16 mmHg.

Producing respiratory failure requiring ventilation following a direct or indirect pulmonary insult.
Overall mortality is 50–60%.

Precipitating factors for ARDS

- Aspiration pneumonia
- Bacteraemia
- Disseminated intravascular coagulation
- Massive blood transfusion
- Long bone/pelvic fractures.

Early oedematous phase progresses to late fibrotic phase with chronic respiratory impairment.

Management

Respiratory support

- Avoid high airway pressures
- Pressure controlled ventilation reverse I:E ratio
- PEEP
- HFJV
- Posture – prone ventilation
- Nitric oxide.

General support

- Nutrition
- Management of the underlying condition.

BLOOD GAS MONITORING

Analysers measure PaO_2, $PaCO_2$ and pH. Bicarbonate and base deficit are calculated values.

Look at PaO$_2$

Calculate alveolar–arterial oxygen difference ({A–a}DO$_2$)

$(A–a)DO_2 = P_AO_2 - P_aO_2$ where

$$P_AO_2 = F_iO_2(P_B - P_AH_2O). \frac{P_ACO_2}{R}$$

P$_B$:   Barometric pressure (760 mmHg)

P$_A$H$_2$O: Alveolar partial pressure of water (47 mmHg)

P$_A$CO$_2$:   Alveolar CO$_2$ – usually P$_a$CO$_2$ is used

$(A–a)DO_2$ is elevated with increasing shunt or ventilation–perfusion mismatch.

Look at P$_a$CO$_2$

• Elevated – respiratory acidosis or corrected metabolic alkalosis
• Low – respiratory alkalosis or corrected metabolic acidosis.

Look at base excess

• Amount of titratable base required to normalise pH assuming a normal P$_a$CO$_2$
• Metabolic acidosis – negative value.

CARDIOVASCULAR FAILURE

This gives rise to shock – inadequate or inappropriate tissue perfusion leading to cellular hypoxia.

Causes

• Pump failure
• Loss of circulating volume
• Maldistribution of circulating volume
• Mechanical obstruction to flow.

Treatment goal

To restore adequate tissue perfusion and oxygenation:

Oxygen delivery = Cardiac output × arterial oxygen content
$$C_aO_2 = Q \times (Hb \times 1.34 \times SpO_2) + (F_iO_2 \times 0.003)$$

Manipulation of F$_i$O$_2$, haemoglobin and cardiac output will alter oxygen delivery.

Measurement of cardiac output

• Thermodilution
   — Intermittent bolus
   — Continuous

- Oesophageal Doppler
- Lithium dilution
- Impedance cardiography.

Also:

Systemic vascular resistance = $\dfrac{MAP - CVP}{Q} \times 82.2$ (dyne.s.cm^{-5})
Normal 1000–1500

Variables are usually indexed for body surface area.

CARDIOGENIC SHOCK

Causes

- Massive infarction
- Acute aortic/mitral regurgitation
- Post cardiac surgery
- Traumatic myocardial contusions.

Effects

- Cold, clammy, sweating, tachycardic, hypotensive, tachypnoeic patient
- Pulmonary oedema but relatively hypovolaemic due to fluid redistribution, diuretics and sweating.

Management

- Oxygen, consider ventilation
- Optimise PCWP (Better guide than CVP, aim for 16–20 mmHg)
- Inotropic support plus vasodilatation (Table 16.1)
- Consider balloon pump.

SEPTIC SHOCK

Both sepsis and non-septic events (trauma, ischaemia, haemorrhage, pancreatitis) can induce the systemic inflammatory response syndrome (SIRS):

- Disseminated macrophage and neutrophil activation
- Mediator release
- Endothelial damage.

SIRS is clinically manifest by two or more of the following:

- Temperature > 38°C or < 36°C
- Heart rate > 90/min
- Resp rate > 20/min or P_aCO_2 < 4.0 KPa
- White cell count > 12 000/mm^3 or < 4000/mm^3.

Table 16.1 Inotropic drugs

Drug	Dose (mcg/kg/min)	Receptor	Effect
Dopamine	0–5	Dopamine	Renal/mesenteric vasodilatation, increased GFR
	5–10	β_1	Increased cardiac output, BP, O_2 consumption
	> 10	α_1	Vasoconstriction
Dobutamine	2.5–15	$\beta_1 > \beta_2$	Increased myocardial contractility
			Reduced left ventricular end diastolic pressure
			Minimal increase in myocardial O_2 consumption
			α action only seen if patient is β-blocked
Adrenaline	0.01–0.2	$\beta_{1+2} > \alpha$	Increased cardiac output (β_1)
			Vasodilatation (β_2)
			α mediated vasoconstriction at higher doses
Enoximone		Phospho-	Vasodilatation ++
Milrinone		diesterase	Increased myocardial contractility
		inhibitors	Minimal increase in myocardial O_2 consumption

When SIRS is due to documented infection with manifest organ hypoperfusion (oliguria, altered mental state, lactic acidosis), and hypotension despite fluid resuscitation (systolic < 90 mmHg or a fall of > 40 mmHg) this meets the criteria for septic shock.

The principal mediators released in septic shock include:

- Activation of the complement system
- Cytokines, TNF, interleukin 1,6,8
- Arachidonic acid metabolites
- Platelet activating factor
- Histamine
- Nitric oxide: TNF and endotoxin stimulate inducible nitric oxide synthase. Prolonged nitric oxide production produces sustained vasodilatation
- Adhesion molecules.

The overall effects of these changes are:

- Vasodilatation
- Arterio-venous shunting
- Increased capillary permeability
- Poor cellular oxygen utilisation
- Myocardial depression.

The end result is cellular hypoxia and the multiple organ dysfunction syndrome.

Special monitoring in septic shock

- Cardiac output and SVR
- Core – peripheral temperature gradient
- Arterial blood gases
- Gastric tonometry – a useful guide to tissue perfusion.

Management

Adequate oxygenation and cardiovascular support
Circulatory support is usually with noradrenaline 0.01–
0.2 mcg/kg/min adjusted according to SVR. Inotropic support may
also be required. Filling should be cautious and to preset limits as
much fluid is lost via leaky capillaries.

Other support

- Treat underlying infection
- Renal support: frusemide or haemofiltration if indicated
- Goal-directed therapy: provide supramaximal oxygen delivery –
  little evidence of long-term benefit.

BRAIN STEM DEATH

Causes

- Head injury
- Intracranial haemorrhage
- Hypoxic injury (cardiac arrest).

Conditions for diagnosis

- Unconscious patient – known irreversible cause of coma
- No drug-induced, metabolic or endocrine cause
- Core temperature greater than 35°C
- **Absent**
  — Brain stem reflexes
  — Pupillary response
  — Corneal reflex
  — Occulo-vestibular reflex
  — Cranial nerve motor response to peripheral stimulation
  — Cough/gag reflex
  — No respiratory effort despite P_aCO_2 > 6.7 KPa with adequate
    oxygenation

  Consider organ donation.

PARENTERAL NUTRITION

Since the work of Studley in 1936 it is accepted that surgical
patients with stigmata of pre-operative malnutrition have an

increased risk of complications. This relates to poor healing and impaired immunity. Starvation and the stress response to trauma and surgery are associated with a catabolic state featuring:

- Insulin resistance mediated partly by high levels of circulating catecholamines
- Cellular protein breakdown leading to
- Negative nitrogen balance (loss of nitrogen from the body).

Enteral nutrition should be provided to all such patients. However this is not possible where:

- Adequate calories cannot be provided enterally (catabolic states, e.g. burns)
- There are reasons for resting the gut (e.g. intrinsic bowel disease, small bowel anastomosis)
- There is gut failure (e.g. malabsorption, diarrhoea, gastric stasis).

Despite many years of the use of TPN in both surgical and ICU groups of patients there is little evidence to suggest any overall benefit.

Parenteral nutrition has seven key constituents:

1. Protein
   - A mix of essential and semi-essential L-amino acids
   - Provide a positive nitrogen balance (about 0.2 g/kg/day of nitrogen)
2. Carbohydrate
   - Provision of greater than 60% of calories as glucose may lead to fatty liver
   - Additional potassium and insulin required which may reduce catabolic response
3. Fat
   - Provides remaining calories
   - Given as the soya bean preparation Intralipid
   - Prevents development of essential fatty acid deficit
   - Provides a source of phosphate
   - Some patients (hepatic disease, pancreatitis) are fat-intolerant developing lipaemic serum
   - Overall energy requirements are about 30 Kcal/kg/day
   - 100–200 Kcal of non-protein energy is provided per gram of nitrogen
4. Electrolytes
   - Sodium, potassium and calcium are corrected on a daily basis
   - Phosphate (30–50 mmol/day) is routinely added as most patients are initially depleted
   - Electrolyte free amino acid solutions are available for hypernatraemic or hyperkalaemic patients
5. Water
   - Daily requirement of about 2 L

6. Trace elements
   - Long-term TPN leads to deficiencies
   - Supplementation includes iron, zinc, manganese, copper, chromium and selenium
7. Vitamins
   - Daily supplementation with vitamins A, D_2, E, K, B complex and C
   - Folate, biotin, nicotinamide and pantothenic acid are added daily.

ROUTE OF ADMINISTRATION

TPN is usually administered centrally, thereby avoiding thrombophlebitis associated with hyperosmolar solutions. A tunnelled silicone catheter placed in the subclavian vein with full aseptic precautions is the route of choice. Solutions with a lower osmolarity (less than 900 mosmol/L) may be administered peripherally. These have lower glucose concentrations (10–20%). Peripheral lines need replacing about every 5 days making long-term use impractical.

Complications

Related to central line

- Insertion complications: arterial puncture, haematoma, pneumothorax, dysrhythmias
- Displacement of tip
- Air embolism
- Thrombosis
- Infection (incidence may be reduced with tunnelled line).

Relating to feed

- Metabolic (high or low levels of sodium, potassium, glucose, phosphate, calcium and magnesium. Also metabolic acidosis) (see Table 16.2)
- Vitamin/trace element deficiencies
- Fluid overload
- Hepatic: elevated liver enzymes (alkaline phosphatase, bilirubin – occasionally producing jaundice, transaminases) due to

Table 16.2 TPN monitoring

Two-hourly	Blood glucose
Daily	Haemoglobin, urea and electrolytes
Three times per week	Liver function tests, calcium, phosphate
Weekly	Magnesium, zinc, nitrogen balance
Monthly	Total iron binding capacity, vitamin B_{12}, folate

provision of excess calories leading to fatty liver or intrahepatic cholestasis from alterations in bile composition. Changes in liver function are usually reversible in adults but may produce chronic liver disease in children

• Intestinal: lack of glutamate and fibre leads to intestinal atrophy. This, combined with glutamate mediated immunity, has been postulated to produce bacterial translocation from the gut leading to sepsis.

Gut protection against stress ulceration should be provided to patients on TPN, i.e. ranitidine or sucralfate.

FURTHER READING

Hinds C J, Watson D 1996 Intensive care, a concise textbook, 2nd edn. W B Saunders, London

Index